Women's Issues in Gastroenterology

Guest Editors

ASYIA AHMAD, MD, MPH
BARBARA B. FRANK, MD

GASTROENTEROLOGY CLINICS OF NORTH AMERICA

www.gastro.theclinics.com

June 2011 • Volume 40 • Number 2

SAUNDERS an imprint of ELSEVIER, Inc.

W.B. SAUNDERS COMPANY

A Division of Elsevier Inc.

Elsevier Inc. • 1600 John F. Kennedy Blvd., Suite 1800 • Philadelphia, Pennsylvania 19103-2899

http://www.theclinics.com

GASTROENTEROLOGY CLINICS OF NORTH AMERICA Volume 40, Number 2
June 2011 ISSN 0889-8553, ISBN-13: 978-1-4557-0451-4

Editor: Kerry Holland
Developmental Editor: Donald Mumford

Gastroenterology Clinics of North America (ISSN 0889-8553) is published quarterly by Elsevier Inc., 360 Park Avenue South, New York, NY 10010-1710. Months of issue are March, June, September, and December. Business and Editorial Offices: 1600 John F. Kennedy Blvd., Suite 1800, Philadelphia, PA 19103-2899. Customer Service Office: 6277 Sea Harbor Drive, Orlando, FL 32887-4800. Periodicals postage paid at New York, NY and additional mailing offices. Subscription prices are $282.00 per year (US individuals), $142.00 per year (US students), $458.00 per year (US institutions), $310.00 per year (Canadian individuals), $558.00 per year (Canadian institutions), $392.00 per year (international individuals), $195.00 per year (international students), and $558.00 per year (international institutions). Foreign air speed delivery is included in all *Clinics* subscription prices. All prices are subject to change without notice. **POSTMASTER:** Send address changes to *Gastroenterology Clinics of North America*, Elsevier Health Sciences Division, Subscription Customer Service, 3251 Riverport Lane, Maryland Heights, MO 63043. Telephone: 1-800-654-2452 (U.S. and Canada); 314-447-8871 (outside U.S. and Canada). Fax: 314-447-8029. E-mail: journalscustomerservice-usa@elsevier.com (for print support); journalsonlinesupport-usa@elsevier.com (for online support).

Reprints. For copies of 100 or more, of articles in this publication, please contact the Commercial Reprints Department, Elsevier Inc., 360 Park Avenue South, New York, New York 10010-1710. Tel. (212) 633-3813, Fax: (212) 462-1935, E-mail: reprints@elsevier.com.

Gastroenterology Clinics of North America is also published in Italian by Il Pensiero Scientifico Editore, Rome, Italy; and in Portuguese by Interlivros Edicoes Ltda., Rua Commandante Coelho 1085, 21250 Cordovil, Rio de Janeiro, Brazil.

Gastroenterology Clinics of North America is covered in *MEDLINE/PubMed (Index Medicus)*, *Excerpta Medica*, *Current Contents/Clinical Medicine*, *Science Citation Index*, *ISI/BIOMED*, and *BIOSIS*.

Printed and bound by CPI Group (UK) Ltd, Croydon, CR0 4YY

Transferred to Digital Print 2011

Contributors

GUEST EDITORS

ASYIA AHMAD, MD, MPH
Associate Professor of Medicine, Division of Gastroenterology and Hepatology, Department of Medicine, Drexel University College of Medicine, Philadelphia, Pennsylvania

BARBARA B. FRANK, MD
Professor of Medicine, Division of Gastroenterology and Hepatology, Department of Medicine, Drexel University College of Medicine, Philadelphia, Pennsylvania

AUTHORS

ASYIA AHMAD, MD, MPH
Associate Professor of Medicine, Division of Gastroenterology and Hepatology, Department of Medicine, Drexel University College of Medicine, Philadelphia, Pennsylvania

HASAN BAYAT, BS
Drexel University College of Medicine, Philadelphia, Pennsylvania

DAWN B. BEAULIEU, MD
Assistant Professor of Medicine, Division of Gastroenterology, Hepatology and Nutrition, Inflammatory Bowl Disease Center, Vanderbilt University, Nashville, Tennessee

BHAVIK M. BHANDARI, MD
Fellow, Division of Gastroenterology and Hepatology, Department of Medicine, Drexel University College of Medicine, Philadelphia, Pennsylvania

CUCKOO CHOUDHARY, MD, FACP
Assistant Professor of Medicine, Division of Gastroenterology and Hepatology, Thomas Jefferson University Hospital, Philadelphia, Pennsylvania

SHEILA E. CROWE, MD, FRCPC
Professor of Medicine, Division of Gastroenterology and Hepatology, University of Virginia, Charlottesville, Virginia

SILVIA DEGLI ESPOSTI, MD
Associate Professor of Medicine (Clinical), The Alpert Medical School of Brown University; Director, Department of Medicine, Center for Women's Gastrointestinal Services, Women & Infants Hospital of Rhode Island, Providence, Rhode Island

GRACE H. ELTA, MD
Professor of Medicine, Division of Gastroenterology, University of Michigan, Ann Arbor, Michigan

CHRISTOPHER W. HAMMERLE, MD
Division of Gastroenterology and Hepatology, University of Virginia,
Charlottesville, Virginia

BRENDA JIMENEZ, MD
Department of Gastroenterology and Hepatology, Cleveland Clinic Florida,
Weston, Florida

SUNANDA KANE, MD, MSPH, FACG, FACP, AGAF
Professor of Medicine, Division of Gastroenterology and Hepatology, Mayo Clinic,
Rochester, Minnesota

JOYANN A. KROSER, MD, FACP, FACG, FAGA
Clinical Associate Professor of Medicine, Division of Gastroenterology and
Hepatology, Department of Medicine, Drexel University College of Medicine,
Philadelphia, Pennsylvania

NOEL M. LEE, MD
Gastroenterology Fellow, Division of Gastroenterology and Hepatology,
University of Wisconsin School of Medicine and Public Health,
Madison, Wisconsin

AYAZ MATIN, MD
Fellow, Division of Gastroenterology and Hepatology, Department of Medicine,
Drexel University College of Medicine, Philadelphia, Pennsylvania

RADHA MENON, MD
Fellow, Division of Gastroenterology and Hepatology, Department of Medicine,
Drexel University College of Medicine, Philadelphia, Pennsylvania

STEPHANIE M. MOLESKI, MD
Gastroenterology Fellow, Division of Gastroenterology and Hepatology, Thomas
Jefferson University Hospital, Philadelphia, Pennsylvania

SCOTT E. MYERS, MD, FACP
Associate Professor of Medicine, Division of Gastroenterology and Hepatology
Department of Medicine; Associate Director, Internal Medicine Residency Program,
Drexel University College of Medicine, Philadelphia, Pennsylvania

NICOLE PALEKAR, MD
Department of Gastroenterology and Hepatology, Cleveland Clinic Florida,
Weston, Florida

ANDRES RIERA, MD
Resident, Division of Internal Medicine, Department of Medicine, Drexel University
College of Medicine, Philadelphia, Pennsylvania

KENNETH D. ROTHSTEIN, MD
Associate Professor and Chief, Division of Gastroenterology and Hepatology,
Department of Medicine, Drexel University College of Medicine,
Philadelphia, Pennsylvania

SUMONA SAHA, MD
Assistant Professor of Medicine, Division of Gastroenterology and Hepatology,
University of Wisconsin School of Medicine and Public Health, Madison,
Wisconsin

DAVID A. SASS, MD, FACP, FACG, AGAF
Associate Professor of Medicine and Surgery, Division of Gastroenterology and Hepatology, Department of Medicine, Drexel University College of Medicine, Philadelphia, Pennsylvania

ALISON SCHNEIDER, MD
Department of Gastroenterology and Hepatology, Cleveland Clinic Florida, Weston, Florida

DHVANI SHAH, BA
The Alpert Medical School of Brown University, Providence, Rhode Island

SAVANNA THOR, DO, MPH
Resident in Internal Medicine, Department of Internal Medicine, Hahnemann University Hospital, Drexel University College of Medicine, Philadelphia, Pennsylvania

DONALD N. TSYNMAN, MD
Resident in Internal Medicine, Department of Internal Medicine, Hahnemann University Hospital, Drexel University College of Medicine, Philadelphia, Pennsylvania

TOBIAS ZUCHELLI, MD
Internal Medicine Resident, Drexel University College of Medicine, Philadelphia, Pennsylvania

DAVID A. SASS, MD, FACP, FACG, AGAF
Associate Professor of Medicine and Surgery, Division of Gastroenterology and Hepatology, Department of Medicine, Drexel University College of Medicine, Philadelphia, Pennsylvania

ALISON SCHNEIDER, MD
Department of Gastroenterology and Hepatology, Cleveland Clinic Florida, Weston, Florida

DHVANI SHAH, BA
The Alpert Medical School of Brown University, Providence, Rhode Island

SAVANNA THOR, DO, MPH
Resident in Internal Medicine, Department of Internal Medicine, Hahnemann University Hospital, Drexel University College of Medicine, Philadelphia, Pennsylvania

DONALD N. TSYNMAN, MD
Resident in Internal Medicine, Department of Internal Medicine, Hahnemann University Hospital, Drexel University College of Medicine, Philadelphia, Pennsylvania

TOBIAS ZUCHELLI, MD
Internal Medicine Resident, Drexel University College of Medicine, Philadelphia, Pennsylvania

Contents

> Irritable bowel syndrome (IBS) is a complex clinical process with multiple pathophysiologic mechanisms. There has recently been a shift in the treatment of patients with severe IBS symptoms to disease-modifying therapies as opposed to symptomatic treatment. Because pathophysiologic differences exist between men and women, so does the efficacy of treatment options. These differences could further explain gender-related differences in disease prevalence and treatment response. A brief discussion of the definition, epidemiology, and diagnostic criteria of IBS is followed by a comprehensive review of the current treatment choices and potential future therapeutic options of IBS in women.

> Irritable bowel syndrome (IBS) is a highly prevalent disorder characterized by nonspecific symptoms that can mimic other common medical conditions. A careful history and physical examination may reveal clues that suggest a coexisting or alternative diagnosis, such as small intestinal bacterial overgrowth or celiac disease (CD). Testing for bacterial overgrowth has limitations, but emerging data suggest that antibiotics may be of some benefit in patients with IBS with diarrhea and bloating. CD seems to have a higher prevalence in patients with IBS. Some patients with IBS may have symptomatic improvement on gluten-restricted diets, without histologic or serologic evidence of CD.

> Nausea and vomiting are common experiences in pregnancy, affecting 70% to 80% of all pregnant women. Various metabolic and neuromuscular factors have been implicated in the pathogenesis of nausea and vomiting of pregnancy (NVP) and hyperemesis gravidarum (HG), an entity distinct from NVP. However, their exact cause is unknown. Consequently, treatment of NVP and HG can be difficult, as neither the optimal targets for treatment nor the full effects of potential treatments on the developing fetus are known. This article reviews the epidemiology, pathology, diagnosis, outcomes, and treatment of NVP and HG.

LIVER

This article briefly discusses gestational physiologic changes and thereafter reviews liver diseases during pregnancy, which are divided into 3 main categories. The first category includes conditions that are unique to pregnancy and generally resolve with the termination of pregnancy, the second category includes liver diseases that are not unique to the pregnant population but occur commonly or are severely affected by pregnancy, and the third category includes diseases that occur coincidentally with pregnancy and in patients with underlying chronic liver disease, with cirrhosis, or after liver transplant who become pregnant.

Hepatitis B virus (HBV) during pregnancy presents unique management challenges. Varying aspects of care must be considered, including the effects of HBV on maternal and fetal health, effects of pregnancy on the course of HBV infection, treatment of HBV during and after pregnancy, and prevention of perinatal infection. Antiretroviral therapy has not been associated with increased risk of birth defects or toxicity, but despite studies designed to elucidate the drug efficacy and safety in affected individuals and the developing fetus, recommendations are inconclusive. Clinicians and patients must make individualized decisions after carefully evaluating the risks and benefits summarized in this article.

Primary biliary cirrhosis is a chronic autoimmune inflammatory disease of the liver with a striking female preponderance. It has an insidious onset and typically affects middle-aged women. The disease manifests gradually with symptoms of fatigue, pruritis, and increased alkaline phosphatase levels on laboratory evaluation. The hallmark of the disease is the circulating antimitochondrial antibody. Histology is characterized by inflammation of the bile ducts, destruction of cholangiocytes, and subsequent cholestasis, progressing to biliary cirrhosis. The standard treatment for primary biliary cirrhosis is ursodeoxycholic acid, which improves survival, but the disease can still lead to cirrhosis and liver failure over decades.

COLONIC

Inflammatory bowel diseases (IBD), namely Crohn disease (CD) and ulcerative colitis (UC), are common in Western society. Because at least half of the patients suffering from these diseases are women, it is important that physicians are aware of their gender-specific needs. There are multiple important concerns for women with UC and CD including issues of body image and sexuality, menstruation, contraception, screening for cervical cancer, matters related to menopause and hormone replacement therapy, osteoporosis, and the overlap seen between IBS and IBD. In this article, we have addressed these important, non–pregnancy-related issues faced by women with IBD.

Crohn disease and ulcerative colitis commonly affect women in their child-bearing years. Fortunately, advances in the field of inflammatory bowel disease have made successful pregnancy outcomes a reality for many women. These advances have led to family planning as a common discussion between gastroenterologists and inflammatory bowel disease patients. Common discussion topics are fertility, conception, medication safety, pregnancy, delivery, and breastfeeding although there are limited available data. Education and patient awareness have become vital factors in successful pregnancy outcomes.

Studies have shown that colorectal cancer (CRC) incidence is equal between men and women. However, several studies have demonstrated lower adenoma detection rates in women than in men. Many questions arise about differences in adenomas, CRC, and screening practices between men and women: should screening be the same for both sexes, are there differences in risk factors in the formation of colon cancer, should special groups of women be screened differently from the general population, are colonoscopies tolerated differently in women and why, and what determines if a woman will undergo colonoscopy? This article reviews these issues.

OTHER

Common gastrointestinal diseases often exhibit geographic, cultural, and gender variations. Diseases previously less common in certain areas of the world have shown a recent increase in prevalence. Industrialization has traditionally been noted as a major cause for this epidemiologic evolution. However, environmental factors such as diet, hygiene, and exposure to infections may play a major role. Moreover, the way one disease presents in a certain location may vary significantly from the way it manifests in another culture or location. This article discusses global variations of inflammatory bowel disease, *Helicobacter pylori*, irritable bowel disease, fecal incontinence, hepatitis B, and hepatocellular cancer.

Women have started to enter gastroenterology (GI) in significant numbers over the past 5 years, although they are still underrepresented compared with the proportion of female graduating medical students. This underrepresentation is most likely caused by the culture of GI where female students and residents have felt undervalued and unwelcome. This type of discrimination is difficult to fight because it is behind the scenes. However, with increasing female role models in GI, this underrepresentation will likely change in the coming years.

Tobias Zuchelli and Scott E. Myers

As the body ages, it undergoes a multitude of changes. Some of these changes are visible, whereas others are not and may be elicited during the patient encounter. Some gastrointestinal issues may be more common in the elderly population and possibly in older women. These issues range from motility disorders, such as fecal incontinence and constipation, to changes in neuropeptide function and its effect on the anorexia of aging. This article comprehensively reviews gastrointestinal issues that commonly afflict the elderly female population.

THE CLINICS ARE NOW AVAILABLE ONLINE!

Access your subscription at:
www.theclinics.com

Preface

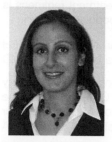 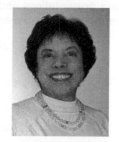

Asyia Ahmad, MD, MPH   Barbara B. Frank, MD
Guest Editors

Over the last few decades there has been an increased awareness that medical disorders in men and woman may present differently and be treated uniquely. As a result, clinicians have recognized that clinical and research initiatives need to explore these gender-specific variations. Discussions of gastrointestinal gender-related issues have lagged behind other fields and may be the result of the previous domination of men within the field of gastroenterology. With the more recent influx of women into gastroenterology, gender-specific gastrointestinal disorders have been increasingly exposed, researched, and discussed.

There are many facets of gastroenterology that have unique gender-based issues. For instance, women with inflammatory bowel disease may deal with altered body image and sexuality, reduced fertility, and an increased incidence of flares around menstruation. Irritable bowel syndrome and primary biliary cirrhosis are conditions with a female preponderance, although it is unclear if estrogen, genetic differences, or varying disclosure rates are responsible for this finding. It has also been recently recognized that men and women have an overall similar risk of colon cancer throughout their lives, although women may present at a later age. The geriatric female population specifically faces anorexia and fecal incontinence, which can be explained by alterations of hormones as well as mechanical changes due to aging.

Pregnancy is an obvious gender-specific condition that may directly lead to gastrointestinal disease such as hyperemesis gravidarum or hepatic disorders, including fatty liver of pregnancy, cholestasis of pregnancy, or eclampsia. Furthermore, pregnant women with inflammatory bowel disease must balance the detrimental effects of disease flares against the potential toxicities of available medical therapies.

A public health approach to a variety of gender-based issues has recently evolved. Initiatives aimed at reducing the maternal-fetal transmission of Hepatitis B have markedly reduced the incidence of this disease. Global variations in diet, hygiene, environmental exposures, and infections have also uncovered cultural and gender differences throughout the world.

Gastroenterol Clin N Am 40 (2011) xiii–xiv
doi:10.1016/j.gtc.2011.04.001
0889-8553/11/$ – see front matter © 2011 Elsevier Inc. All rights reserved.

gastro.theclinics.com

This edition of *Gastroenterology Clinics of North America* discusses a plethora of gender-related gastrointestinal issues that have been mentioned above. Knowledge of gender-specific gastrointestinal disease presentations and treatment regimens is essential to thoroughly and effectively treat our diverse patient population.

Asyia Ahmad, MD, MPH
Barbara B. Frank, MD

Division of Gastroenterology and Hepatology
Drexel University College of Medicine
219 North Broad Street, 5th Floor
Philadelphia, PA 19107, USA

E-mail addresses:
asyia.ahmad@drexelmed.edu (A. Ahmad)
Barbara.Frank@drexelmed.edu (B.B. Frank)

Treatment of Irritable Bowel Syndrome in Women

Donald N. Tsynman, MD[a], Savanna Thor, DO, MPH[a],
Joyann A. Kroser, MD[b],*

KEYWORDS

• Irritable bowel syndrome • Women • Treatment

Irritable bowel syndrome (IBS) has been defined as a functional bowel disorder in which abdominal pain or discomfort is associated with defecation or a change in bowel habits, along with features of unsatisfactory defecation. Characterized by cramping, abdominal pain, bloating, constipation, or diarrhea, IBS affects an estimated 58 million individuals in the United States. It is considered among the most frequent causes of outpatient gastroenterology consultations in the Western world[1] and statistically one of the most common functional gastrointestinal (GI) disorders worldwide.

EPIDEMIOLOGY AND PREVALENCE

It has been frequently noted that women bear much of the burden of IBS, with twice as many women as men seeking treatment for IBS in the United States.[2,3] Whether the increased prevalence in female patients means that women are more willing than men to report IBS-related symptoms, or if it means that women are biologically predisposed to IBS is still not clear. However, there are associations between the diagnosis of IBS and psychiatric diagnoses, such as anxiety and depression, and pain syndromes, such as fibromyalgia, chronic fatigue syndrome, and migraine headaches, all of which are seen more frequently women.[4] A population-based study evaluating the prevalence of IBS symptoms among healthy university students supported this increased prevalence seen in the general public, with 15.7% prevalence in women compared with 7.7% prevalence in men (odds ratio [OR], 2.2; 95% confidence interval [CI], 1.7–2.9; P<.0001). In particular, constipation-predominant IBS (IBS-C) was more

The authors have nothing to disclose.

[a] Department of Internal Medicine, Hahnemann University Hospital, Drexel University College of Medicine, Broad and Vine Street, Philadelphia, PA 19104, USA

[b] Department of Gastroenterology and Hepatology, Drexel University College of Medicine, 219 North Broad Street, 5th floor, Philadelphia, PA 19107, USA

* Corresponding author.

E-mail address: joyann.kroser@drexelmed.edu

frequently associated with women than with men (OR, 6.4; 95% CI, 4.1–9.7; $P<.001$).[5] Subsequent studies have also reported that women with IBS had a lower quality of life (QoL) score and reported more fatigue, depressed mood, and levels of anxiety, and less positive self-esteem and well-being compared with men with IBS,[4] underlying the need for further review of the impact of IBS in the female population.

COST OF IBS

The prevalence of IBS is best exemplified by the significant economic burden exerted on the health care system by the syndrome. The mean annual direct health care costs for IBS have been shown to be upward of $5000 per patient with annual average out-of-pocket expenses of over $400 per year.[6] Health care costs of IBS and associated productivity losses attributed to IBS symptoms have previously been shown to be around $30 billion annually.[7]

DIAGNOSIS

This highly prevalent condition is best diagnosed by assessing the constellation of symptoms with which patients present to their physicians. Because some critics have previously questioned whether IBS and other functional GI disorders truly exist because they do not have defining structural features, the Rome Foundation fostered the use of symptom-based criteria for universal use.[8] The use of these Rome criteria (**Box 1**) has led to a standardization of diagnosis in the field, which has made demographic and treatment reviews, such as this article, more accurate.

Based on these specific symptoms, IBS can further be classified into a diarrhea-predominant (IBS-D), IBS-C, or a mixed-type disease (IBS-mixed). These specifications of disease symptoms, along with the aforementioned Rome criteria, have created standardization in diagnosis. With this clarification, recent data suggest that gender differences absolutely exist in the symptoms, pathophysiology, and response to certain treatments in IBS.[9] For example, female IBS patients are more likely to be constipated and complain of abdominal distention and extraintestinal symptoms

---

Box 1
IBS Rome III Criteria

Twelve weeks or more in the past 12 months of abdominal pain or discomfort that has two out of three features

- Relieved with defecation
- Associated with a change in frequency of stool
- Associated with a change in consistency of stool

Supportive, but not essential features to diagnosis include

- Abnormal stool frequency (>3/day or <3/week)
- Abnormal stool form >25% of all defecations
- Abnormal stool passage (straining, urgency, feeling of incomplete evacuation) >25% of all defecations
- Passage of mucus >25% of all defecations

Data from Drossman DA, Corazziari E, Delavaux M, et al. Rome III: the functional gastrointestinal disorders. McLean (VA): Degnon Associates; 2006.

than male counterparts. With such specific differences in the disease process, the purpose of this article is to highlight the issues specifically facing women with IBS, including potential differences in etiology, proper management, and current and potential future treatment options.

DIFFERENCES IN PATHOPHYSIOLOGY AND ETIOLOGY

Because IBS is a chronic, relapsing, and frequently lifelong condition of unknown cause,[10] abnormalities of GI visceral sensation, motility, autonomic function, bacterial flora, and immunity have all been cited as possible mechanisms to explain this multi-faceted disease process.[11] Subsequently, however, many studies have shown that the etiology of IBS is likely not from a single cause but rather represents an integrated response to a variety of complex biologic and psychosocial factors.[12] This has led to the current understanding of IBS as a disorder of brain–gut interactions with both physical and psychosocial components.[12,13]

Although the precise etiology and role of motility anomalies in IBS may still be in question, researchers have long believed that distorted motility patterns of the rectum, colon, and small bowel are the primary reason for the abdominal pain experienced by IBS patients.[14] As such, an important consideration specific to this theory of etiology is gender differences in gut transit. Studies have previously elucidated slower gut transit time in females as opposed to males[4] and there has been an attempt to correlate this with the aforementioned disparity of disease prevalence in the female population.

Additionally, studies involving balloon distention of the bowel have confirmed that visceral hypersensitivity with a lower threshold for pain occurs in IBS patients compared with healthy counterparts, confirming a brain–gut interaction.[15] There are also gender differences in processing visceral perception in IBS patients. Whereas male IBS patients show greater activation of the cognitive area, central sympathetic area, and inhibition of limbic regions of the brain in response to visceral stimulation, female IBS patients display greater activation of affective and autonomic regions of the central nervous system.[16]

It has also been postulated that there may be a role for hormonal dysregulation that affects pain perception, which may account for some differences in prevalence seen in premenopausal women. Women are most commonly diagnosed with IBS between their second and fifth decade of life. In addition, women with GI symptoms report an increase in symptoms at the time of their menstrual period in 35% of women without IBS and 50% of women with IBS.[17,18] Hormonal modulation of GI motility has also been elucidated in some studies, with variations in lower esophageal sphincter pressure reported in pregnancy[19] and a slower rate of gastric emptying in menstruating women compared with similar-aged men.[20] Although slower gut transit time has been demonstrated in female patients, whether this difference is purely a function of the menstrual cycle remains unclear.

Just as pathophysiologic differences exist between men and women, so does the efficacy of treatment options. These differences could further explain gender-related differences in disease prevalence as related to the pathophysiology and treatment responses in the illness, further solidifying the need for disease reviews such as this one specific to the female population.

THERAPEUTIC OPTIONS
General Considerations

It is impossible to identify a single agent that acts on all the mechanisms of action of IBS, because of their complexity. The use of dietary fiber, laxatives, antidiarrheal agents, and antispasmodics as first-line therapies has been limited by marginal therapeutic benefits, side effects, and even exacerbations of IBS symptoms. This article focuses on those pharmacologic therapies that take aim at specific pathophysiologic mechanisms of IBS with attention to gender-specific findings.

Antidepressants

Selective serotonin reuptake inhibitors

Given that IBS is associated with psychiatric disorders, such as anxiety and depression, and pain syndromes, such as fibromyalgia, it has been postulated that antidepressants could have a role in treatment of patients with IBS symptoms. Beyond the treatment benefit for the comorbid diseases, selective serotonin reuptake inhibitors (SSRIs) and tricyclic antidepressants have been shown to improve IBS symptoms, independently of effect on anxiety and depression scores. Serotonin, or 5-hydroxytryptamine (5-HT), is a neurotransmitter that is largely stored in the enterochromaffin cells of the gut and plays a critical part in the motility, sensation, and secretion of the GI tract.[21] A study by Talley and colleagues[22] comparing imipramine, citalopram, and placebo demonstrated significant improvement in Bowel Symptom Severity Rating Scale distress and Bowel Symptom Severity Rating Scale disability in the imipramine (a tricyclic antidepressant) group compared with both placebo and citalopram (an SSRI) after 12 weeks of treatment. There were, however, no significant differences in the global adequate relief symptom end point between the antidepressants and placebo, which is a suggested end point for irritable bowel symptoms. This study, unfortunately, had a large drop-out rate in the imipramine group (50%) despite having similar side effects between the groups, which may limit its applicability to female patients. Most of the patients in this study (76% of the citalopram group, 67% of the imipramine group, and 75% of the placebo group) had IBS-D, which may explain why the citalopram group did not receive any benefit because SSRIs can increase intestinal transit, and thus potentially exacerbate symptoms in this particular group of patients.

Amitriptyline

Studies have demonstrated the effect of amitriptyline on symptoms of IBS that do not correlate with baseline anxiety and depression scores[23] and affect GI pain at lower doses than their antidepressant effects,[24] subsequently suggesting an alternate mechanism of action. The mechanism of action of amitriptyline is likely multifactorial, with altered gut motility, reduced ororectal transit time, and an alteration of visceral sensitivity. Most of these studies are relatively small and have used more typical antidepressant level dosing (between 50 and 75 mg/day).[25] However, an Iranian study used low-dose amitriptyline to determine its effectiveness in patients with IBS-D. Fifty-four patients, who met inclusion criteria for IBS-D and passed an initial 2-week lactose-free diet, were randomized to receive amitriptyline, 10 mg daily, or placebo for a 60-day treatment period. Although there was no significant improvement in the mean number of symptoms at the end of the first month of treatment, there was improvement noted at the end of the second month of treatment (2 vs 0.8; $P = .01$).[26] There was also an increase in the percentage of complete responders (defined as absence of all symptoms) in the amitriptyline group compared with placebo (63% vs 26%; $P = .01$) in the intention-to-treat analysis.

Amitriptyline may also have a role in decreasing pain sensitivity by influencing central activation pathways. A study of 19 women compared amitriptyline with placebo for a 4-week treatment period, then crossed over to the alternate treatment, and evaluated activation of the anterior cingulate cortex, the area of the brain that responds to noxious stimuli, and patient pain ratings during rectal distention.[23] This study demonstrated decreased activation of the anterior cingulate cortex noted on MRI images of the amitriptyline patients, although no significant difference was found in the pain ratings of patients with amitriptyline. Although no improvement in symptoms was noted with amitriptyline in this short but well-designed study, extending the treatment period, as is often needed with depression, may demonstrate if patients would receive any clinically significant benefit as has been shown with other longer studies.

Antibiotics

Neomycin

Because the putative role of small intestine bacterial overgrowth in the pathogenesis of IBS has grown, studies to determine the therapeutic value of antibiotics in IBS become more crucial. It has been demonstrated that up to 84% of IBS patients have positive lactulose breath tests.[27,28] Studies comparing neomycin with placebo have shown that symptoms significantly improve in those patients treated with neomycin, and this symptom improvement is correlated with improvement in lactulose breath test results. Furthermore, a study by Pimental and colleagues[29] demonstrated that although global improvement in IBS symptoms was noted in the neomycin group compared with placebo, the patients that were methane producers on lactulose breath testing had more improvement than hydrogen producers when treated with neomycin. The etiology of this association is unclear but it is postulated that improvement in symptoms may be secondary to improved colonic transit, decreasing methane production by bacterial overgrowth. It is known that some antibiotics, such as erythromycin and neomycin, have been demonstrated to increase GI motility; thus, the role of these antibiotics may be multiple in improving intestinal transit and decreasing bacterial overgrowth through bactericidal actions.

Rifaximin

Rifaximin has also been used in suspected small intestine bacterial overgrowth cases. Rifaximin is a broad-spectrum antibiotic with in vitro activity against gram-positive and gram-negative aerobes and anaerobes, with minimal systemic absorption. It also has some activity against *Clostridium difficile*. A double-blinded randomized control trial (RCT) of 87 patients compared rifaximin with placebo in patients with IBS. Study participants were randomized to a 10-day course of treatment of rifaximin, 400 mg three times daily, versus placebo, and followed-up for 10 weeks. The rifaximin group had mean global improvement scores of 36.4% (standard deviation, 31.46%) compared with 21% (standard deviation, 22.08%) for the placebo group after 10 weeks ($P = .02$).[30] The presence of these large standard deviations limits the ability to generalize these findings to all IBS patients; thus, further larger studies are needed to evaluate the effectiveness of this antibiotic. Adverse events were most commonly abdominal pain, constipation, and bad taste in the mouth, but were not statistically different from the placebo group; therefore, patient compliance with rifaximin should not be of significant concern.

Serotonin Receptor Medications

Alosetron

Alosetron, a selective 5-HT$_3$ receptor antagonist, has been demonstrated to improve IBS symptoms in women with severe IBS-D. However, despite a study by Chang and colleagues,[31] which also demonstrated improvement in symptoms in men, its efficacy in men is still in question. A multicenter RCT of 801 women[32] recruited patients with nonconstipated IBS by Rome II criteria and randomized them to alosetron, 1-mg tablets twice daily, for a 12-week treatment versus placebo and examined bowel urgency symptoms. The alosetron group demonstrated improvement in the median proportion of days (0.57 in placebo vs 0.73 in the alosetron group; P<.001) with satisfactory control of bowel urgency over the 12-week period. Bowel urgency has been cited as one of the more difficult symptoms to treat in IBS.[33] Patients in the alosetron group were also significantly more likely to report moderate or substantial global improvement in symptoms (P<.001). Several serious adverse events in the alosetron group were noted, including one case each of ischemic colitis, cholecystitis, pneumonia, diverticulitis, headache, migraine, and ankle fracture.

A study by Krause and colleagues[34] compared different doses of alosetron (0.5 mg daily, 1 mg once daily, 1 mg twice daily, and placebo) to determine the optimal dose maximizing benefit while limiting adverse effects. All of the alosetron groups had statistically significant improvement in global improvement scores compared with placebo but the percentage of patients with adverse events increased with dosage, particularly with constipation. This study, unfortunately, had a large drop-out rate, with completion rates ranging between 52% (in the alosetron twice-daily group) and 66% (in the alosetron 0.5-mg daily group). One patient in the 0.5-mg daily alosetron group did develop ischemic colitis, which was thought to be related to the medication. Thus, despite apparent efficacy and decreased occurrence of adverse events with lower doses of alosetron, there is still no currently established safe dose to prevent ischemic colitis.

Chey and colleagues[35] further evaluated the long-term safety and efficacy of alosetron in a study of 814 women with severe IBS-D symptoms, demonstrating adequate relief rate in 51.6% in the alosetron group compared with 40.9% in the placebo group (P = .005) over a 48-week treatment period with a number-needed-to-treat of 9 (95% CI, 6–30). No serious adverse events, including ischemic colitis, occurred in this study, the first with a relatively long treatment period. Adverse events were constipation, nausea, vomiting, abdominal pain, and diarrhea. This suggests that alosetron may be used as a long-term medication, although whether there is an increase in relapse of IBS symptoms after discontinuation of long-term use of this medication has not been studied.

In its branded form (Lotronex), alosetron does carry a black box warning. As per FDA recommendations, prescribing physicians must enroll in the Prometheus Prescribing Program for Lotronex attesting to their understanding of treatment risks and benefits to decrease the risk of serious adverse events. This has certainly added to the possible lack of popularity of the drug (Table 1).[31,32,34–39]

Tegaserod

Tegaserod, a selective 5-HT$_4$ receptor agonist, has been shown to have efficacy in the treatment of IBS-C in women. In a multicenter, double-blind, RCT of 661 women with IBS-C and IBS-mixed randomized to tegaserod or placebo, patients had satisfactory relief of IBS symptoms in both the IBS-mixed and IBS-C groups when treated with tegaserod.[40] This is one of the first trials to focus on IBS-mixed patients, who may constitute 30% to 50% of IBS patients but have been underrepresented in many of the studies.[41,42] Adverse events to tegaserod were mostly limited to diarrhea and abdominal pain. A large, multinational study used repeated treatment design and demonstrated improvement in symptoms in IBS-C with both first and repeated treatment with tegaserod. Improvement in QoL scores, improved work productivity, and higher levels of patent satisfaction compared with placebo were also significant findings.[43]

Table 1
RCTs comparing alosetron to placebo

Study (Reference)	Location	Design	Treatment Length	IBS Subtype	Women	N	% Responders Placebo Versus Control (at Treatment Completion)	Ischemic Colitis (N)
Krause et al,[34] 2007	Tennessee, North Carolina	RCT	12 weeks	IBS-D	100%	705	50.8% 0.5 mg daily, 48% 1 mg daily, 42.9% 1 mg bid, 30.7% placebo	1
Chey et al,[35] 2004	Multinational	RCT	48 weeks	80% IBS-D	100%	714	52.1% vs 43.9%	0
Lembo et al,[32] 2001	Massachusetts, Kentucky, North Carolina	RCT	12 weeks	98% IBS-D	100%	801	76% vs 44%	1
Chang et al,[31] 2005	United States and Canada	RCT	12 weeks	IBS-D	0%	662	49.8% vs 39.8%	1
Camilleri et al,[37] 2001	104 sites across United States	RCT	12 weeks	71% IBS-D	100%	626	60% vs 41%	0
Camilleri et al,[38] 2000	119 sites across United States	RCT	12 weeks	71% IBS-D	100%	647	41% vs 29%	1

Seven large randomized control trials that compare placebo with alosetron treatment. Most of the trials focused on IBS-D predominant patients, and most focused on women. The studies by Krause and coworkers and Lembo and coworkers focused on global improvement of symptoms as end points, whereas the other studies have adequate relief of IBS pain and discomfort as their end points. Given that the fear of ischemic colitis has been a concern in prescribing alosetron, the last column reports the events of ischemic colitis in these studies. It is, however, worth noting that many of these studies required patients with normal colonoscopy or flexible sigmoidoscopy results before enrollment, which may eliminate some patients who may potentially be more likely to develop ischemic colitis.

Information from the aforementioned studies on tegaserod and alosetron demonstrates an increased efficacy of the treatments for women compared with men that further highlights the aforementioned differences in pathophysiology between the genders. This may be caused by inherent differences in visceral hypersensitivity and pain perception, but other gender differences also may have a role. Alterations in drug clearance may, for example, impact the efficacy of medication treatment because men and women have differences in drug metabolism and different body sizes and adipose content, which may cause variations in the systemic level of the drug and thus change the effective dosing on the patient.

On March 30, 2007, the US Food and Drug Administration (FDA) requested that Novartis withdraw tegaserod, marketed as Zelnorm, from shelves secondary to a proposed relationship between prescriptions of the drug and increased risks of heart attack or stroke. An analysis of data collected on over 18,000 patients demonstrated adverse cardiovascular events in 13 of 11,614 patients treated with Zelnorm (a rate of 0.11%) compared with 1 of 7031 patients treated with placebo (a rate of 0.01%).[44] Novartis alleges all of the affected patients had preexisting cardiovascular disease or risk factors for such, and further alleges that no causal relationship between tegaserod use and cardiovascular events has been demonstrated. On the same day as the FDA announcement, Novartis Pharmaceuticals Canada announced that it was suspending marketing and sales of the drug in Canada in response to a request from Health Canada. However, some manufacturers in India, such as Cipla, still have generic tegaserod available in their listings and some online merchants may be selling the drug. In a large cohort study based on a US health insurance database, no increase in the risk of cardiovascular events was found with tegaserod treatment.[36]

Renzapride

Renzapride is a novel mixed $5-HT_4$ receptor full agonist and $5-HT_3$ receptor antagonist, which has been shown in some small studies to improve GI motility and increase GI transit rates, and thus is a potential treatment for IBS-C. A large, double-blinded phase IIb RCT in England of 510 men and women with IBS modified to IBS-C form compared placebo with 1 mg, 2 mg, or 4 mg per day renzapride treatment for 12 weeks.[45] Although there was a dose-dependent trend showing improvement in abdominal pain and discomfort during weeks 5 to 12 of treatment, these results did not reach statistical significance. A post hoc analysis was performed in the female patients (which accounted for 89% of the subjects) and showed a greater average weekly treatment difference from placebo in the subgroup of females compared with the overall group (12% vs 8%, respectively). This study was limited by the large drop-out rate of participants (197 [38.6%] of 510). However, 51% of the discontinuation was reportedly secondary to adverse events. Adverse events most commonly noted were diarrhea, headache, abdominal pain, aggravated constipation, nausea, dyspepsia, and vomiting. Consequently, studies evaluating the effect of renzapride should be repeated in women to determine whether a therapeutic benefit exists.

Renzapride was under development by Alizyme of the United Kingdom. However, as of April 23, 2008, all further development of the medication was ceased by Alizyme citing a Phase III trial in the United States that did not show enough efficacy over placebo to justify further study.[46]

Hormonal Receptor Modulators

Leuprolide

Hormonal modulation has been postulated to play a role in IBS symptoms, because IBS is more common in women in their premenopausal years and because of the fact that women with IBS have reported an increase in their symptoms during their menstrual cycles. Thus, an Italian study randomized young premenopausal women with menstrual-related increases in IBS symptoms to leuprolide acetate (LAD; a gonadotropin-releasing hormone agonist) plus tibolone (a synthetic compound with estrogenic, androgenic, and progestogenic properties), LAD plus placebo, or placebo and subsequently evaluated the severity of bowel symptoms and QoL scores using validated surveys at baseline and after 6 months of treatment. It was found that IBS symptoms and QoL scores significantly improved in the LAD plus tibolone and LAD groups compared with placebo.[47] However, the LAD plus placebo group had significantly decreased bone mineral density scores compared with the other two groups, although it is unclear if this will manifest in any clinical significance. No fractures were observed during this study period, but long-term administration of this drug could yield a potential risk in female patients. It is unclear if the mechanism of drug action is related to mood regulation and thus decreasing mood-based symptom perception. This study also uses validated questionnaires to assess symptoms and is the first study to evaluate the addition of tibolone to gonadotropin-releasing hormone as a treatment for IBS in women. Tibolone has previously been used in postmenopausal women to prevent bone loss. This pharmacologic therapy may be used in young premenopausal women with increased IBS symptoms during menses. Because adverse events were not specifically reported in this article, it is unknown what the potential side effects may prove to be because of the medication.

Leuoprolide was initially approved in the injection form by the FDA on April 9, 1985, specifically for the use of advanced prostate cancer, and with the many aforementioned ongoing studies, its use for treatment of IBS remains strictly off-label.

Pexacerfront

Pexacerfront is a selective antagonist of corticotrophin-releasing factor 1 (CRF_1) receptor. CRF is a mediator of the stress response in the brain–gut axis and has been demonstrated in animal models to alter GI function.[48] A double-blind study in 39 women with IBS-D, however, randomized to 50/25 mg pexacerfront versus 100/50 mg pexacerfront did not find any statistically significant differences in colonic transit time or secondary end points (number of stools, ease of passage, bloating, gas, urgency or abdominal pain) between placebo and pexacerfront groups.[49] The results of this study are in contrast to prior study results, which demonstrated that CRF agonists affect gut motility by decreasing transit times and increasing stool frequency. CRF_1 inhibition by the selective antagonist pexacerfront was hypothesized to increase transit time and decrease diarrheal symptoms. Future studies may need to evaluate increased doses, medication duration, or different CRF receptor subtype localization to determine whether this pathway can be used effectively in female patients with IBS-D.

Developed by Bristol-Myers Squibb with the premise of treating anxiety disorders, Pexacerfont remains in the clinical stages of development and its use is not FDA approved for IBS at the time of publication.

Supplementation of Specific Dietary Components

Fiber

Dietary fiber may be considered primarily the storage and cell wall polysaccharides of plants that cannot be hydrolyzed by human enzymes.[50] A simpler definition for dietary fiber is specifically nonstarch polysaccharides derived from plant foods that are poorly digestible by human enzymes.[51] Fiber can further be divided based on water solubility into soluble fiber and insoluble fiber.

Soluble fiber retains water and turns to a viscous gel during digestion. These viscous solutions delay gastric emptying and small intestinal absorption and are eventually fermented in the proximal colon by bacteria to a greater extent than insoluble fiber.[52] The active metabolites of this fermentation are short-chain fatty acids and gas (including carbon dioxide, hydrogen, and methane). Examples of soluble fiber are found specifically in foods including oat bran, barley, nuts, seeds, beans, lentils, peas, and some fruits and vegetables.

Insoluble fiber includes cellulose, hemicelluloses, and lignins.[49] These sources have less of an effect on the viscosity of intestinal contents. Their physiologic effect is to hold onto water and increase the size and bulk of stool because they are poorly fermented.[51] Insoluble fiber seems to speed the passage of foods through the stomach and intestines and, by adding bulk to the stool, can make bowel movement passage easier. It is found in such foods as wheat bran, vegetables, and whole grains.

Some of these fiber sources are used as the basis for many of the products termed "bulking agents" and often sold as supplements. Metamucil and Konsyl, for example, are largely psyllium seed. Benefiber is partially hydrolyzed guar gum. The largely artificial products available commercially include Citrucel and Fibercon. Citrucel is composed of methylcellulose and semisynthetic fiber that is nonfermentable. Calcium polycarbophil is a purely synthetic fiber also resistant to bacterial degradation.

The proposed mechanism of action for fiber in the treatment of IBS and constipation is the acceleration of oral–anal transit and a decrease in intracolonic pressures,[53] either as a direct effect or by binding bile salts. The short-chain fatty acids and gaseous products of soluble fiber metabolism decrease gut transit time and have been postulated consequently to decrease intracolonic pressure. In contrast, insoluble fiber has been thought to decrease colonic transit secondary to the change in stool viscosity.[54] Although both types of fiber have been studied in IBS patients, the soluble fibers studied have generally included psyllium, partially hydrolysed guar gum, oligosaccharides, and calcium polycarbophil. Products rich in insoluble fiber that have been studied are wheat bran, corn bran, and defatted ground flaxseed. The results of these studies exploring the effect of different types of fiber on GI transit have been conflicting.[55]

Depending on the source (National Cancer Institute, American Gastroenterological Association, or American Heart Association), dietary fiber recommendations are generally in the range of 20 to 35 g/day per healthy individual.[50] Various surveys, however, have shown that the mean dietary fiber intake in the adult population of the United States is in the range of 11.1 to 13.3 g/day.[56] This observation was widely believed to be the primary cause of IBS.[57] That conviction has been slow to change despite numerous studies to the contrary spurred on by reports that cereal fiber worsened symptoms in 55% of secondary care IBS patients[58] and 22% of primary care IBS patients.[59] Nevertheless, fiber supplementation has remained the most extensively and carefully studied dietary treatment for IBS.

The use of fiber or bulking agents for treatment of IBS has been reviewed in two meta-analyses,[60,61] four systematic reviews,[54,62–64] and two comprehensive narrative reviews.[65,66] The reviews uniformly concluded that fiber either has no efficacy for treatment of IBS or possible limited benefits for patients who have IBS-C. Soluble fiber showed a tendency to greater global symptom improvement than insoluble fiber.[67–69] One review found that insoluble fiber worsened symptoms.[68] An additional meta-analysis[50] concluded that although wheat bran was not effective for treating IBS, the soluble fibers, such as psyllium, were likely effective. In contrast to the large number of studies of fiber supplementation, few studies have examined the effect of increasing fiber intake in the form of ordinary food.[70] These have reported improvement of IBS symptoms on both high- and low-fiber diets, a result often attributed to a placebo effect.[71] Consequently, the information has been conflicting at best and has led to little standardization in the way of official recommendations.

Systematic reviews of clinical trials of fiber for IBS have found no clear beneficial effects for fiber supplementation or bulking agents in female patients. The American College of Gastroenterology Functional Gastrointestinal Disorders Task Force's recommendations are that fiber is appropriate for the treatment of constipation but may not be recommended for the sole treatment of IBS.[72] A similar more recent meta-analysis of therapies for IBS does not recommend the use of bulking agents except as an adjuvant therapy.[73]

Although dietary fiber or bulking agents do not seem to be useful as sole treatment of IBS, they may have a limited initial role in empiric therapy depending on the patient's symptom complex, especially if constipation is the most significant symptom. The basic principles for using fiber therapy in this manner, based on limited efficacy and known potential adverse effects of worsening or causing abdominal discomfort and bloating, are to give an adequate trial, to evaluate the results early and periodically, and to start with a low dose and increase slowly. Physicians and dieticians should use insoluble fiber and soluble fiber carefully.[74] Methods for increasing fiber intake must be individualized. One proposed method is to add additional portions of fruits and vegetable. If constipation is not improved, or if the diet cannot be tolerated or followed, a trial of soluble fiber can be instituted. Recommendations for IBS-D patients are even less clear, although some authorities use a trial of increasing soluble fiber with psyllium or partially hydrolyzed guar gum.[75]

Fiber is commonly used in the treatment of patients with IBS; but despite a large number of trials, many with design limitations, benefits are unproved and patient tolerance may be a problem. Because most patients in all the studies evaluated are female, there may be a limited role for the careful use of dietary fiber or bulking agents in the management of some patients with IBS, especially if constipation is the dominant concern.

Probiotics

Probiotics are defined as live microorganisms that, when administered in adequate amounts, confer a health benefit to the host.[76] Although they have been used throughout history in the management of a variety of medical disorders, any actual evidence of their possible health benefits has been limited until recently. Probiotics can occur naturally in fermented foods, such as yogurt, buttermilk, sour poi, and miso. Pure and mixed cultures of potentially beneficial organisms have been added to foods or ingested in tablets, capsules, or liquids and have subsequently provided the basis for most of the scientific studies.[77]

Many mechanisms by which probiotics may improve IBS symptoms have been postulated.[78] Up to 25% of patients date the onset of their problem from a GI infection,[79] and evidence has accumulated to indicate the presence of an inflammatory response in the GI mucosa in IBS.[80,81] Additionally, the observation that IBS may be exacerbated by antibiotics,[82] coupled with reports of abnormal colonization of the small bowel in some patients,[27,28] suggests that it is possible that alterations in the bacterial flora of the gut may be of relevance.

Probiotics reportedly bind to small and large bowel epithelium and produce substances with antibiotic properties that may inhibit attachment and invasion by pathogenic organisms.[83,84] Probiotics may also modulate GI luminal immunity by changing the cytokine and cellular milieu from a proinflammatory to an antiinflammatory state.[85] They also convert undigested carbohydrates into short-chain fatty acids, which act as nutrients for the cells of the colon and alter gut motility. Therefore, it has been theorized that probiotics may lead to symptomatic improvements in patients with IBS, and it has been speculated that each individual bacterial strain or a combination of strains may affect select subclasses of symptoms in the IBS patient population.[86]

These findings formed the basis for a study examining the antiinflammatory properties of *Bifidobacterium infantis* in a large-scale, multicenter, clinical trial of women with IBS. Peripheral blood monocytes were extracted from IBS patients and healthy volunteers. The levels of cytokines interleukin (IL)-10 and IL-12 were assessed both at baseline and after treatment with either *B infantis* or *Lactobacillus salivarius*. At baseline the ratio of IL-10/IL-12 was significantly lower in the IBS population. After treatment with *B infantis*, these cytokine levels returned to levels consistent with those observed in controls and the IL-10/IL-12 ratio normalized.[87] These findings seem to support the theory that the mechanism for symptomatic improvement shown in patients receiving *B infantis* in the study seems to be down-regulation of a proinflammatory state. The study also showed that *B infantis*, delivered in a convenient formulation over a 4-week period, is a safe and effective treatment for patients with mild to moderate IBS symptoms and has the distinct advantage that it can be given to patients with IBS, which is characterized by either diarrhea or constipation.

Two recently published metaanalyses[78,88] and two comprehensive narrative reviews[89,90] further explored the use of probiotics in the treatment of IBS in the female population. All concluded that probiotics may be useful but confirmed that there are many variables affecting the results, such as the type, dose, and formulation of bacteria comprising the probiotic preparation; the outcome measured; and the size and characteristics of the IBS population studied.

Although clinical evidence of efficacy is now beginning to emerge, a review of available trials emphasizes the importance of clear definition of strain selection, dose, and viability.[91] Other probiotics may prove beneficial in the future; however, further studies are necessary before their use can be categorically recommended.

Turmeric

Turmeric is a member of the ginger family and its extract, curcumin, has antiinflammatory effects. In a partially blinded, randomized, 8-week trial of oral turmeric in 207 individuals with IBS (most of whom were female), overall symptoms improved more than 65%.[92] However, there was no placebo control and, therefore, no conclusions can be drawn from this study. Another double-blinded, placebo-controlled trial also examined the role of turmeric in patients, predominantly female, with IBS. In this study, the global assessment of changes in IBS symptoms and psychological stress caused by IBS did not differ significantly among the various treatment arms.[93] This additional study confirmed that turmeric did not show any therapeutic benefit over placebo in patients and hence the addition of this herb as a dietary supplement to IBS patients, female or male, cannot be firmly recommended.

Dietary Restrictions

Several studies report that IBS patients consider their symptoms to be related to certain foods because their symptoms often follow eating.[94–96] However, postprandial symptoms in IBS are not included in Rome III criteria,[97] and adverse reactions to food were reported to have a weak association in a factor analysis study.[98] Still, it is unavoidable that patients presenting with IBS ask their physicians for alimentary advice regarding dietary restrictions and limitations to decrease IBS symptoms. Consequently, different aspects of the relationship that could exist between dietary restrictions and IBS have repeatedly been studied and reviewed.

A recent review of the dietary habits of IBS patients has shown that IBS patients try a wide variety of diets.[99] However, the value of exclusion diets in IBS has repeatedly been questioned.[100] Although double-blind, placebo-controlled in vivo challenge is considered the gold standard in the diagnosis of food intolerance, these studies are hampered by both false-positive and false-negative reactions, mainly because of the fact that subjective symptoms still represent the basic premises for diagnosis.

A recent population-based case control study with a large control group used questionnaires to specifically explore nutritional limitations and restrictions as possible treatment and causes of symptoms in female IBS patients. Fatty foods (including fast food), certain vegetables, and dairy products were reported to cause significantly more GI complaints among both female and male IBS patients compared with their controls.[101] In addition, grilled or fried, hot and spicy food, coffee or tea, fruit and juices, sweets, and cakes also caused more GI problems among both female and male IBS patients compared with their control groups. Although the hypothesis of the study was that gender differences may exist in the types of foods resulting in worsened symptoms in IBS patients and would lead to different general dietary recommendations for female and male IBS patients in primary care, no significant differences were found.

Differences were, however, found in how female IBS patients responded to the belief that their symptoms were worsened by certain foods. Female IBS patients reported more changes in their dietary habits because of their GI problems than men with the disease compared with their controls. Most women and men who changed their dietary habits because of GI problems did, however, report some improvement in their symptoms.

Although food is certainly not responsible for all IBS symptoms, dietary manipulation targeted to individual IBS patients could help them to keep some control of well-being. A gastroenterologist should always start by taking a dietary history in any patient manifesting symptoms of IBS. Certain summarizing dietary advice can also be given. This ensures that recommendations of dietary restrictions are not misinterpreted and that important nutrients are not omitted based on recommendations made in the media or by nonmedical practitioners.

In patients with IBS-D, the intake of sugars, such as fructose and sorbitol, needs to be assessed and advice given regarding reduction of the intake of apple juice, soft drinks, and sugarless chewing gum.[102] Also, in IBS-D patients, it could be useful to assess the patient's intake of coffee and use of other stimuli. In cases of lactose intolerance, it is important to identify sources of lactose other than in dairy products (eg, food preservative and drug additives) and teach patients to carefully study product labels in this respect.[103]

Dietary restrictions can be recommended as adjuvant treatment in patients with either IBS-C or IBS-D. However, sole treatment with dietary limitations has not proved to be helpful in patients with true IBS, nor have recommendations specific to female IBS patients. Physicians should be willing and able to make dietary recommendations to their IBS patients but understand that dietary restrictions alone may not completely improve symptoms in all patients.

Herbals and Medicinals

Because a cure does not exist for IBS and conventional medicines provide only some relief of symptoms,[104] alternative medicine seems to be a potential source of benefit for many patients.[105] In the United States, an estimated 20% of patients with IBS have consulted an alternative health care provider (including homeopaths, naturopaths, and acupuncturists). Additionally, 29% of IBS patients report active use of an alternative medicine.[106] Because the use of alternative medicines in IBS patients is increasing in popularity, research in this field to specifically evaluate alternative approaches to IBS has also increased. Also of note, female IBS patients are more prone to use alternative medicine than are patients with other GI conditions.[107] Remedies being taken include herbal preparations, such as St John's wort (SJW), peppermint, and Chinese herbs. Safety is a common concern with herbal medicines. A systematic review of 22 RCTs of herbal medicines for IBS symptoms reported that adverse events occurred in 2.97% of patients (95% CI, 2.04%–3.90%), none of which was considered serious.[108] As noted by the authors of these trials, it is important to remind the IBS patient interested in herbal preparations that most of these trials were of poor quality and might have underreported adverse events. Consequently, it can only be recommended that clinicians should weigh the potential benefits and uncertainties of these therapies when advising patients about their use.

St John's wort

The herbal preparation of SJW, *Hypericum perforatum*, is known to effectively treat patients with mild-to-moderate depression with a reported 70% treatment response rate.[109] Although the mechanism of action of SJW has not been clearly delineated, it is postulated to exert an effect on serotonin pathways.[110] Aside from its neurologic effects, because 95% of serotonin is contained and released by the enterochromaffin cells of the GI tract,[111] manipulation of serotonin and its receptors has been shown to also affect gut function.[112] The frequent association of IBS with depression and the potential effect of SJW as an inhibitor of serotonin uptake have provided researchers rationale to evaluate its clinical effects on patients specifically with IBS.

Until a recent placebo-controlled, randomized, double-blind study,[113] no previous exploration of the clinical efficacy of SJW in IBS patients had been undertaken. The clinical efficacy in controlling IBS symptoms of 450 mg by mouth twice daily over 12 weeks was compared with a parallel control group. Of the 225 participants screened for eligibility for the study, 70 were randomized and began the treatment phase of the study. Eighty-six percent of participants were women. Overall, 29% had IBS-C, 37% had IBS-D, and 31% had IBS-mixed. Both groups reported decreases in overall bowel symptom score from baseline, with the placebo arm having significantly lower scores at 12 weeks compared with the SJW group. These patterns of improvement were mirrored in the secondary end points with the placebo group faring better than the SJW-treated group. Significant differences were observed at Week 12 for the IBS-D group and the portion of patients reporting adequate relief of IBS symptoms during the last 4 weeks of therapy.

Consequently, this pioneering study did not show that SJW had any benefit over placebo, and placebo seemed to work better for control of IBS symptoms. Although severity of symptoms was evaluated by a baseline bowel symptoms score questionnaire, the improvement obtained with the placebo was of similar magnitude to the improvement reported in the SJW group. Although the number of participants in the study limits its power and conclusion, the results do not support the use of SJW in IBS and may even suggest that its use should be discouraged in this setting.

Peppermint

An oil extract of the peppermint plant, *Mentha piperita*, has been used to treat stomach upset for millennia. Peppermint oil may alleviate IBS symptoms, including abdominal discomfort. The mechanism of action of peppermint has been extensively studied and it has been found to relax intestinal smooth muscle cells by interfering with calcium channels.[114,115] A fair, although limited, number of trials have been used to specifically assess the value of peppermint in female patients with IBS.

Of the short-term trials that show a positive correlation with peppermint use and a decrease in symptoms of IBS in females, the daily use of three to six enteric-coated capsules containing 0.2 to 0.4 mL of peppermint oil each has been found to improve IBS symptoms.[116–118] These observations are supported by two meta-analyses.[119,120] The first was based on five trials that suggested efficacy of the medicinal herb. However, although most of the patients studied were female, the use of heterogeneous diagnostic criteria and symptom scores weakened the power of the findings in this trial.[119] Another review of four small trials, also with mostly female patients, found overall symptom improvement with peppermint oil (OR 2.7; 95% CI, 1.6–4.8).[120] Another trial examined the role of peppermint in 110 patients who were prescreened for celiac disease and lactose intolerance. In this group, patients took four capsules daily for 4 weeks and symptoms were improved in 75% of those taking peppermint oil compared with 38% of those taking placebo ($P<.01$). The strict inclusion criteria in this study limit the extrapolation of the results, but peppermint oil may be considered as an adjunct therapy for all female patients with IBS.

Peppermint oil capsules are often specifically enteric-coated to prevent gastroesophageal reflux. Patients should be reminded not to chew the capsules. Perianal burning and nausea have been reported side effects.[121]

Tong xie yao fang

Tong xie yao fang is an herbal formula commonly used in traditional Eastern medicine. A meta-analysis of different variations of this formula included 12 Chinese studies examining its use in patients with IBS.[122] Studying a patient population that was predominantly female, the study preliminarily found tong xie yao fang formulations to be more effective than placebo (relative risk, 1.35; 95% CI, 1.21–1.50). However, it is important to note that the trials were heterogeneous and essentially of poor quality. Additionally, the formulations of tong xie yao fang were not standardized and the doses used were inconsistent. Among an additional three trials that used different traditional Chinese medical herbal formulas containing the ingredients of tong xie yao fang, two demonstrated efficacy[123,124] but the other did not.[125] These studies again suffered from the same deficiencies as the ones mentioned in the meta-analysis.

Mind Body Therapeutics

As has been demonstrated, IBS is a disorder with physical, psychological, and social components, which interact in complex and heterogeneous ways. The patient's perception of symptoms has been shown to be just as important as the physical nature of the symptoms themselves. These perceptions and understandings of the illness have been purported to have an equally important impact on a patient's functioning and QoL. It is postulated that this interaction is why IBS has previously been associated with a high prevalence of depression and anxiety, especially in the female population of patients. Some individuals develop unhelpful beliefs and behaviors regarding eating and bowel function, which may exacerbate physical symptoms, make them more distressing, and increase their impact on functioning. For these reasons, an evaluation of mind body medicine with a useful overview of psychological aspects and possible therapies for the treatment of IBS in women is necessary.[126]

Cognitive behavioral therapy

Because there is no specific medical treatment approach for IBS that works for all patients, physicians have turned to the evaluation of psychological therapies to provide relief for their patients.[127] Although the evidence is based on small, often poorly designed studies, cognitive-behavioral therapy (CBT) is one of the most studied of the mind–body therapeutics.

Patients undergoing CBT are trained to recognize and correct thoughts and behaviors that amplify symptoms or undermine well-being. This is combined with psychological strategies for coping with symptoms and illness to allow the patient to exert greater control over symptoms.[12,128] Five controlled trials have evaluated CBT in the treatment of IBS with mixed results.[129–133] Although all trials had mostly female patients, none of the trials found that women reported more success in their symptom management than their male counterparts. Three trials used individualized CBT with thought correction techniques, with the largest (N = 431) trial demonstrating that 12 weekly sessions improved symptoms more than did simply providing patients with information to recognize symptoms and triggers (response rate to therapy 70% vs 37%; $P = .0001$).[129] Of the two smaller trials, one found CBT to be equivalent to a relaxation technique[130] and the other was limited by a dropout rate of more than 50%.[132] The remaining two trials used group CBT; one (N = 45) found that symptoms and well-being improved more with CBT than a wait-list control,[132] but the other (N = 188) found that group CBT was not superior to psychoeducational support.[132] Although initially optimistic, the information from these studies is in no way uniform in recommendations regarding the use of CBT for female patients with IBS.

However, because of the lack of harm with CBT, psychological interventions can be considered for most patients with IBS. The specific intervention used can depend on many factors, including patients' preference, cost, and the availability of trained providers. Clinicians trained in CBT can consider providing it to their IBS patients but patients should be aware that CBT is certainly not a panacea and they may benefit from also continuing with traditional therapies.

Hypnotherapy

The field of hypnotherapy was initially pioneered by the mid-nineteenth century Scottish physician James Braid to evaluate eye and muscular conditions during what he termed the state of "nervous-sleep."[134] It is Braid's early evaluation of hypnotherapy that today forms the basis for the use of therapeutic suggestions to help patients deal with physiologic ailments.

Gut-directed hypnotherapy is a specific technique that combines suggestions related to emotional well-being and intestinal health. It is hypothesized that hypnotherapy could provide benefit for IBS, by affecting parts of the brain that experience abdominal pain or influence the movement of the bowel. Studies evaluating this type of hypnotherapy have involved mostly female patients, accurately representing the greater prevalence of the syndrome in this population.

Its use in IBS was first reported in a small trial of 30 patients, in which improvements in symptoms were greater after 7 weekly sessions of hypnotherapy than they were with supportive psychotherapy alone.[135] This was one of four trials identified in a Cochrane review of hypnotherapy in IBS.[136] The other three trials were also positive compared with medical treatment controls.[137–139] In the largest trial, 81 IBS patients in primary care received either five weekly sessions and self-hypnosis audiotapes daily or no treatment (neither medical nor psychological).[140] Patients, most of whom were female, who received hypnotherapy had a greater decline in symptom scores at 3 months (mean change in score of 13 out of 100 points vs 4.5 points in the control group; $P = .008$). It is important to note, however, that overall QoL scores did not reach statistical significance. Other systematic reviews have yielded similar borderline positive results,[140,141] with one review reporting an outlier of 87% as the median response rate to hypnosis treatment.[142]

As safety and potential long-term benefits add to the appeal of hypnotherapy for adjuvant therapy in IBS,[143] documented clinical experience by experts in the field suggests that some patients are more "hypnotizable" than others.[144] There is no mention in the literature if women are more susceptible to the benefits of hypnotherapy than men. Additionally, results of the included studies need to be interpreted with caution because of small size and methodologic limitations. Consequently, because of the essentially benign nature of therapy and lack of harm, it is reasonable to advise patients to consider a trial with a therapist trained in gut-directed hypnotherapy to augment other therapies that have already been initiated by their gastroenterologist.

Potential Future Therapeutic Options

As more and more patients continue to flood gastroenterology offices with new and challenging cases of IBS, so does the expanse of potential therapeutic options in females continue to increase. The trend of targeting GI motility agents and tachykinins, and hormonal modulation, and the interest in reducing inflammatory reactions in IBS will surely continue.

Tachykinins are biologically active peptides that affect bowel function, and include substance P and neurokinin A. Tachykinins also play a role in inflammatory conditions, such as IBS. A cholecystokinin-1 antagonist, dexloxiglumide, evaluated in a small study of 36 women, was associated with accelerated gastric emptying and slower ascending colon emptying.[145] This cholecystokinin inhibitor, however, did not demonstrate an improvement in symptom relief in this study; however, cholecystokinin-1 gene polymorphisms are a potential target for therapeutics, which should be evaluated in future studies. Linaclotide, a minimally adsorbed, guanylate cyclase, type-C receptor agonist demonstrated an increase in complete spontaneous bowel movements compared with placebo,[146] and will likely be a tool in the arsenal of IBS-C treatment in the future in addition to the currently FDA-approved lubiprostone (a type-2 chloride channel activator that increases intestinal secretions) for IBS constipation in women.[147] Neurotrophin-3 is an injectable prokinetic, which has been shown to increase GI motility in animal studies,[148] and is currently being evaluated in small human trials. Substance P binds the neurokinin receptor NK1, which is involved with bowel nociception. Neurokinin A binds the neurokinin receptor NK2, involved in bowel motility and smooth muscle contractility. Nepadutant, a NK2 antagonist, has been shown to reduce bowel motility in healthy volunteers, whereas current studies of nepadutant focus on patients with IBS.[149] Chromogranin A levels have also been shown to be elevated in patients with IBS-D, which may be of use in determining in the future which patients would benefit from octreotide.[150] Whether or not these therapeutics deliver clinically significant changes in global relief from IBS symptoms remains to be determined.

Given that there has been some evidence that the menstrual cycle in females has some effect on prepulse inhibition of the startle reflex,[151] further studies on the potential effect of oral contraceptives on prepulse inhibition and IBS should also be investigated. In addition, because variations during the menstrual cycle may exacerbate IBS symptoms, using oral contraceptives to maintain more consistent hormonal levels may potentially decrease symptomatology. There is also some conflicting evidence that GI symptoms may actually increase in women after menopause,[152] which may promote the use of hormone replacement in these IBS patients. Additionally, because there was no significant reduction in bowel symptoms with selective CRF_1 as opposed to animal studies, future studies targeting CRF_1 or CRF_2 antagonists may identify their role in treating patients with IBS-D.

Because there are postulated mechanisms of toxins involved in the pathogenesis of IBS, an oral, nonabsorbed, carbon-based derivative has been studied as a potential adsorbant of bacterial toxins and bile acids. A RCT demonstrated increased responders with AST-120 compared with placebo during this 8-week study.[153] This continues to demonstrate the trend of targeting mechanisms of inflammation in the pathogenesis of IBS.

SUMMARY

IBS is a complex clinical process with multiple pathophysiologic mechanisms, particularly in women. There has recently been a shift in the treatment of patients with severe IBS symptoms with disease-modifying therapies opposed to symptomatic treatment. There are growing data to support the use of many of the newer therapeutics in female patients whose IBS symptoms are resistant to conventional therapies. Some of the newer medications that have been studied and show promise include both the serotonin and hormone receptor modulators. Because menstruating women have been shown to have more variability their symptoms, it may prove daunting to treat their variable disease courses with standard medications. Given that female IBS patients are more likely to have comorbid conditions of anxiety, depression, and pain syndromes, it seems that psychopharmaceuticals, CBT, and hypnotherapy would be of particular success in these patients. Lastly, the role of education of IBS patients regarding their disease process should be emphasized in all patients because, unfortunately, there remains no single panacea for this complex highly prevalent disorder.

REFERENCES

1. Spiller R, Aziz Q, Creed F, et al. Guidelines on the irritable bowel syndrome: mechanism and practical management. Gut 2007;56:1770–98.
2. American College of Gastroenterology Functional Gastrointestinal Disorders Task Force. Evidence-based position statement on the management of irritable bowel syndrome in North America. Am J Gastroenterol 2002;97(Suppl 11): S1–5.
3. Lee OY, Mayer EA, Schmulson M, et al. Gender-related differences in IBS symptoms. Am J Gastroenterol 2001;96:2184–93.
4. Chang L, Heitkemper MM. Gender differences in irritable bowel syndrome. Gastroenterology 2002;123:1686–701.
5. Shiotani A, Miyanishi T, Takahashi T. Sex differences in irritable bowel syndrome in Japanese university students. J Gastroenterol 2006;41:562–8.
6. Nyrop KA, Palsson OS, Levy RL, et al. Costs of health care for irritable bowel syndrome, chronic constipation, functional diarrhoea and functional abdominal pain. Aliment Pharmacol Ther 2007;26:237–48.
7. Martin BC, Ganguly R, Pannicker S, et al. Utilization patterns and net direct medical cost to Medicaid of irritable bowel syndrome. Curr Med Res Opin 2003;19:771–80.
8. Drossman DA, Corazziari E, Delavaux M, et al. Rome III: the functional gastrointestinal disorders. McLean (VA): Degnon Associates; 2006.
9. Mayer EA, Berman S, Change L, et al. Sex-based differences in gastrointestinal pain. Eur J Pain 2004;8:451–63.
10. Dalrymple J, Bullock I. Diagnosis and management of irritable bowel syndrome in adults in primary care: summary of NICE guidance. BMJ 2007;336:556–8.

11. Spiller R. Clinical update: irritable bowel syndrome. Lancet 2007;369:1586–8.
12. Hayee B, Forgacs I. Psychological approach to managing irritable bowel syndrome. BMJ 2007;334:1105–9.
13. Drossman DA. The functional gastrointestinal disorder and the Rome III process. Gastroenterology 2006;130:1377–90.
14. Saad RJ, Chey WD. Recent developments in the therapy of irritable bowel syndrome. Expert Opin Investig Drugs 2008;17:117–30.
15. Dom SD, Palsson OS, Thiwan SI, et al. Increased colonic pain sensitivity in irritable bowel syndrome is the result of increased tendency to report pain rather than increased neurosensory sensitivity. Gut 2007;156:1202–9.
16. Naliboff BF, Berman S, Chang L, et al. Sex-related differences in IBS patients: central processing of visceral stimuli. Gastroenterology 2003;124:1738–47.
17. Heitkemper MM, Jarrett M. Pattern of gastrointestinal and somatic symptoms across the menstrual cycle. Gastroenterology 1992;102:505–13.
18. Ouyang A, Wrzos HF. Contribution of gender to pathophysiology and clinical presentation of IBS: should management be different in women? Am J Gastroenterol 2006;101:S602–9.
19. Bainbridge ET, Nicholas SD, Newton JR, et al. Gastrooesophageal reflux in pregnancy. Altered function of the barrier to reflux in asymptomatic women during early pregnancy. Scand J Gastroenterol 1985;19:85–9.
20. Knight LC, Parkman HP, Brown KL, et al. Delayed gastric emptying and decreased antral contractility in normal premenopausal women compared with men. Am J Gastroenterol 1997;92:968–75.
21. Camilleri M. Serotonin in the gastrointestinal tract. Curr Opin Endocrinol Diabetes Obes 2009;16:53–9.
22. Talley NJ, Kellow JE, Boyce P, et al. Antidepressant therapy (Imipramine and Citalopram) for irritable bowel syndrome: a double-blind, randomized, placebo-controlled trial. Dig Dis Sci 2008;53:108–15.
23. Morgan V, Pickens D, Gautam S, et al. Amitriptyline reduces rectal pain related activation of the anterior cingulate cortex in patients with irritable bowel syndrome. Gut 2005;54:601–7.
24. Halpert A, Dalton CB, Diamant NE, et al. Clinical response to tricyclic antidepressants in functional bowel disorders is not related to dosage. Am J Gastroenterol 2005;100:664–71.
25. Rajagopalan M, Kurian G, John J. Symptom relief with amitriptyline in the irritable bowel syndrome. J Gastroenterol Hepatol 1998;13:738–41.
26. Vahedi H, Merat S, Momtahen S, et al. Clinical trial: the effect of amitiptyline in patients with diarrhoea-predominant irritable bowel syndrome. Aliment Pharmacol Ther 2008;27:678–84.
27. Pimental M, Chow EJ, Lin HC. Eradication of small intestinal bacterial overgrowth reduces symptoms of irritable bowel syndrome. Am J Gastroenterol 2000;95:3503–6.
28. Pimental M, Chow EJ, Lin HC. Normalization of lactulose breath testing correlates with symptom improvement in irritable bowel syndrome: a double-blind, randomized, placebo-controlled study. Am J Gastroenterol 2003;98:412–9.
29. Pimental M, Chatterjee S, Chow EJ, et al. Neomycin improves constipation-predominant irritable bowel syndrome in a fashion that is dependent on the presence of methane gas: subanalysis of a double-blind randomized controlled study. Dig Dis Sci 2006;51:1287–301.

30. Pimental M, Park S, Mirocha J, et al. The effect of a nonabsorbed oral antibiotic (Rifaximin) on the symptoms of the irritable bowel syndrome. Ann Intern Med 2006;145:557–63.
31. Chang L, Ameen VZ, Dukes GE, et al. A dose-ranging, phase II study of the efficacy and safety of alosetron in men with diarrhea-predominant IBS. Am J Gastroenterol 2005;100:115–23.
32. Lembo T, Wright RA, Bagby B, et al. Alosetron controls bowel urgency and provides global symptom improvement in women with diarrhea-predominant irritable bowel syndrome. Am J Gastroenterol 2001;96:2662–70.
33. Chang L. Current perspectives in irritable bowel syndrome. Presented at the Fourth National Forum on Women's Issues in Gastroenterology and Hepatology. Philadelphia, June 4, 2010.
34. Krause R, Ameen V, Gordon SH, et al. A randomized, double-blind, placebo-controlled study to assess efficacy and safety of 0.5 mg and 1 mg alosetron in women with severe diarrhea-predominant IBS. Am J Gastroenterol 2007; 102:1709–19.
35. Chey WD, Chey WY, Heath AT, et al. Long-term safety and efficacy of alosetron in women with severe diarrhea-predominant irritable bowel syndrome. Am J Gastroenterol 2004;99:2195–203.
36. Loughlin J, Quinn S, Rivero E, et al. Tegaserod and the risk of cardiovascular ischemic events. J Cardiovasc Pharmacol Ther 2010;15(2):151–7.
37. Camilleri M, Chey WY, Mayer EA, et al. A randomized controlled clinical trial of the serotonin type 3 receptor antagonist alosetron in women with diarrhea-predominant irritable bowel syndrome. Arch Intern Med 2001;161: 1733–40.
38. Camilleri M, Northcutt AR, Kong S, et al. Efficacy and safety of alosetron in women with irritable bowel syndrome: a randomised, placebo-controlled trial. Lancet 2000;355:1035–40.
39. Bardhan KD, Bodemar G, Geldof H, et al. A double-blind, randomized, placebo-controlled dose-ranging study to evaluate the efficacy of alosetron in the treatment of irritable bowel syndrome. Aliment Pharmacol Ther 2000; 14:23–34.
40. Chey WD, Pare P, Viegas A, et al. Tegaserod for female patients suffering from IBS with mixed bowel habits or constipation: a randomized controlled trial. Am J Gastroenterol 2008;103:1217–25.
41. Drossman DA, Morris CB, Hu Y, et al. A prospective assessment of bowel habit in irritable bowel syndrome in women: defining an alternator. Gastroenterology 2005;128:580–9.
42. Mearin F, Balboa A, Badia X, et al. Irritable bowel syndrome subtypes according to bowel habit: revisiting the alternating subtype. Eur J Gastroenterol Hepatol 2003;15:165–72.
43. Tack J, Muller-Lissner S, Bytzer P, et al. A randomized controlled trial assessing the efficacy and safety of repeated tegaserod therapy in women with irritable bowel syndrome with constipation. Gut 2005;54:1707–13.
44. Novartis Pharmaceutical. Zelnorm [Online PDF]. Available at: http://web. archive.org/web/20070410024119/; http://www.zelnorm.com/Zelnrom_PR_US_ 330_Final_12_1007.pdf. Archived 2007-04-10. Accessed December 30, 2010.
45. George AM, Meyers NL, Hickling RI. Clinical trial: renzapride therapy for constipation-predominant irritable bowel syndrome: multicentre, randomized, placebo-controlled, double-blind study in primary healthcare setting. Aliment Pharmacol Ther 2008;27:830–7.

46. Alizyme pls. Results from renzapride [Online Press-Release]. Available at: http://www.alizyme.com/alizyme/media/press/show.jsp?ref=128. Archived 2008-04-23. Accessed December 30, 2010.

47. Palomba S, Orio F, Manguso F, et al. Leuprolide acetate treatment with and without coadministration of tibolone in premenopausal women with menstrual cycle-related irritable bowel syndrome. Fertil Steril 2005;83(4):1012–9.

48. Tache Y, Monnikes H, Bonaz B, et al. Role of CRF in stress-related alterations of gastric and colonic motor function. Ann N Y Acad Sci 1993;697:233–43.

49. Sweetser S, Camilleri M, Linker Nord SJ, et al. Do corticotropin releasing factor-1 receptors influence colonic transit and bowel function in women with irritable bowel syndrome? Am J Physiol Gastrointest Liver Physiol 2009;296:1299–306.

50. Marlett JA, McBurney MI, Slavin JL. Position of the American Dietetic Association: health implications of dietary fiber. J Am Diet Assoc 2002;102:993–1000.

51. Floch MH, Narayan R. Diet in the irritable bowel syndrome. J Clin Gastroenterol 2002;35(Suppl 1):S45–52.

52. Spiller RC. Pharmacology of dietary fibre. Pharmacol Ther 1994;62:402–27.

53. Camilleri M, Heading RC, Thompson WG. Consensus report: clinical perspectives, mechanism, diagnosis and management of irritable bowel syndrome. Aliment Pharmacol Ther 2002;16:1407–30.

54. Bijkerk CJ, Muris JW, Knottnerus JA, et al. Systematic review: the role of different types of fiber in the treatment of irritable bowel syndrome. Aliment Pharmacol Ther 2004;19:245–51.

55. Hebden JM, Blackshaw E, D'Amato M, et al. Abnormalities of GI transit in bloated irritable bowel syndrome: effect of bran on transit and symptoms. Am J Gastroenterol 2002;97:2315–20.

56. Lanza E, Jones DY, Block E, et al. Dietary fiber intake in the US population. Am J Clin Nutr 1987;46:790–7.

57. Bijkerk CJ, de Wit NJ, Stalman WA, et al. Irritable bowel syndrome in primary care. The patients' and doctors' views on symptoms, etiology and management. Can J Gastroenterol 2003;17:363–8.

58. Miller V, Lea R, Agrawal A, et al. Bran and irritable bowel syndrome: the primary-care perspective. Dig Liver Dis 2006;33:737–40.

59. Lea R, Whowell PJ. The role of food intolerance in irritable bowel syndrome: the primary-care perspective. Dig Liver Dis 2006;38:737–40.

60. Ford AC, Talley NJ, Spiegel BM, et al. Effect of fibre, antispasmodics, and peppermint oil in the treatment of irritable bowel syndrome: systematic review and meta-analysis. BMJ 2008;337:a2313.

61. Lesbros-Pantoflickova D, Michetti P, Fried M, et al. Meta-analysis: the treatment of irritable bowel syndrome. Aliment Pharmacol Ther 2004;20:1253–69.

62. Brandt LK, Bjorkman D, Fennerty MB, et al. Systematic review on the management of irritable bowel syndrome in North America. Am J Gastroenterol 2002;97:S7–26.

63. Quartero AO, Meineche-Schmidt V, Muris J, et al. Bulking agents, antispasmodic and antidepressant medication for the treatment of irritable bowel syndrome. Cochrane Database Syst Rev 2005;2:CD003460.

64. Jailwala J, Imperiale TH, Kroenke K. Pharmacologic treatment of the irritable bowel syndrome: a systematic review of randomized, controlled trials. Ann Intern Med 2000;133:136–47.

65. Zuckerman MJ. The role of fiber in the treatment of irritable bowel syndrome: therapeutic recommendations. J Clin Gastroenterol 2006;40:104–8.

66. Akehurst R, Kaltenthaler E. Treatment of irritable bowel syndrome: a review of randomized controlled trials. Gut 2001;48:272–82.

67. Prior A, Whowell PJ. Double blind study of ispaghula in irritable bowel syndrome. Gut 1987;28:1510–3.

68. Kumar A, Kumar N, Vij JC, et al. Optimum dosage of ispaghula husk in patients with irritable bowel syndrome: correlation of symptom relief with whole gut transit time and stool weight. Gut 1987;28:150–5.

69. Villagrasa M, Boix J, Humbert P, et al. Aleatory clinical study comparing otilonium bromide with a fiber-rich diet in the treatment of irritable bowel syndrome. Ital J Gastroenterol 1991;23(Suppl 1):67–70.

70. Fowlie S, Eastwood M, Prescott R. Irritable bowel syndrome: assessment of psychological disturbance and its influence on the response to fibre supplementation. J Psychosom Res 1992;36:175–80.

71. Parisi GC, Zilli M, Miani MP, et al. High-fiver diet supplementation in patients with IBS: a multicenter, randomized open trial comparison between wheat bran diet and partially hydrolyces guar gum. Dig Dis Sci 2002;47:1697–704.

72. Burden S. Dietary treatment of irritable bowel syndrome: current evidence and guidelines for future practice. J Hum Nutr Diet 2001;14:231–41.

73. Paineau D, Payen F, Panserieu D, et al. The effects of regular consumption of short-chain fructo-oligosacccharides on digestive comfort of subject with minor function bowel disorders. Br J Nutr 2008;99:311–8.

74. Bernstein CN. The placebo effect for gastroenterology: tool or torment. Clin Gastroenterol Hepatol 2006;4:1302–8.

75. Karamanolis G, Tack J. Nutrition and motility disorders. Best Pract Res Clin Gastroenterol 2006;20:485–505.

76. O'Sullivan MA, O'Morain CA. Bacterial supplementation in the irritable bowel syndrome. A randomised double-blind placebo-controlled crossover study. Dig Liver Dis 2000;32:294–301.

77. Sen S, Mullan MM, Parker TJ, et al. Effect of *Lactobacillus plantarum* 299v on colonic fermentation and symptoms of irritable bowel syndrome. Dig Dis Sci 2002;47:2615–20.

78. Nikfar S, Rahimi R, Rahimi F, et al. Efficacy of probiotics in irritable bowel syndrome: a meta-analysis of randomized, controlled trials. Dis Colon Rectum 2008;51:1776–80.

79. Chadwick B, Chen W, Shu D, et al. Activation of the mucosal immune system in irritable bowel syndrome. Gastroenterology 2002;123:1972–9.

80. Gonsalkorale WM, Perrey C, Pravica V, et al. Interleukin 10 genotypes in irritable bowel syndrome: evidence for an inflammatory component? Gut 2003;52:91–3.

81. Barbara G, Stanghellini V, De Giorgio R, et al. Activated mast cells in proximity to colonic nerves correlate with abdominal pain in irritable bowel syndrome. Gastroenterology 2004;126:693–702.

82. Maxwell PR, Rink E, Kumar D, et al. Antibiotics increase functional abdominal symptoms. Am J Gastroenterol 2002;97:104–8.

83. Johansson ML, Molin G, Jeppsson B, et al. Administration of different *Lactobacillus* strains in fermented oatmeal soup: in vivo colonization of human intestinal mucosa and effect on the indigenous flora. Appl Environ Microbiol 1993;59:15–20.

84. Pathmakanthan S, Li C, Cowie J, et al. *Lactobacillus plantarum* 299: beneficial in vitro immunomodulation in cells extracted from inflamed human colon. J Gastroenterol Hepatol 2004;19:166–73.

85. O'Mahony L, McCarthy J, Kelly P, et al. *Lactobacillus* and *Bifobacterium* in irritable bowel syndrome: symptom responses and relationship to cytokine profiles. Gastroenterology 2005;128:541–51.

86. Floch MH. Use of diet and probiotic therapy in the irritable bowel syndrome. J Clin Gastroenterol 2005;39:S243–6.

87. Whorwell PJ, Altringer L, Morel J, et al. Efficacy of an encapsulated probiotic *Bifidobacterium infantis* 35624 in women with IBS. Am J Gastroenterol 2006;101: 1581–90.

88. McFarland LV, Dublin S. Meta-analysis of probiotics for the treatment of irritable bowel syndrome. World J Gastroenterol 2008;14:2650–61.

89. Wilhelm SM, Brubaker CM, Varcak EA, et al. Effectiveness of probiotics in the treatment of irritable bowel syndrome. Pharmacotherapy 2008;28:496–505.

90. Spiller R. Review article: probiotics and prebiotics in irritable bowel syndrome. Aliment Pharmacol Ther 2008;28:385–96.

91. Quigley EM, Flourie B. Probiotics and irritable bowel syndrome: a rationale for their use and an assessment of the evidence to date. Neurogastroenterol Motil 2007;19:166–72.

92. Bundy R, Walker AF, Middleton RW, et al. Turmeric extract may improve irritable bowel syndrome symptomology in otherwise healthy adults: a pilot study. J Altern Complement Med 2004;10:1015–8.

93. Brinkhaus B, Hentschel C, Von Keudell C, et al. Herbal medicine with curcuma fumitory in the treatment of irritable bowel syndrome: a randomized, placebo-controlled, double-blind clinical trial. Scand J Gastroenterol 2005;40:936–43.

94. Lacy BE, Weiser K, Noddin L, et al. Irritable bowel syndrome: patients attitudes, concerns and level of knowledge. Aliment Pharmacol Ther 2007;25:1329–41.

95. Simren M, Mansson A, Langklide AM, et al. Food-related gastrointestinal symptoms in irritable bowel syndrome. Digestion 2001;63:108–15.

96. Halpert A, Dalton CB, Palsson O, et al. What patients know about irritable bowel syndrome and what they would like to know. National survey on patient educational needs in IBS and development and validation of patient educational needs questionnaire (PEQ). Am J Gastroenterol 2007;102:1972–82.

97. Whitehead WE, Drossman DA. Validation of symptom-based diagnostic criteria for irritable bowel syndrome: a critical review. Am J Gastroenterol 2010;105: 814–20.

98. Whitehead WE, Crowell MD, Bosmajian L, et al. Existence of irritable bowel syndrome supported by factor analysis of symptoms in two community samples. Gastroenterology 1990;98:336–40.

99. Rees GA, Davies GI, Parker M, et al. Gastrointestinal symptoms and diet of members of an irritable bowel self-help group. J R Soc Health 1994;114:182–7.

100. McKee AM, Prior A, Whorwell PJ. Exclusion diets in irritable bowel syndrome: are they worthwhile? J Clin Gastroenterol 1987;9:526–8.

101. Faresjo A, Johansson S, Faresjo T, et al. Sex differences in dietary coping with gastrointestinal symptoms. Eur J Gastroenterol Hepatol 2010;22:327–33.

102. Muller-lissner SA, Kaatz V, Brandt W, et al. The perceived effect of various food and beverages on stool consistency. Eur J Gastroenterol Hepatol 2005;17: 109–12.

103. Saito YA, Locket GR III, Weaver AL, et al. Diet and functional gastrointestinal disorders: a populations-based case-control study. Am J Gastroenterol 2005; 100:2743–8.

104. Drossman DA, Camilleri M, Mayer EA, et al. AGA technical review on irritable bowel syndrome. Gastroenterology 2002;123:2108–31.

105. Koloski NA, Talley NJ, Huskic SS, et al. Predictors of conventional and alternative health care seeking for irritable bowel syndrome and functional dyspepsia. Aliment Pharmacol Ther 2003;17:841–51.
106. Jarrett ME, Heitkempre MM, Hertig V, et al. Alternative health care practices in women with irritable bowel syndrome. Gastroenterology 1999;116:A1012.
107. Kong SC, Hurlstone DP, Pocock CY, et al. The incidence of self-prescribed oral complimentary and alternative medicine use by patients with gastrointestinal diseases. J Clin Gastroenterol 2005;39:138–41.
108. Shi K, Tong Y, Shen JG, et al. Effectiveness and safety of herbal medicines in the treatment of irritable bowel syndrome: a systematic review. World J Gastroenterol 2008;14:454–62.
109. Linde K, Berner MM, Kriston L. St John's wort for major depression. Cochrane Database Syst Rev 2008;3:CD000448.
110. Franklin M, Chi J, McGavin C, et al. Neuroendocrine evidence for dopaminerfic actions of hypericum extract in healthy volunteers. Biol Psychiatry 1999;46:581–4.
111. Gershon MN, Tack J. The serotonin signaling system: from basic understanding to drug development for functional GI disorders. Gastroenterology 2007;132:397–414.
112. Jackson JL, O'Malley PG, Tomkins G, et al. Treatment of functional gastrointestinal disorders with antidepressant medications: a meta-analysis. Am J Med 2000;108:65–72.
113. Saito YA, Rey E, Almazar-Elder AE, et al. A randomized, double-blind, placebo-controlled trial of St. John's wort for treating irritable bowel syndrome. Am J Gastroenterol 2010;105:170–7.
114. Kligler B, Chaudhary S. Peppermint oil. Am Fam Physician 2007;75:1027–30.
115. Hills JM, Aaronson PI. The mechanism of action of peppermint oil on gastrointestinal smooth muscle. Gastroenterology 1991;101:55–65.
116. Cappello G, Spezzaferro M, Grossi L, et al. Peppermint oil in the treatment of irritable bowel syndrome: a prospective double blind placebo-controlled randomized trial. Dig Liver Dis 2007;39:530–6.
117. Liu JH, Chen GH, Yeh HZ, et al. Enteric-coated peppermint-oil capsules in the treatment of irritable bowel syndrome: a prospective, randomized trial. J Gastroenterol 1997;32:765–8.
118. Merat S, Khalili S, Mostajabi P, et al. The effect of enteric-coated, delayed-release peppermint oil on irritable bowel syndrome. Dig Dis Sci 2010;55:1385–90.
119. Pittler MH, Ernst E. Peppermint oil for irritable bowel syndrome: a critical review and meta-analysis. Am J Gastroenterol 1998;98:1131–5.
120. Spanier JA, Howden CW, Jones MP. A systematic review of alternative therapies in the irritable bowel syndrome. Arch Intern Med 2003;163:265–74.
121. Lawson MJ, Knight RE, Tran K, et al. Failure of enteric-coated peppermint oil in the irritable bowel syndrome: a randomized double-blind crossover study. J Gastroenterol Hepatol 1988;3:235–8.
122. Bian Z, Wu T, Liu L, et al. Effectiveness of the Chinese herbal formula tong xie yao fang for irritable bowel syndrome: a systematic review. J Altern Complement Med 2006;12:401–7.
123. Bensoussan A, Talley NJ, Hing M, et al. Treatment of irritable bowel syndrome with Chinese herbal medicine: a randomized controlled trial. JAMA 1999;282:1585–9.
124. Wang G, Li TQ, Wang L, et al. Tong-xie-ning, a Chinese herbal formula, in treatment of diarrhea-predominant irritable bowel syndrome: a prospective,

randomized, double-blind, placebo-controlled trial. Chin Med J (Engl) 2006;119: 2114–9.

125. Leung WK, Wu JC, Liang SM, et al. Treatment of diarrhea-predominant irritable bowel syndrome with traditional Chinese herbal medicine: a randomized placebo-controlled trial. Am J Gastroenterol 2006;101:1574–80.

126. Hutton JM. Issues to consider in cognitive-behavioral therapy for irritable bowel syndrome. Eur J Gastroenterol Hepatol 2008;20:249–51.

127. Ross-Morris R, McAlpine L, Didsbury LP, et al. A randomized controlled trial of a cognitive behavioral therapy-based self-management intervention for irritable bowel syndrome in primary care. Psychol Med 2010;40:85–94.

128. Palsson OS. Should we incorporate psychological care into the management of IBS? Nat Clin Pract Gastroenterol Hepatol 2006;3:474–5.

129. Drossman DA, Toner BB, Whitehead WE, et al. Cognitive-behavioral therapy versus education and desipramine versus placebo for moderate to severe functional bowel disorders. Gastroenterology 2003;125:19–31.

130. Boyce PM, Talley NJ, Balaam B, et al. A randomized controlled trial of cognitive behavior therapy, relaxation training, and routine clinical care for the irritable bowel syndrome. Am J Gastroenterol 2003;98:2209–18.

131. Kennedy T, Jones R, Darnley S, et al. Cognitive behavior therapy in addition to antispasmodic treatment for irritable bowel syndrome in primary care: randomized controlled trial. BMJ 2005;331:435.

132. Van Dulmen AM, Fennis JF, Bleijenberg G. Cognitive-behavioral group therapy for irritable bowel syndrome: effects and long-term follow-up. Psychosom Med 1996;58:508–14.

133. Blanchard EB, Lackner JM, Sanders K, et al. A controlled evaluation of group cognitive therapy in the treatment of irritable bowel syndrome. Behav Res Ther 2007;45:633–48.

134. Braid J. Practical essay on the curative agency of neuro-hypnotism. London: J. Churchill Press; 1843.

135. Whorwell PJ, Prior A, Faragher EB. Controlled trial of hypnotherapy in the treatment of severe refractory irritable-bowel syndrome. Lancet 1984;2:1232–4.

136. Webb AN, Kukuruzovic RH, Catto-Smith AG. Hypnotherapy for treatment of irritable bowel syndrome. Cochrane Database Syst Rev 2007;4:CD005110.

137. Galovski TE, Blanchard EB. The treatment of irritable bowel syndrome with hypnotherapy. Appl Psychophysiol Biofeedback 1998;23:219–32.

138. Palsson OS, Turner MJ, Johnson DA, et al. Hypnosis treatment for severe irritable bowel syndrome: investigation of mechanism and effects on symptoms. Dig Dis Sci 2002;47:2605–14.

139. Roberts L, Wilson S, Singh S, et al. Gut-directed hypnotherapy for irritable bowel syndrome: piloting a primary care-based randomized controlled trial. Br J Gen Pract 2006;56:115–21.

140. Wilson S, Maddison T, Roberts L, et al. Birmingham IBS Research Group. Systematic review: the effectiveness of hypnotherapy in the management of irritable bowel syndrome. Aliment Pharmacol Ther 2006;24:769–80.

141. Gholamrezaei A, Ardestani SK, Emami MN. Where does hypnotherapy stand in the management of irritable bowel syndrome? A systematic review. J Altern Complement Med 2006;12:517–27.

142. Whitehead WE. Hypnosis for irritable bowel syndrome: the empirical evidence of therapeutic effects. Int J Clin Exp Hypn 2006;54:7–20.

143. Gonsalkorale WM, Miller V, Afzal A, et al. Long term benefits of hypnotherapy for irritable bowel syndrome. Gut 2004;52:1623–9.

144. Gonsalkorale WM, Houghton LA, Whorwell PJ. Hypnotherapy in irritable bowel syndrome: a large-scale audit of a clinical service with examination of factors influencing responsiveness. Am J Gastroenterol 2002;97:954–61.

145. Cremonini F, Camilleri M, McKinzie S, et al. Effect of CCK-1 antagonist, dexloxiglumide, in female patients with irritable bowel syndrome: a pharmacodynamic and pharmacogenomic study. Am J Gastroenterol 2005;100:652–63.

146. Andresen V, Camilleri M, Busciglio IA, et al. Effect of 5 days Linaclotide on transit and bowel function in females with constipation-predominant irritable bowel syndrome. Gastroenterology 2007;133:761–8.

147. Camilleri M, Bharucha AE, Ueno R, et al. Effect of a selective chloride channel activator, lubiprostone, on gastrointestinal transit, gastric sensory, and motor functions in healthy volunteers. Am J Physiol Gastrointest Liver Physiol 2006; 290:G942–7.

148. Chai N, Dong L, Zong-Fang L, et al. Effects of neurotrophins on gastrointestinal myoelectric activities of rats. World J Gastroenterol 2003;9(8):1874–7.

149. Lecci A, Capriati A, Maggi CA. Tachykinin NK2 receptor antagonists for the treatment of irritable bowel syndrome. Br J Pharmacol 2004;141:1249–63.

150. Sidhu R, McAlindon ME, Leeds JS, et al. The role of serum chromogranin A in diarrhoea predominant irritable bowel syndrome. J Gastrointestin Liver Dis 2009;18(1):23–6.

151. Kilpatrick LA, Ornitz E, Ibrahimovic H, et al. Sex-related differences in prepulse inhibition of startle in irritable bowel syndrome (IBS). Biol Psychol 2010;84: 272–8.

152. Cain KC, Jarrett ME, Burr RL, et al. Gender differences in gastrointestinal, psychological, and somatic symptoms in irritable bowel syndrome. Dig Dis Sci 2009;54:1542–9.

153. Tack JF, Harris M, Proksch S, et al. AST-120 (spherical carbon adsorbent) improves pain and bloating in a randomized, double-blind, placebo-controlled trial in patients with non-constipating irritable bowel syndrome (IBS). Presented at Digestive Disease Week (DDW) 2010. New Orleans, May 1, 2010. Abstract S1298.

When to Reconsider the Diagnosis of Irritable Bowel Syndrome

Christopher W. Hammerle, MD, Sheila E. Crowe, MD, FRCPC*

KEYWORDS

• Irritable bowel syndrome • Celiac disease • Food intolerance
• Small intestinal bacterial overgrowth

A 33-year-old woman presents for a second opinion after recently being diagnosed with irritable bowel syndrome (IBS) by her primary care physician. She
never had gastrointestinal problems until going on a vacation to South America
2 years ago. During the trip, both she and her husband had an episode of food
poisoning from which he recovered uneventfully within several days. However,
since that time she has had persistent abdominal cramping, bloating, and intermittent episodes of diarrhea. After reading about IBS on the Internet, she altered her
diet to include more fresh fruits and vegetables and began taking fiber supplements. Despite these dietary modifications, she has had little symptomatic
improvement. Her medical history is notable for 2 miscarriages and anemia. In
your office her physical examination is normal, and the results of a recently
ordered complete blood cell count and comprehensive metabolic panel are
normal except for a mildly elevated mean corpuscular volume. Does this patient
have IBS, or are there clues in her presentation to suggest an alternative or coex-
isting diagnosis, such as small intestinal bacterial overgrowth (SIBO) or Celiac
disease (CD)? How do we best approach this case?

IRRITABLE BOWEL SYNDROME

Irritable bowel syndrome (IBS) is a chronic gastrointestinal (GI) tract disorder of
unknown origin characterized by abdominal pain and altered bowel habits in the
absence of detectable biochemical or structural abnormalities.[1] IBS is one of the
most common functional GI disorders with an estimated prevalence of 10% to 15%
in Western adult populations.[2-4] Although only a minority of patients with IBS seek

The authors have nothing to disclose.
Division of Gastroenterology and Hepatology, University of Virginia, PO Box 800708,
Charlottesville, VA 22908-0708, USA
* Corresponding author.
E-mail address: scrowe@virginia.edu

medical care,[5] they account for a large percentage of referrals to gastroenterologists and use a substantial portion of health care resources.[6,7] Direct and indirect costs of IBS are staggering, reaching up to $30 billion per annum in the United States alone.[8–10]

IBS occurs in both genders; however, women are affected roughly in the ratio of 2:1 and tend to seek medical care more often than men.[11] The onset of symptoms occurs most frequently before the age of 50 years; however, all ages are affected and symptoms can persist well into advancing years.[3] IBS is commonly subdivided into different phenotypes depending on the most prevalent bowel habit: diarrhea-predominant IBS (IBS-D), constipation predominant (IBS-C), and mixed features (IBS-M). The prevalence of each subtype has been shown to vary in different studies, but overall, IBS-D or IBS-M may be slightly more common.[12–14] Comorbid symptoms and disorders are common with IBS, particularly in patients with severe symptoms and those seen in referral practices. Psychiatric comorbidities are estimated to occur in about 60% of patients with IBS presenting to gastroenterology clinics and in up to 70% of those seen in tertiary referral centers.[15] Health-related quality-of-life scores are lower in patients with IBS than healthy controls and are similar to other chronic medical disorders, such as asthma, gastroesophageal reflux, and end-stage renal disease.[16,17]

The pathophysiology of IBS is incompletely understood, although it is considered to be a multifactorial disorder arising from dysregulation in the brain-gut axis as well as interactions between genetics,[18,19] motor and sensory dysfunction,[20,21] dysregulated intestinal immunity,[22] and psychosocial abnormalities.[23,24] Recent data suggest that patients with IBS may have increased hydrogen gas production in their small bowel.[25,26] This observation has led some clinicians to hypothesize a role for small intestinal bacterial overgrowth (SIBO) in the pathogenesis of IBS and propose treating patients with antibiotics, especially those with symptoms of bloating and diarrhea.[27] Although still controversial, this approach is gaining popularity and at present is the subject of much research and debate. Postinfectious IBS (PI-IBS) is a well-described subtype of IBS that can present de novo following a bacterial or viral gastroenteritis. It tends to occur more often in women and with time, usually develops into an IBS-D phenotype.[28,29] Although a recent study concluded that PI-IBS likely accounts for only a small subset of IBS cases,[30] its existence argues for a strong association between environmental triggers and intestinal inflammation in the development of symptoms in certain at-risk individuals.

On further questioning, it was found that our patient's bloating and diarrhea is generally worse following meals and seems to be particularly bad after consuming dairy products. She is always fatigued and has gained 20 pounds (9 kg) since the onset of her symptoms. She denies any rectal bleeding and has no family history of colorectal cancer. At this point, do we have enough information to diagnose her with IBS? What additional studies, if any, should be performed?

DIAGNOSING IBS

In clinical practice, IBS symptoms are often heterogeneous and can masquerade as several other medical conditions. Because of this ambiguity, it is common for both general practitioners and gastroenterologists to order an array of expensive and invasive tests before the correct diagnosis is eventually made.[31] National guidelines discourage this approach and recommend using clinical grounds to diagnose IBS without pursuing an exhaustive investigation to rule out organic disease. The American Gastroenterological Association's current recommendations are to use patient symptoms supplemented with a narrow set of laboratory studies such as a complete blood cell count (CBC), erythrocyte sedimentation rate (ESR), and thyroid function tests in select populations.[3] The American College of Gastroenterology (ACG) advises against routine serologic tests, stool studies, and abdominal imaging in patients with typical IBS symptoms and no alarm features (weight loss, anemia, family history of colorectal cancer, inflammatory bowel disease, or Celiac disease [CD]) because of a low likelihood of uncovering organic disease.[11] In patients with IBS-D or IBS-M, serologic tests for CD should be ordered, and a colonoscopy should be performed for patients with alarm features to rule out other diseases. Patients older than 50 years who are diagnosed with IBS should also undergo a colonoscopy for screening for colon cancer, if not already performed.

There have been several symptom-based IBS criteria developed over the past few decades, but in general, they have not proven very practical for routine clinical use. The first of these criteria were put forth by Manning and colleagues[32] in 1978 and included abdominal pain relieved by defecation, presence of frequent loose stools, passage of mucus, and abdominal distension as key symptoms of the disorder. In 1984, the Kruis criteria were developed that expanded on Manning's by suggesting that patients with IBS should have a 2-year duration of symptoms in addition to a physical examination with negative results and normal results in serologic tests, including a CBC and ESR.[33] The Rome criteria were developed in 1988 and have since undergone 3 iterations. Though frequently used in research studies, the Rome criteria are relatively cumbersome to use in daily practice, with a sensitivity and specificity that is not perfect for diagnosing IBS. Recognizing the limitations and shortcomings of the current IBS criteria, the ACG Task Force on Irritable Bowel Syndrome has suggested a simpler and more concise definition: "Abdominal pain or discomfort that occurs in association with altered bowel habits over a period of at least 3 months."

Given the patient's young age, lack of "alarm signs," and laboratory studies with negative results, you provide reassurance that this is less likely another condition and more likely a functional disorder such as IBS. During this office visit, you check her thyroid-stimulating hormone levels given her weight gain and fatigue and find them to be normal. For now you recommend that she need not have any further diagnostic testing. You instruct her to try a lactose-free diet and to keep a strict diet diary for the next 4 weeks to see if there are any obvious triggers for her symptoms. You plan to see her back in clinic in 1 month to see how she is doing.

ROLE OF DIET IN IBS

Many patients with IBS think that diet plays an important role in their disorder and that avoiding certain foods can improve symptoms.[34–37] Although the importance of diet in IBS remains debated, studies have shown that approximately two-thirds of patients with IBS report worsening of symptoms after a meal.[38] A frequently heard clinical narrative is the sudden overwhelming urge to defecate within several minutes of eating. Although many patients assume this implies a food allergy, there are several other mechanisms that may account for these symptoms, including abnormal gas handling, abnormal colonic fermentation, psychosocial factors, intolerances to certain foods, and exaggeration of normal physiologic processes.

Adverse reactions to specific foods are reported in up to 45% of the general population and in up to 70% of individuals with IBS.[35,39] These foods are often referred to as trigger foods, the most common of which are milk, wheat-containing products, fructose, caffeine, and certain types of meats. True immunoglobulin (Ig) E-mediated food allergies (eg, peanut or shellfish allergies) are rare and occur in only 1% to 4% of adults.[40] There is no strong evidence to suggest that allergic food reactions play a significant role in IBS. In a study by Zar and colleagues,[41] the presence of IgG4 antibodies to wheat was reported in 60% of patients with IBS compared with 27% of healthy controls. Another study demonstrated that patients with IBS had a substantial improvement in symptoms on elimination of specific foods to which they had IgG antibodies and had a marked worsening of symptoms on reintroduction of those foods.[42] These results have not been widely replicated and controlled trials of elimination diets have been much more disappointing. In addition, detection of IgG antibodies to food is no longer considered a reliable diagnostic test for food allergy.[43] Slow-onset immune responses to food (occurring over days to weeks) resulting from mucosa-based mast cells, T lymphocytes, and eosinophils may have a role in IBS symptoms, although the evidence is scant and still controversial. Examples of this type of immune response include CD (see later discussion), eosinophilic gastroenteropathies, and food protein–induced enterocolitis syndrome. Evidence to suggest a role for this type of allergic reaction in IBS comes from the discovery of increased mast cell and eosinophil counts in close proximity to the enteric nerves within the mucosa of patients with IBS.[44] Further evidence is needed to support this theory.

Poorly absorbed carbohydrates have been studied for their role in the development of IBS symptoms. Lactose is a disaccharide that is poorly digested and absorbed in most adults around the world. The true prevalence of lactose intolerance is unknown due in part to the varying incidence within different racial and ethnic populations and to the different definitions used for intolerance and malabsorption. Native American, Asian, and black populations have the highest reported rates of lactose intolerance (80%–90%), whereas the lowest rates are reported among Caucasians living in northern Europe, Australia, and North America (5%–10%). Individuals with lactose intolerance report abdominal distension, bloating, excess gas production, and diarrhea following the ingestion of milk and ice cream. Several studies have investigated lactose intolerance in IBS, and the available data are conflicting. Although some studies have shown no difference in the prevalence of lactose intolerance in IBS than that in the general population,[45] others have demonstrated that anywhere from 40% to 80% of patients with IBS report significant symptom improvement on a lactose-restricted diet.[46,47] It remains unclear whether the latter finding is because of true lactase deficiency or intolerance to another component in the restricted diet. Nonetheless, these 2 conditions share a very similar set of symptoms and can exist simultaneously in the same patient. Patients should be encouraged to keep a food diary to assess the relationship between symptoms and dairy intake, and if a consistent association is identified, consumption of milk, ice cream, and soft cheeses should be avoided or at least minimized.

Fructose is another poorly absorbed carbohydrate that has been implicated in the development of IBS symptoms. It is found in the diet as free fructose (fruits and honey), long polymers called fructans (wheat-containing products and onions), and the disaccharide, sucrose (table sugar). The consumption of fructose over the past 2 decades has increased dramatically as a result of the ubiquitous introduction of high-fructose corn syrup into food. Even in an average American diet, the amount of fructose ingested on a daily basis is sufficient to cause GI symptoms in healthy individuals.[48] In a retrospective study, 38% of patients with IBS had significant improvement in pain, belching, bloating, and diarrhea when fructose was restricted.[49] In another uncontrolled unblinded study, 46 of 48 patients who adhered to a strict fructose-restricted diet had a marked improvement in most of their IBS symptoms.[50] When fructose and other nonabsorbed carbohydrates such as galactans are poorly absorbed in the small bowel, they are fermented by luminal bacteria into hydrogen, carbon dioxide, and short-chain fatty acids. These byproducts increase the osmotic load and levels of gas within the gut and act as a laxative leading to symptoms of bloating and diarrhea. There are several other dietary components, such as high fat and caffeine, and nonabsorbed carbohydrates and sugar alcohols, that are likely responsible for symptoms experienced by patients with IBS, but randomized controlled trials are currently lacking.

Fiber is one of the best studied yet most misunderstood dietary components in IBS. It has long been held that inadequate amounts of dietary fiber are responsible for the symptoms in IBS. Despite many systematic reviews and meta-analyses showing otherwise, this notion has been slow to change among practitioners, and patients with IBS are still counseled to increase the amount of insoluble fiber in their diets. The use of insoluble fiber as a bulking agent in IBS-D has been reviewed. Although the study populations were largely heterogeneous and the studies varied significantly in their methods, fiber was uniformly shown to have either no efficacy in IBS or only minimal effect in IBS-C (soluble fiber only).[51]

Many patients both with and without IBS complain of adverse reactions to foods. Studies on diet in IBS are often difficult to interpret because of inadequate controls, poor methodology, heterogeneous populations, and a large placebo effect. Postprandial symptoms likely occur for several reasons including food intolerances, abnormal motility and gas handling, and psychosocial factors. True allergies to foods are possibly important for a small subset of patients but should probably be considered only in individuals with a history of atopy, allergic rhinitis, and/or asthma. In general, it is worth attempting a limited exclusion of food based on a diet dairy, understanding that the likelihood of complete sustained improvement is probably less than 20%. Focusing on foods that trigger symptoms within 1 to 3 days of ingestion will probably provide the highest yield, and patients should be instructed to pay particular attention to the ingestion of lactose, fructose, and high amounts of fat and caffeine.

After eliminating dairy products for 1 month, her symptoms have not improved, and a diet diary did not help identify any obvious food triggers. Over-the-counter antidiarrheal agents reduce her postprandial diarrhea, but her bloating and abdominal distension continue to be her biggest complaint. She has a great deal of flatulence, which has become socially embarrassing for her. These symptoms generally worsen throughout the day, and by dinner she is unable to fit into her pants comfortably. You order a measurement of vitamin B_{12} and folic acid levels given her macrocytosis and a suspicion for SIBO. What is the yield of testing for bacterial overgrowth in IBS? Should we just treat empirically?

SIBO AND IBS

Over the last several decades, there has been an increased interest in the role of SIBO in the pathogenesis of IBS. In addition to the substantial overlap in symptoms between these 2 disorders, there are several lines of evidence that provide support for this hypothesis. Bacterial overgrowth has long been known to disrupt epithelial absorption and secretion, but recent data also suggest that SIBO may be an important activator of mucosa-based immunity.[52,53] Activation of proinflammatory cytokines by bacteria may alter epithelial cellular function, enhance nociceptive pain signaling, and alter intestinal motility—all purported pathophysiologic mechanisms in IBS. Bloating, abdominal distension, and excessive gas production are symptoms reported in up to 80% of patients with IBS.[54,55] In fact, although the data are conflicting, there is evidence that patients with IBS produce and expel significantly more hydrogen gas than normal healthy controls.[25,56] There is also evidence that these patients have increased amounts of small-intestinal gas on abdominal radiographs; however, there is not a strong correlation between these findings and the presence of symptomatic bloating.[26,57] It has been subsequently suggested that the bloating and diarrhea in patients with IBS with excessive gas are caused by the overgrowth of the fermenting bacteria in the small bowel.

Under normal circumstances, the small intestine is a relatively sterile environment consisting of mostly gram-positive and, within the terminal ileum, gram-negative bacteria numbering between 10^5 and 10^8 colony-forming units (CFUs) per milliliter. In the colon, bacterial counts increase markedly (10^{12} CFUs/mL), and the composition changes primarily to gram-negative bacteria, anaerobes, and enterococci. The bacterial count in the small bowel is maintained by normal peristalsis, gastric acid and mucus secretion, secretory IgA levels and an intact ileocecal valve. Predisposing conditions to the development of SIBO include altered gut anatomy (blind loops, surgical removal of ileocecal valve, small bowel diverticula), abnormal motility (scleroderma, diabetes), and decreased GI defense mechanisms (hypochlorhydria, immunodeficiency). In SIBO, abnormal migration of bacteria proximally into the small intestine results in premature fermentation of substrates, fat malabsorption, and consumption of carbohydrates and nutrients such as vitamin B_{12}.

SIBO is defined by the presence of more than 10^5 CFUs/mL of colonic type bacteria in aspirates obtained from the proximal small bowel. Although many agree that direct aspiration and culture represents the gold standard for SIBO, there are several potential problems with this diagnostic approach, including the observation that SIBO is primarily a distal small bowel process that may not be adequately detected through proximal jejunal aspirates. In addition, there is no standardized approach in selecting an area of bowel to retrieve samples for analysis, anaerobes are difficult to collect and preserve without affecting total bacterial colony counts, and many if not most laboratories are not well versed in the correct method of counting and culturing bowel bacteria. In a recent systematic review of all the diagnostic tests for SIBO, no test was found to be appropriately validated, including the gold standard culture technique.[58] Given the limitations of the gold standard, clinicians often rely on hydrogen breath tests to diagnose SIBO. These tests exploit the fact that bacterial fermentation of carbohydrates is the only source of hydrogen gas in the body.[59] Hydrogen gas is readily absorbed from the gut lumen into the circulation and can be measured in breath samples in ppm. The lactulose hydrogen breath test (LHBT) is conducted by administering an oral 10-g dose of lactulose (a nonabsorbed sugar) and measuring breath samples for the presence of hydrogen gas every 15 minutes. In SIBO, an early detectable increase in hydrogen gas production corresponds to lactulose fermentation in the small bowel, followed shortly by a second increase that is attributable to normal colonic fermentation. This double peak is 1 of 3 criteria used to define an abnormal LHBT result. Other positive criteria include an increase in hydrogen of more than 20 ppm before 90 minutes and/or an absolute increase from baseline of 20 ppm by 180 minutes. Other carbohydrates, such as glucose or dextrose, can also be used for hydrogen breath testing.

In their pivotal 2000 study, Pimentel and colleagues laid the groundwork for the SIBO-IBS hypothesis by showing that most patients with IBS (78%) have SIBO based on the results of LHBT.[27] They also demonstrated that when these patients are treated with antibiotics and SIBO eradication is confirmed with LHBT, they have sustained symptomatic improvement. Since these data were published, several subsequent studies, including a large meta-analysis in 2009,[60] have failed to demonstrate such a robust association. In their meta-analysis, Ford and colleagues evaluated 12 studies and 1912 subjects and found that the prevalence of SIBO in subjects meeting the diagnostic criteria for IBS was between 4% and 64% depending on the type of test and the criteria used to define a positive test.[60] For the LHBT, 6 studies with 964 subjects were evaluated and the pooled prevalence of SIBO in patients meeting IBS criteria was 54% (95% confidence interval [CI], 32–76). However, there was substantial heterogeneity among all the studies, making interpretation somewhat difficult (**Fig. 1**). In a 2007 Swedish study, 162 patients with IBS defined by Rome II criteria were tested for SIBO using jejunal aspirates and cultures. The prevalence of a positive test result was only 4% (95% CI, 2–6) when a value of more than 10^5 CFUs/mL was used.[61] Some of the large differences in these findings have been argued to be the result of the poor test characteristics of the LHBT, possibly because of lactulose fermentation by gastric and oral flora or perhaps because of the effects of rapid transit times in some individuals (giving false-positive results). Whatever the reason for these discrepancies, the LHBT is likely not the best diagnostic test for SIBO and will probably be supplanted by more accurate tests in the future. More importantly, however, the pathologic consequences of SIBO in IBS have not yet been fully elucidated, and despite some positive data regarding the use of antibiotics for IBS, it is not entirely clear what do the antibiotics treat.[62,63] Most recently, a double-blind placebo-controlled study by Pimentel and colleagues[64] showed that administration of rifaximin at a dose of 550 mg 3 times daily for 2 weeks led to significant improvement in global IBS symptoms (40.7% vs 31.7%, P<.001) and bloating (40.2% vs 30.3%, P<.001) when compared with placebo. In the authors' practice, a short empirical course of antibiotics (neomycin, rifaximin, or doxycycline) is administered, which serves both a diagnostic and therapeutic role, with the understanding that this approach is not something that is universally agreed on.

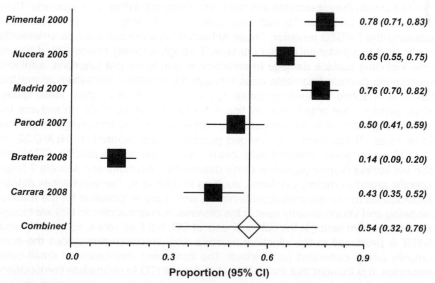

Fig. 1. Prevalence of a positive LHBT in subjects meeting diagnostic criteria for IBS. Meta-analysis of 6 studies with proportion plot with 95% CI. Open diamond represents combined data. (*Reproduced from* Ford AC, Spiegel BM, Talley NJ, et al. Small intestinal bacterial overgrowth in irritable bowel syndrome: systematic review and meta-analysis. Clin Gastroenterol Hepatol 2009;7(12):1282; with permission.)

She returns to your office now having tried an empirical 2-week course of rifaximin for SIBO but is still without improvement. Her vitamin B_{12} and folate levels were normal. Her best friend has CD and suggested that she try a gluten-free diet (GFD), which she plans to initiate within the next few days. Given her ongoing symptoms, you opt to expand your workup to include iron studies, stool studies for Giardia lamblia, and detection of tissue transglutaminase (tTG) and immunoglobulin (Ig) A. What is the prevalence of CD in patients with IBS, and are there individuals who should be routinely screened?

CD, GLUTEN SENSITIVITY, AND IBS

CD is a chronic inflammatory enteropathy of the small bowel that occurs in genetically susceptible individuals who are exposed to gluten. Patients develop a varying degree of intestinal inflammation, ranging from a mild intraepithelial lymphocytosis to a marked subepithelial mononuclear infiltration leading to total villous atrophy and malabsorption. The prevalence of CD in North America is approximately 1% and has been increasing over the past several decades in part because of better detection through serologic testing.[65–67] Symptoms of CD include bloating, abdominal pain, and diarrhea and can strongly mimic those of IBS. A recent systematic review and meta-analysis by Ford and colleagues[68] found that in patients meeting criteria for IBS, there was a more than 4-fold higher likelihood of having biopsy-proved CD than in controls without IBS. Whether these findings truly reflect an increased association between these 2 clinical entities remains a matter of some debate.

The pathophysiologic mechanisms causing CD are complex and occur as a result of exposure to dietary gluten, a storage protein of wheat, barley, and rye. Gluten is partially cleaved in the upper GI system, resulting in a variety of smaller peptide sequences, some of which are immunogenic to patients with CD. In genetically susceptible individuals, certain peptides invoke an innate immune response when they interact with the enterocytes and cell populations within the lamina propria. These cells generate interleukin 15 that can activate intraepithelial lymphocytes (IELs) expressing the NKG2D receptor. These activated IELs are cytotoxic to enterocytes and can lead to substantial cellular damage. Through a variety of postulated mechanisms, including surface damage to enterocytes and leaky cell junctions, additional immunogenic peptide fragments pass through the intestinal epithelium where they initiate the adaptive immune response. Once in the lamina propria, these gluten-derived peptides are acted upon by tissue transglutaminase (tTG), an enzyme that deamidates glutamine to form negatively charged and highly immunogenic glutamic acid residues. These negatively charged peptides are presented via HLA-DQ2 and HLA-DQ8 on antigen-presenting cells located within the lamina propria. $CD4^+$ cells within the lamina propria recognize these deamidated peptides and secrete T helper 1–specific proinflammatory cytokines, such as interferon γ. These cytokines activate myofibroblasts to secrete metalloproteinases, which are responsible for the mucosal remodeling and villous atrophy seen in the disease. Autoantibodies to tTG are thought to be an important factor in the pathogenesis of CD, but their role is not entirely clear. IgA-tTG is produced in the intestinal mucosa and circulates throughout the body, eventually being deposited just beneath the basement membrane of small-bowel enterocytes. It is thought that the ability of IgA-bound tTG to deamidate immunogenic peptides is enhanced and that it modulates intestinal cell behavior by increasing proliferation and permeability.

Several populations are at increased risk for developing CD. Whereas some of these higher-risk groups should be routinely screened, others should probably be tested for CD only when symptoms appear because currently available evidence suggests that early diagnosis and treatment in asymptomatic patients is not associated with better outcomes.[69] Patients with unexplained iron deficiency anemia have a much higher prevalence of CD than the general population, with rates ranging from 5% in asymptomatic patients to 15% in symptomatic patients. Because of this intense association, current recommendations from the American Gastroenterological Association are to screen this population whether or not GI symptoms are present. Family members of patients with CD are also at increased risk of developing CD, although the role of routine screening is less clear. Studies of at-risk first-degree relatives show prevalence rates of biopsy-proved CD, ranging from 10.3% to 20.0%, but this number may approach 40% if subtle mucosal lesions are included.[70] Other higher-risk categories include type 1 diabetes mellitus (1%–11%), Down syndrome (12%), microscopic colitis (15%–27%), chronic fatigue syndrome (2%), osteoporosis (1%–3%), abnormal liver enzymes (1.5%–9.0%), and autoimmune thyroid disease (5%). The usefulness of routine screening in any of these populations is not known, but clinicians should be aware of their associations and consider testing at any point GI symptoms develop. Furthermore, if any of these patients presents for an upper endoscopy for any indication, biopsies of the small bowel should be routinely obtained.

CD diagnosis has been greatly facilitated by the availability of accurate serologic tests that detect the presence of endomysial antibodies (EMAs) and tTG antibodies (**Table 1**). EMA detection is an immunofluorescence study that stains for IgA antibodies using either monkey esophagus or human umbilical vein as tissue substrate. It is a rather laborious test to perform and has the downside of being observer dependent. Nonetheless, the specificity of IgA-EMA is 100% with either tissue substrate, and the test has a sensitivity ranging between 90% and 97%. The IgA-tTG assay is an operator-independent enzyme-linked immunosorbent assay that uses substrate derived from guinea pig liver or human recombinant red cells (the latter is currently used by most commercial laboratories). The assay's accuracy has been shown to vary depending on the substrate used, but overall, its sensitivity and specificity are excellent ranging from 90% to 97% and 95% to 98%, respectively.[71] IgA-tTG assay is currently recommended as the initial test to screen for the presence of CD. IgG-tTG has proved to be of limited diagnostic value in adult patients with CD and

Table 1
Diagnostic accuracy of serologic tests for CD

Test	Sensitivity	Specificity
AGA IgA	<80%	≈80%–90%
AGA IgG	Variable, likely <80%	Nonspecific
EMA IgA	96%–97% ME, 90% HUV	100% ME, HUV
tTG IgA	90% GP, 98% HR	95% GP, 98% HR
tTG IgG	40% (higher in IgA deficiency)	98%

Summary of sensitivity and specificity values for AGA IgA, AGA IgG, EMA IgA, tTG IgA, and tTG IgG antibodies for detecting histologic changes of CD in adults. These values are based on data presented at the 2004 National Institutes of Health Consensus Conference on Celiac Disease and summarized in the publication by Rostom and colleagues.[71] Based on these data, the recommendation was made not to use AGAs in adults based on lower accuracy and instead tTG IgA was recommended as the preferred serologic test for screening and diagnosing CD.

Abbreviations: AGA, antigladin antibody; GP, guinea pig; HR, human recombinant; HUV, human umbilical vein; ME, monkey esophagus.

Data from Rostom A, Dube C, Cranney A, et al. The diagnostic accuracy of serologic tests for celiac disease: a systematic review. Gastroenterology 2005;128(4 Suppl 1):S38–46.

is currently used only for those with selective IgA deficiency because the sensitivity is reported to be much higher in this subset of the population. Antigliadin antibody (AGA) assays are no longer routinely used in adult populations as a screening test because of their inferior sensitivity and specificity; however, they still have a role in children. More recently, the presence of IgA and IgG antibodies to deamidated gliadin peptides has been shown to have excellent sensitivity (around 97%) and specificity (around 100%). This assay is not yet routinely used in clinical practice, but as more prospective data becomes available, detection of deamidated gliadin peptide antibodies either alone or combined with tTG-IgA may become the screening test of choice for CD.[72] The performance characteristics of all available diagnostic tests for CD were reevaluated recently in a large meta-analysis by van der Windt and colleagues.[73] In their evaluation of 16 studies (N = 6085), pooled estimates for IgA anti-EMAs (8 studies) were 0.90 (95% CI, 0.80–0.95) for sensitivity and 0.99 (95% CI, 0.98–1.00) for specificity. Pooled estimates for IgA anti-tTG antibodies (7 studies) were 0.89 (95% CI, 0.82–0.94) for sensitivity and 0.98 (95% CI, 0.95–0.99) for specificity. The IgA and IgG AGAs showed variable results, especially for sensitivity (range, 0.46–0.87 and range, 0.25–0.93; respectively).

Intestinal biopsies are the gold standard for the diagnosis of CD and must be performed to confirm a positive serologic test result before starting a patient on a lifelong gluten-free diet (GFD). The one exception is for patients with biopsy-proved dermatitis herpetiformis, the diagnosis of CD is assured and small-bowel biopsies are not required. In all other cases, the diagnosis requires identification of characteristic histologic findings, such as crypt hyperplasia, villous blunting, and increased IEL counts, within the small intestinal mucosa. The degree of damage is typically graded according to a scoring system that was devised by Marsh and colleagues[74] in 1992 and subsequently modified in 1999.[75] Endoscopic findings are quite specific for the diagnosis of CD and can include flattened intestinal folds, or notched or scalloped folds (Fig. 2). In many cases, the gross appearance of involved portions of the small intestine may be normal, reflecting the lower sensitivity of endoscopic findings, and therefore, if CD is a possible diagnosis, small-bowel biopsies must be performed. There are

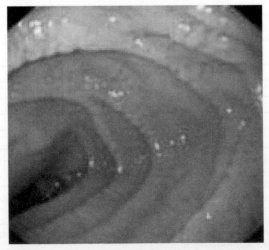

Fig. 2. Endoscopic findings in CD. A representative endoscopic image demonstrating scalloping (or notching) of the folds in the duodenum, which is characteristic of CD.

limitations with the current gold standard. False-positive results can occur as the result of conditions that mimic the histologic changes of CD as seen in peptic duodenitis, giardia infection, bacterial overgrowth, or tropical sprue. False-negative results can occur as a result of the patchy nature of the disease, subtle histologic findings (such as Marsh I or II), or predominantly distal disease. In order to overcome some of these pitfalls, 4 to 6 biopsy samples must be routinely taken, including at least 1 from the duodenal bulb, and the histology should be reviewed by an expert pathologist.[69] Generally, once the diagnosis is confirmed by a small-bowel biopsy and there is an appropriate clinical and serologic response, it is not required to repeat the endoscopy to evaluate for regression of disease. Once a patient starts a GFD and symptoms improve, serologic test results will typically begin to revert to normal over a period of 6 to 12 months.

Her tTG and IgA levels are normal. Her ferritin level is also normal, and her stool study is negative for Giardia. Her symptoms have improved somewhat over the past month on a GFD, and she is convinced that she has CD despite her negative serologic test results. She is not interested in having an endoscopy. You test her for the HLA-DQ2/DQ8 gene, and she is not a carrier of either allele. What is the likelihood that this patient could still have CD? How accurate is dietary gluten withdrawal for diagnosing CD?

The association between CD and the HLA-DQ2 and HLA-DQ8 haplotypes has been well established. Approximately 95% of patients with CD express the DQ2 haplotype, whereas the remaining 5% are positive for DQ8.[76–78] The presence of these alleles provides near 100% sensitivity for CD and has a very high negative predictive value (ie, patients who test negative for DQ2 or DQ8 have an extremely low likelihood of having or developing CD). However, up to 40% of the general North American population carries some combination of these alleles, which makes the specificity for CD fairly low (**Fig. 3**). In clinical practice, testing for DQ2/DQ8 is useful in some settings. In cases in which a family member has proved CD, DQ2/DQ8 testing can be used to screen other family members to determine their susceptibility for developing CD and to guide the need for further serologic and endoscopic testing. Serologic and

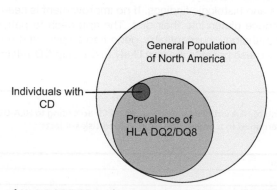

Fig. 3. Prevalence of HLA-DQ2/DQ8 in the general population and in CD. The outer circle represents the proportion of North Americans without HLA-DQ2 or HLA-DQ8 gene, whereas the lighter-shaded inner circle represents the subset that bear these genes. The inner small area includes those who are predicted to have CD, representing up to 1% of the population and 2% to 3% of the genetically at-risk subset. (*Adapted from* Kagnoff MF. Celiac disease: pathogenesis of a model immunogenetic disease. J Clin Invest 2007;117:43; with permission.)

histologic tests have less utility in patients who already follow a GFD, so in circumstances in which a patient is unable or unwilling to reintroduce gluten into their diet, genetic testing provides a very useful screening tool. It may also be useful in equivocal cases such as early-stage disease with minimal histologic changes and in those with only a weakly increased tTG-IgA level. In patients unwilling to undergo an upper endoscopy to confirm the diagnosis, a negative genetic test result can reassure the patient and physician that the likelihood of CD is very low (**Table 2**).

In a subset of individuals, IBS symptoms improve on withdrawal of dietary gluten despite lacking the classic CD phenotype. There may be several explanations for this finding, including the very large placebo effect seen with virtually all types of IBS therapies. In a study by Campanella and colleagues,[79] 180 patients who had been previously improperly diagnosed with CD were studied as gluten was removed and reintroduced into their diets. GI symptoms improved in 64.7% of patients with CD and 75% of patients without CD after gluten withdrawal (P = NS), and reintroduction of gluten led to symptom exacerbation in 71.4% of patients with CD and 54.2% of patients without CD (P = NS). Other explanations for their improvement include the possible inadvertent exclusion of other non–gluten-based nutrients and food sources that could act as potential symptom triggers in these patients. Some patients with IBS may fall into the less well-defined category of gluten sensitivity (GS). The term gluten sensitivity has been coined to describe a subset of patients who do not present with typical CD symptoms or small-bowel pathology, but who express some degree of intolerance to gluten. Patients with GS are often positive for both HLA-DQ2/DQ8 and CD serologic findings, they frequently cluster in families with CD, and they often present with extraintestinal manifestations of CD. In a study of 102 patients with IBS-D, 58% of patients with IBS carrying either HLA-DQ2 or HLA-DQ8 also had positive IgA-AGA or IgA-tTG antibodies in duodenal aspirates and higher IEL counts compared with 15% of patients with IBS lacking the HLA-DQ2 allele.[80] Although there is likely a pathophysiologic basis for some of their symptoms, the management of GS is unclear at present. Some patients may respond to a GFD (especially in those who possess at-risk haplotypes), but it is difficult to predict who is likely to benefit. In patients with atypical symptoms and negative serologic findings, but with minimal enteropathy, a GFD trial is probably warranted. For these patients, follow-up in 3 to 6 months (and potential rebiopsy) would be reasonable to see if there is any improvement in symptoms and histologic findings. If no improvement is seen, they can probably safely reintroduce gluten into their diet. The approach to patients with GS but without intestinal pathology, susceptibility gene haplotypes, and negative serologic findings is unclear. These patients are less likely to develop CD-related complications

Table 2
Risk of CD according to HLA antigen status. The risk of CD according to HLA-DQ2 and HLA-DQ8 expression as determined in a population of increased-risk subjects

Haplotype	Risk of CD
General population	≈1%
DQ2+/DQ2+	×28.28
DQ2+/DQ8+	×11.78
DQ8+/DQ8+	×8.42
DQ2–/DQ8–	×0.16

Data from Pietzak MM, Schofield TC, McGinniss MJ, et al. Stratifying risk for celiac disease in a large at-risk United States population by using HLA alleles. Clin Gastroenterol Hepatol 2009;7(9):966–71.

and can probably liberalize their GFD. As time goes on and the pathophysiologic spectrum of CD becomes better understood, it is hoped that new diagnostic and therapeutic approaches will emerge for these patients.

At this point, all of her blood tests have been normal. She neither responded to a trial of lactose restriction nor showed any improvement following a short course of antibiotics. She did not have any HLA-DQ CD susceptibility genes, and her tTG-IgA and total IgA levels were normal. At this point, you explain to her that she most likely has IBS with a component of gluten sensitivity. You agree with her modified diet but encourage her to loosen her gluten restriction knowing that her risks of CD-related complications are low. Six months later she returns to your office continuing to do well on a partially GFD and plans to see you back only on an as-needed basis.

SUMMARY

IBS is a very common disorder that lacks specific biochemical, structural, and radiographic findings. Complicating the diagnosis is the number of other medical conditions, such as food intolerances, SIBO, and CD, that can mimic or coexist with IBS. A careful history and physical examination are paramount to establishing an accurate diagnosis and avoiding unnecessary tests. Food intolerances are reported by many patients with IBS, so it is worthwhile attempting to illicit specific trigger foods (especially lactose and fructose), keeping in mind that this approach may help only a percentage of patients with IBS. There are currently limitations to the diagnostic tests available for SIBO, and treatments of this disorder have not been well studied. Nonetheless, a short trial of antibiotics may be useful, especially in patients with known risk factors for bacterial overgrowth. CD is not rare in North America and affects roughly 1 in 100 individuals. CD should be suspected in any individual with IBS-D. Other high-risk populations should be tested for CD on a case-by-case basis. Diagnostic tests for CD perform well but have some limitations. Not all patients who respond to gluten withdrawal have CD, but some may have a component of GS. These patients can usually liberalize their gluten restrictions and do very well on a partially GFD.

REFERENCES

1. Longstreth GF, Thompson WG, Chey WD, et al. Functional bowel disorders. Gastroenterology 2006;130(5):1480–91.
2. Drossman DA, Li Z, Andruzzi E, et al. U.S. householder survey of functional gastrointestinal disorders. Prevalence, sociodemography, and health impact. Dig Dis Sci 1993;38(9):1569–80.
3. Drossman DA, Camilleri M, Mayer EA, et al. AGA technical review on irritable bowel syndrome. Gastroenterology 2002;123(6):2108–31.
4. Cremonini F, Talley NJ. Irritable bowel syndrome: epidemiology, natural history, health care seeking and emerging risk factors. Gastroenterol Clin North Am 2005;34(2):189–204.
5. Drossman DA, Sandler RS, McKee DC, et al. Bowel patterns among subjects not seeking health care. Use of a questionnaire to identify a population with bowel dysfunction. Gastroenterology 1982;83(3):529–34.
6. Thompson WG, Heaton KW, Smyth GT, et al. Irritable bowel syndrome in general practice: prevalence, characteristics, and referral. Gut 2000;46(1):78–82.
7. Schuster MM. Defining and diagnosing irritable bowel syndrome. Am J Manag Care 2001;7(Suppl 8):S246–51.

8. Longstreth GF, Wilson A, Knight K, et al. Irritable bowel syndrome, health care use, and costs: a U.S. managed care perspective. Am J Gastroenterol 2003; 98(3):600–7.

9. Talley NJ, Gabriel SE, Harmsen WS, et al. Medical costs in community subjects with irritable bowel syndrome. Gastroenterology 1995;109(6):1736–41.

10. Sandler RS, Everhart JE, Donowitz M, et al. The burden of selected digestive diseases in the United States. Gastroenterology 2002;122(5):1500–11.

11. American College of Gastroenterology Functional Gastrointestinal Disorders Task Force. Evidence-based position statement on the management of irritable bowel syndrome. Am J Gastroenterol 2002;97(Suppl 11):S1–5.

12. Saito YA, Schoenfeld P, Locke GR 3rd. The epidemiology of irritable bowel syndrome in North America: a systematic review. Am J Gastroenterol 2002; 97(8):1910–5.

13. Andrews EB, Eaton SC, Hollis KA, et al. Prevalence and demographics of irritable bowel syndrome: results from a large web-based survey. Aliment Pharmacol Ther 2005;22(10):935–42.

14. Hungin AP, Chang L, Locke GR, et al. Irritable bowel syndrome in the United States: prevalence, symptom patterns and impact. Aliment Pharmacol Ther 2005;21(11):1365–75.

15. Lydiard RB. Irritable bowel syndrome, anxiety, and depression: what are the links? J Clin Psychiatry 2001;62(Suppl 8):38–45 [discussion: 46–7].

16. Gralnek IM, Hays RD, Kilbourne A, et al. The impact of irritable bowel syndrome on health-related quality of life. Gastroenterology 2000;119(3):654–60.

17. Frank L, Kleinman L, Rentz A, et al. Health-related quality of life associated with irritable bowel syndrome: comparison with other chronic diseases. Clin Ther 2002;24(4):675–89 [discussion: 674].

18. Morris-Yates A, Talley NJ, Boyce PM, et al. Evidence of a genetic contribution to functional bowel disorder. Am J Gastroenterol 1998;93(8):1311–7.

19. Levy RL, Jones KR, Whitehead WE, et al. Irritable bowel syndrome in twins: heredity and social learning both contribute to etiology. Gastroenterology 2001; 121(4):799–804.

20. Kellow JE, Eckersley CM, Jones MP. Enhanced perception of physiological intestinal motility in the irritable bowel syndrome. Gastroenterology 1991;101(6): 1621–7.

21. Serra J, Azpiroz F, Malagelada JR. Impaired transit and tolerance of intestinal gas in the irritable bowel syndrome. Gut 2001;48(1):14–9.

22. Chadwick VS, Chen W, Shu D, et al. Activation of the mucosal immune system in irritable bowel syndrome. Gastroenterology 2002;122(7):1778–83.

23. Whitehead WE, Crowell MD. Psychologic considerations in the irritable bowel syndrome. Gastroenterol Clin North Am 1991;20(2):249–67.

24. Lydiard RB, Falsetti SA. Experience with anxiety and depression treatment studies: implications for designing irritable bowel syndrome clinical trials. Am J Med 1999;107(5A):65S–73S.

25. King TS, Elia M, Hunter JO. Abnormal colonic fermentation in irritable bowel syndrome. Lancet 1998;352(9135):1187–9.

26. Koide A, Yamaguchi T, Odaka T, et al. Quantitative analysis of bowel gas using plain abdominal radiograph in patients with irritable bowel syndrome. Am J Gastroenterol 2000;95(7):1735–41.

27. Pimentel M, Chow EJ, Lin HC. Eradication of small intestinal bacterial overgrowth reduces symptoms of irritable bowel syndrome. Am J Gastroenterol 2000;95(12): 3503–6.

28. Marshall JK. Post-infectious irritable bowel syndrome following water contamination. Kidney Int Suppl 2009;(112):S42–3.
29. Spiller R, Garsed K. Postinfectious irritable bowel syndrome. Gastroenterology 2009;136(6):1979–88.
30. Borgaonkar MR, Ford DC, Marshall JK, et al. The incidence of irritable bowel syndrome among community subjects with previous acute enteric infection. Dig Dis Sci 2006;51(5):1026–32.
31. Spiegel BM, Farid M, Esrailian E, et al. Is irritable bowel syndrome a diagnosis of exclusion? a survey of primary care providers, gastroenterologists, and IBS experts. Am J Gastroenterol 2010;105(4):848–58.
32. Manning AP, Thompson WG, Heaton KW, et al. Towards positive diagnosis of the irritable bowel. Br Med J 1978;2(6138):653–4.
33. Kruis W, Thieme C, Weinzierl M, et al. A diagnostic score for the irritable bowel syndrome. Its value in the exclusion of organic disease. Gastroenterology 1984;87(1):1–7.
34. Jarrett M, Visser R, Heitkemper M. Diet triggers symptoms in women with irritable bowel syndrome. The patient's perspective. Gastroenterol Nurs 2001;24(5):246–52.
35. Monsbakken KW, Vandvik PO, Farup PG. Perceived food intolerance in subjects with irritable bowel syndrome—etiology, prevalence and consequences. Eur J Clin Nutr 2006;60(5):667–72.
36. Halpert A, Dalton CB, Palsson O, et al. What patients know about irritable bowel syndrome (IBS) and what they would like to know. National Survey on Patient Educational Needs in IBS and development and validation of the Patient Educational Needs Questionnaire (PEQ). Am J Gastroenterol 2007;102(9):1972–82.
37. Lacy BE, Weiser K, Noddin L, et al. Irritable bowel syndrome: patients' attitudes, concerns and level of knowledge. Aliment Pharmacol Ther 2007;25(11):1329–41.
38. Simren M, Mansson A, Langkilde AM, et al. Food-related gastrointestinal symptoms in the irritable bowel syndrome. Digestion 2001;63(2):108–15.
39. Nanda R, James R, Smith H, et al. Food intolerance and the irritable bowel syndrome. Gut 1989;30(8):1099–104.
40. Sicherer SH, Sampson HA. Food allergy: recent advances in pathophysiology and treatment. Annu Rev Med 2009;60:261–77.
41. Zar S, Benson MJ, Kumar D. Food-specific serum IgG4 and IgE titers to common food antigens in irritable bowel syndrome. Am J Gastroenterol 2005;100(7):1550–7.
42. Atkinson W, Sheldon TA, Shaath N, et al. Food elimination based on IgG antibodies in irritable bowel syndrome: a randomised controlled trial. Gut 2004;53(10):1459–64.
43. Stapel SO, Asero R, Ballmer-Weber BK, et al. Testing for IgG4 against foods is not recommended as a diagnostic tool: EAACI Task Force Report. Allergy 2008;63(7):793–6.
44. Guilarte M, Santos J, de Torres I, et al. Diarrhoea-predominant IBS patients show mast cell activation and hyperplasia in the jejunum. Gut 2007;56(2):203–9.
45. Farup PG, Monsbakken KW, Vandvik PO. Lactose malabsorption in a population with irritable bowel syndrome: prevalence and symptoms. A case-control study. Scand J Gastroenterol 2004;39(7):645–9.
46. Vernia P, Ricciardi MR, Frandina C, et al. Lactose malabsorption and irritable bowel syndrome. Effect of a long-term lactose-free diet. Ital J Gastroenterol 1995;27(3):117–21.

47. Goldstein R, Braverman D, Stankiewicz H. Carbohydrate malabsorption and the effect of dietary restriction on symptoms of irritable bowel syndrome and functional bowel complaints. Isr Med Assoc J 2000;2(8):583–7.
48. Beyer PL, Caviar EM, McCallum RW. Fructose intake at current levels in the United States may cause gastrointestinal distress in normal adults. J Am Diet Assoc 2005;105(10):1559–66.
49. Choi YK, Kraft N, Zimmerman B, et al. Fructose intolerance in IBS and utility of fructose-restricted diet. J Clin Gastroenterol 2008;42(3):233–8.
50. Shepherd SJ, Gibson PR. Fructose malabsorption and symptoms of irritable bowel syndrome: guidelines for effective dietary management. J Am Diet Assoc 2006;106(10):1631–9.
51. Ford AC, Talley NJ, Spiegel BM, et al. Effect of fibre, antispasmodics, and peppermint oil in the treatment of irritable bowel syndrome: systematic review and meta-analysis. BMJ 2008;337:a2313.
52. Shanahan F. Irritable bowel syndrome: shifting the focus toward the gut microbiota. Gastroenterology 2007;133(1):340–2.
53. Barbara G, Stanghellini V, Brandi G, et al. Interactions between commensal bacteria and gut sensorimotor function in health and disease. Am J Gastroenterol 2005;100(11):2560–8.
54. Chang L, Lee OY, Naliboff B, et al. Sensation of bloating and visible abdominal distension in patients with irritable bowel syndrome. Am J Gastroenterol 2001; 96(12):3341–7.
55. Ringel Y, Williams RE, Kalilani L, et al. Prevalence, characteristics, and impact of bloating symptoms in patients with irritable bowel syndrome. Clin Gastroenterol Hepatol 2009;7(1):68–72 [quiz: 63].
56. Sen S, Dear KL, King TS, et al. Evaluation of hydrogen excretion after lactulose administration as a screening test for causes of irritable bowel syndrome. Eur J Gastroenterol Hepatol 2002;14(7):753–6.
57. Chami TN, Schuster MM, Bohlman ME, et al. A simple radiologic method to estimate the quantity of bowel gas. Am J Gastroenterol 1991;86(5):599–602.
58. Khoshini R, Dai SC, Lezcano S, et al. A systematic review of diagnostic tests for small intestinal bacterial overgrowth. Dig Dis Sci 2008;53(6):1443–54.
59. Simren M, Stotzer PO. Use and abuse of hydrogen breath tests. Gut 2006;55(3): 297–303.
60. Ford AC, Spiegel BM, Talley NJ, et al. Small intestinal bacterial overgrowth in irritable bowel syndrome: systematic review and meta-analysis. Clin Gastroenterol Hepatol 2009;7(12):1279–86.
61. Posserud I, Stotzer PO, Bjornsson ES, et al. Small intestinal bacterial overgrowth in patients with irritable bowel syndrome. Gut 2007;56(6):802–8.
62. Pimentel M, Park S, Mirocha J, et al. The effect of a nonabsorbed oral antibiotic (rifaximin) on the symptoms of the irritable bowel syndrome: a randomized trial. Ann Intern Med 2006;145(8):557–63.
63. Sharara AI, Aoun E, Abdul-Baki H, et al. A randomized double-blind placebo-controlled trial of rifaximin in patients with abdominal bloating and flatulence. Am J Gastroenterol 2006;101(2):326–33.
64. Pimentel M, Lembo A, Chey WD, et al. Rifaximin therapy for patients with irritable bowel syndrome without constipation. N Engl J Med 2011;364(1):22–32.
65. Fasano A, Berti I, Gerarduzzi T, et al. Prevalence of celiac disease in at-risk and not-at-risk groups in the United States: a large multicenter study. Arch Intern Med 2003;163(3):286–92.

66. Lohi S, Mustalahti K, Kaukinen K, et al. Increasing prevalence of coeliac disease over time. Aliment Pharmacol Ther 2007;26(9):1217–25.
67. Rubio-Tapia A, Kyle RA, Kaplan EL, et al. Increased prevalence and mortality in undiagnosed celiac disease. Gastroenterology 2009;137(1):88–93.
68. Ford AC, Chey WD, Talley NJ, et al. Yield of diagnostic tests for celiac disease in individuals with symptoms suggestive of irritable bowel syndrome: systematic review and meta-analysis. Arch Intern Med 2009;169(7):651–8.
69. Rostom A, Murray JA, Kagnoff MF. American Gastroenterological Association (AGA) Institute technical review on the diagnosis and management of celiac disease. Gastroenterology 2006;131(6):1981–2002.
70. Tursi A, Brandimarte G, Giorgetti GM, et al. Effectiveness of the sorbitol H2 breath test in detecting histological damage among relatives of coeliacs. Scand J Gastroenterol 2003;38(7):727–31.
71. Rostom A, Dube C, Cranney A, et al. The diagnostic accuracy of serologic tests for celiac disease: a systematic review. Gastroenterology 2005;128(4 Suppl 1): S38–46.
72. Volta U, Granito A, Parisi C, et al. Deamidated gliadin peptide antibodies as a routine test for celiac disease: a prospective analysis. J Clin Gastroenterol 2010;44(3):186–90.
73. van der Windt DA, Jellema P, Mulder CJ, et al. Diagnostic testing for celiac disease among patients with abdominal symptoms: a systematic review. JAMA 2010;303(17):1738–46.
74. Marsh MN. Gluten, major histocompatibility complex, and the small intestine. A molecular and immunobiologic approach to the spectrum of gluten sensitivity ('celiac sprue'). Gastroenterology 1992;102(1):330–54.
75. Rostami K, Kerckhaert J, Tiemessen R, et al. Sensitivity of antiendomysium and antigliadin antibodies in untreated celiac disease: disappointing in clinical practice. Am J Gastroenterol 1999;94(4):888–94.
76. Sollid LM, Thorsby E. The primary association of celiac disease to a given HLA-DQ alpha/beta heterodimer explains the divergent HLA-DR associations observed in various Caucasian populations. Tissue Antigens 1990;36(3):136–7.
77. Wong RC, Steele RH, Reeves GE, et al. Antibody and genetic testing in coeliac disease. Pathology 2003;35(4):285–304.
78. Vader W, Stepniak D, Kooy Y, et al. The HLA-DQ2 gene dose effect in celiac disease is directly related to the magnitude and breadth of gluten-specific T cell responses. Proc Natl Acad Sci U S A 2003;100(21):12390–5.
79. Campanella J, Biagi F, Bianchi PI, et al. Clinical response to gluten withdrawal is not an indicator of coeliac disease. Scand J Gastroenterol 2008;43(11):1311–4.
80. Wahnschaffe U, Ullrich R, Riecken EO, et al. Celiac disease-like abnormalities in a subgroup of patients with irritable bowel syndrome. Gastroenterology 2001; 121(6):1329–38.

Nausea and Vomiting of Pregnancy

Noel M. Lee, MD, Sumona Saha, MD*

KEYWORDS

• Nausea • Vomiting • Pregnancy • Hyperemesis gravidarum

Nausea and vomiting are common experiences in pregnancy, affecting 70% to 80% of all pregnant women. Although most women with nausea and vomiting of pregnancy (NVP) have symptoms limited to the first trimester, a small percentage have a prolonged course with symptoms extending until delivery. Women with severe nausea and vomiting during pregnancy may have hyperemesis gravidarum (HG), an entity distinct from NVP, which if left untreated may lead to significant maternal and fetal morbidity.

Various metabolic and neuromuscular factors have been implicated in the pathogenesis of NVP and HG; however, their exact cause is unknown. Consequently, treatment of NVP and HG can be difficult, as neither the optimal targets for treatment nor the full effects of potential treatments on the developing fetus are known. This article reviews the epidemiology, pathology, diagnosis, outcomes, and treatment of NVP and HG.

EPIDEMIOLOGY

It is estimated that 70% to 80% of pregnant women experience NVP.[1] In the United States and Canada this translates to approximately 4 million and 350,000 women who are affected each year, respectively.[2]

NVP is found more often in Western countries and urban populations, and is rare among Africans, Native Americans, Eskimos, and most Asian populations.[3] Only a few studies have examined the racial distribution of NVP in a given population with conflicting results. One such study from Canada of 367 women found that Asians and blacks were less likely to report symptoms of NVP than Caucasians. Sociodemographic factors did not account for the racial/ethnic variation in disease prevalence, suggesting that genetic and/or cultural factors may be at play.[4] However, in a study from the United States, 89% of 2407 pregnant women reported symptoms of NVP. Prevalence of NVP was highest in non-Hispanic black and Hispanic women.

University of Wisconsin School of Medicine and Public Health, Division of Gastroenterology and Hepatology, UW Medical Foundation Centennial Building, 1685 Highland Avenue, Room 4224, Madison, WI 53705, USA
* Corresponding author.
E-mail address: ssaha@medicine.wisc.edu

Gastroenterol Clin N Am 40 (2011) 309–334
doi:10.1016/j.gtc.2011.03.009
0889-8553/11/$ – see front matter © 2011 Elsevier Inc. All rights reserved.

HG is rare in comparison with NVP, occurring in 0.3% to 2% of all pregnancies.[5] The incidence appears to vary with ethnicity[6] and ranges between 3 and 20 per 1000 pregnancies.[7]

Risk Factors

Data from the Collaborative Perinatal Project, one of the largest studies to date of pregnant women, found NVP to be more common in younger women, primigravidas, women with less than 12 years of education, nonsmokers, and obese women.[8] Increased risk of NVP in the first trimester has also been reported in women with multiple gestation as compared with women with singleton pregnancies (87% vs 73%, $P<.01$).[9]

NVP has been associated with low income levels and part-time employment status.[10] Housewives have also been found to be at increased risk, whereas women with white collar occupations appear to be protected.[11] Whether employment status is a true risk factor for NVP or a confounder, however, remains unclear, as affected women may cease employment because of their symptoms. Similarly, their decision to not work outside the home may be attributable to multiparity and the need to care for other children.[12]

Maternal genetics also appear to serve as risk factors for NVP. Data from a large Norwegian twin population show higher use of nausea medication in pregnancy among female monozygotic twins compared with female dizygotic twins.[13] In addition, higher levels of nausea have been found in women who had mothers who experienced trouble with nausea in their pregnancy.[14] A personal history of NVP has also been shown to be a risk factor for NVP in subsequent pregnancies[14]; however, this finding has not been consistent across studies.[15]

Other risk factors for NVP include a personal history of motion sickness, due possibly to a common vestibular mechanism,[16] and history of migraine headaches.[17] Women who have a history of nausea when taking estrogen-containing oral contraceptives also appear to be at an increased risk for NVP.[18]

Location of the corpus luteum may also serve as risk factor for NVP. Ultrasound studies have shown that pregnant women experience more nausea and vomiting when the corpus luteum is present in the right ovary.[19] This condition may be caused by differences in venous drainage between the left and right ovary and a higher concentration of sex steroids when the corpus luteum is on the right side.[20]

A higher daily intake of total fat, especially saturated fat, prior to pregnancy increases the risk of hospitalization for NVP.[21] Smoking before pregnancy and vitamin use before and/or in early pregnancy are associated with a decreased risk for NVP.[18] Maternal alcohol consumption prior to conception has also been found to be protective for NVP.[11]

Risk factors for HG are similar to those of NVP and include nulliparity, multiple gestations, trophoblastic disease, HG in prior pregnancy, fetal abnormalities such as triploidy, trisomy 21, and hydrops fetalis.[22] Family history of HG is also a risk factor, with approximately 28% of women reporting a history of HG in their mothers and 19% reporting that their sisters had similar symptoms.[23] Additional risk factors include married or partnered status and age older than 30 years. Cigarette smoking, as in NVP, may be protective.[24]

Maternal body mass index has been evaluated as a risk factor for HG, with inconclusive results. In a study by Depue and colleagues,[25] obesity increased the risk for HG by 50%. Work by Cedergren and colleagues,[26] however, found that a low body mass index (<20 kg/m^2) was associated with a 40% higher risk of HG and that obesity decreased the risk of hospitalization for HG. A more recent study of 33,647 women in Norway found that being either underweight or overweight increased the risk for HG, but only in nonsmokers.[27] It is postulated that underweight women with low body mass indices have low prepregnant estrogen levels and thus may have an exaggerated response during the first trimester when estrogen levels surge.[28] By contrast, in obese women fat deposits may neutralize placental factors thought to contribute to the pathogenesis of HG.[26]

With regard to fetal gender, an association between HG and female gender of the fetus has been found in several studies. Using data from the Swedish Medical Birth Registry, Kallen[29] found HG to be overrepresented in 3068 pregnancies when the infant was a girl. Similarly, in a study of pregnant women hospitalized with HG in the first trimester, the odds of having a female infant were 50% higher in cases than in healthy pregnant controls (odds ratio 1.5, 95% confidence interval [CI] 1.4–1.7).[30]

PATHOGENESIS
Metabolic and Hormonal Factors

Although the exact pathogenesis of NVP and HG are unknown, it is widely accepted that gestational vomiting results from various metabolic and endocrine factors, many of placental origin. The most implicated factor is human chorionic gonadotropin (hCG). This link between hCG and NVP is based largely on the temporal relationship between the peak of NVP and the peak of hCG production, both of which occur between 12 and 14 weeks' gestation. In addition, nausea and vomiting are often worse in pregnant women with conditions associated with elevated hCG levels, such as molar pregnancies, multiple gestations, and Down syndrome.[12] Higher urinary hCG[31] and serum hCG levels have also been found in women with NVP compared with those who are asymptomatic.[32] Furthermore, a study by Goodwin and colleagues[33] found that concentrations of hCG correlated positively with the severity of nausea and vomiting in women with HG.

Despite the multitude of studies linking hCG to NVP and HG, others have found no relationship between serum hCG in pregnant women during the first trimester and the frequency or intensity of nausea and vomiting. In a study by Soules and colleagues,[34] even in a subset of women with molar pregnancies in whom levels of hCG in women were 5 to 10 times higher than in controls, no correlation was found. Furthermore, studies have found high levels of hCG to be associated with fetal growth retardation and preterm delivery[35] whereas NVP appears to be protective for preterm delivery, making it unlikely for hCG to be the sole contributor to the pathogenesis of NVP.

It is postulated that varying biologic forms (ie, isoforms) of hCG may explain the variability between hCG levels and nausea and vomiting in normal and sick populations.[36] Each hCG isoform has a unique half-life and potency at the luteinizing hormone (LH) and thyroid-stimulating hormone (TSH) receptor. Isoforms without the carboxy-terminal portion have shorter half-lives but more are more powerful stimulants of both the LH and TSH receptors. Different isoforms of hCG are likely the result of genetic factors or long-term environmental changes and may explain the differences in HG prevalence found among populations. In addition to isoform variation, hCG receptor mutations may also explain some of the variability in the relationship between NVP and hCG.[36]

The ovarian hormones, estrogen and progesterone have also been implicated in the pathogenesis of NVP and HG. It is known that some women experience nausea when taking oral contraceptives. Furthermore, states of high estrogen concentration such as low parity and high maternal body mass index have been associated with a higher incidence of HG.[25] Estrogen is thought to contribute to HG by stimulating the production of nitric oxide via nitric oxide synthetase, which in turn relaxes smooth muscle, slowing gastrointestinal transit time and gastric emptying.

Jordan and colleagues[37] reported a significant association between hyperemesis gravidarum and a history of intolerance to oral contraceptives. Using a more quantitative approach, Depue and colleagues[25] found mean levels of total estradiol to be 26% higher and mean levels of sex hormone binding–globulin binding capacity to be 37% higher in patients with HG than in control subjects after adjusting for gestational age. It is important to bear in mind, however, that like the relationship between hCG and NVP, the relationship between estrogen levels and NVP has been inconsistent across studies.[32] A review of 17 studies showed a positive association between NVP and estrogen in only 5 studies.[38] Furthermore, estrogen levels peak in the third trimester of pregnancy, whereas HG tends to improve during late pregnancy.[39]

Progesterone in combination with estrogen may also have a role in NVP. Progesterone decreases smooth muscle contractility, and may alter gastric emptying and lead to increased nausea and vomiting. Using elastogastrography after a standard meal, Walsh and colleagues[40] showed that the same slow-wave gastric rhythm disruption found in women with NVP could be evoked in nonpregnant women by progesterone alone or in combination with estradiol in doses that reproduce levels in pregnancy. Other studies, however, have not found any significant difference between progesterone levels in women with or without NVP.[25]

The role of placental prostaglandin E_2 (PGE_2) has also been evaluated in the pathogenesis of NVP, due to its effect on gastric smooth muscle.[41] hCG stimulates placental PGE_2, and like hCG peaks between 9 and 12 weeks of gestation. North and colleagues[42] quantified maternal serum PGE_2, and found levels to be higher during periods of nausea and vomiting in 18 women in early pregnancy than during asymptomatic periods. These investigators also evaluated maternal levels of interleukin-1β and tumor necrosis factor α (TNF-α) levels, and found both to be similar during symptomatic and asymptomatic periods.

Because of its role in chemotherapy-induced nausea and vomiting, serotonin has also been hypothesized to contribute to NVP. A study by Borgeat and colleagues,[43] however, did not show any difference in serotonin levels among pregnant women with HG, asymptomatic pregnant women, and nonpregnant women. In addition, a randomized controlled trial comparing the serotonin 5-HT$_3$ receptor antagonist, ondansteron, with promethazine found no significant difference in symptom control.[44]

Due to the cross-reactivity between hCG and the TSH receptor, thyroid dysfunction has also been studied as a possible mechanism for NVP and HG development. In fact, abnormal results of thyroid function are found in two-thirds of women with HG.[33] This "biochemical thyrotoxicosis" is characterized by suppressed TSH and slightly elevated free T4. Despite these laboratory abnormalities, women with HG are generally euthyroid with no history of prior thyroid diseases, absent goiter, and negative antithyroid antibodies.[45] Furthermore, studies have not found a relationship between thyroid dysfunction and the severity of symptoms,[46] and almost all women with HG have normal TSH levels by 20 weeks' gestation without any intervention.[47]

Recently, a relationship between the hormone leptin and HG has been proposed. Increased serum leptin levels during pregnancy, possibly the result of increased total fat mass and the placenta production, have been found to be significantly higher in patients with HG when compared with healthy pregnant controls.[48,49] Leptin may contribute to HG by increasing hCG secretion by the paracrine action of the placenta or by decreasing appetite and promoting more severe nausea and vomiting. It is noteworthy, however, that prospective cohort studies have not found a statistically significant difference in serum leptin levels in HG between cases and controls.[50,51]

Immune system dysregulation has also been proposed to occur in women with HG. Increased concentrations of fetal cell free DNA have been found in mothers' serum,[52] causing a hyperactive maternal immune response and trophoblast damage. Furthermore, the normal shift in pregnancy wherein T-helper cell types move into T-helper cell type 1 is more exaggerated in women with HG.[53] This in turn leads to increased release of interleukin-4 as well as TNF-α, both of which have been linked to HG.[54] Adenosine, which attenuates TNF-α, has also been found to be increased in HG. Likewise, Il-6, IgG, IgM, complement levels, and lymphocyte counts have been found to be increased in HG.[55–57] One cannot precisely define the role of these immunologic factors, however, because in starvation states the immune system is usually suppressed, not activated; thus, perhaps the boost in immune factors seen in HG could be an attempt to limit the progression of HG.[39]

Other hormones including TSH, growth hormone, prolactin, adrenocortical-stimulating hormone, cortisol, LH, and follicle-stimulating hormone have also been evaluated, and are not considered to contribute to the pathogenesis of NVP.[58]

Helicobacter pylori

An increased incidence of infection with *Helicobacter pylori* has been observed in women with HG and is now considered to play a role in its pathogenesis. Frigo and colleagues[59] found that 90.5% of women with HG were *H pylori* IgG positive, compared with 46.5% of controls. Bagis and colleagues[60] used the gold standard test, histologic examination of the mucosal biopsy, and found that 95% of HG patients tested positive for *H pylori* compared with 50% of controls. These investigators also found higher *H pylori* densities in the gastric antrum and corpus in HG patients, suggesting a possible relationship between *H pylori* density and the severity of symptoms.

A systematic review from 2007 evaluating 14 case-control trials from 1966 to 2007 found a significant association between maternal *H pylori* infection and HG in 10 studies. Odds ratios in the studies varied from 0.55 to 109.33.[61] Similarly, an updated systematic review and meta-analysis from 2009 of 25 studies found a pooled odds ratio of 3.32 (95% CI: 2.25–4.90) for *H pylori* infection in women with HG.[62] Of note, high heterogeneity among studies was found in both reviews.

Infection with *H pylori* in pregnancy may occur because of steroid hormone–induced changes in gastric pH[63] and/or increased susceptibility due to changes in humoral and cell-mediated immunity.[64] However, there is no clear evidence that pregnancy predisposes to de novo *H pylori* infection. On the contrary, it has been suggested that *H pylori* may exacerbate hormone-induced changes in the nerve and electric functioning of the stomach, and thereby increase the risk for infected women to be at the more severe end of the spectrum of nausea and vomiting.[61]

Although the association between *H pylori* and HG is intriguing, it is important to note that infection does not necessarily correlate with symptoms. In fact, most infected women are asymptomatic.[39] In a study by Weyermann and colleagues,[65] 23% of 898 postpartum mothers were positive for *H pylori* by ^{13}C-urea breath test; however, positivity did not correlate with symptoms of nausea, vomiting, or reflux symptoms during pregnancy. Similarly, Wu and colleagues[66] found 69% of pregnant women to be seropositive for *H pylori* compared with 50% in the general population; however, they did not find any correlation between antibody status and gastrointestinal symptoms.

Why *H pylori* cannot be precisely linked to NVP and HG has been attributed to several factors. First, most studies used antibody testing to assess for infection. However, serologic testing for *H pylori* cannot distinguish between active infection and past infection,[67] and active versus past infection may produce different effects on symptoms. Second, most studies have not assessed and/or accounted for the *H pylori* strain. Cytotoxin-associated gene A (CagA) protein is a marker for increased peptic ulcers and is linked to a more aggressive strain of *H pylori*.[68] Only a single study included in the 2009 meta-analysis assessed for CagA pathogenicity. In this study by Xia and colleagues,[69] CagA positivity was more prevalent in patients with HG.

Treatment eradicates *H pylori* in the majority of patients; however, currently there are no guidelines for the evaluation or treatment of *H pylori* during pregnancy, as the subsequent alleviation of symptoms of HG has not been widely studied. Case reports and cases series suggest that treatment and eradication of *H pylori* can decrease nausea and vomiting in pregnancy and should be considered in patients with intractable symptoms.[70] Larger studies, however, are needed to determine if and when treatment should be initiated during pregnancy given the concerns of drug safety. At present, experts recommend that after pregnancy and lactation have been completed, patients should be treated with triple therapy for 2 weeks.[71]

Gastrointestinal Dysmotility

Alterations in lower esophageal sphincter (LES) resting pressure and esophageal peristalsis have been linked to NVP. Although these changes are more typically associated with heartburn in pregnancy, gastroesophageal reflux disease (GERD) may produce atypical symptoms such as nausea,[72] and contribute to NVP. Estrogen and progesterone are the likely mediators of esophageal dysmotility in pregnancy, wherein estrogen serves as a primer and progesterone causes LES relaxation.[73]

Changes in gastric rhythmic activity may also contribute to NVP. Normal gastric myoelectric activity results in slow-wave propagation from the proximal body to the distal antrum at a rate of 3 cycles per minute (cpm). Rhythm disturbance, either increased or decreased slow-wave propagation, is associated with nausea.[71] Using elastogastrography (EGG), Koch and colleagues[74] demonstrated that individuals with normal slow-wave activity were less likely to complain of nausea during pregnancy. By contrast, individuals with higher or lower rates were more likely to complain of nausea. Similarly, Riezzo and colleagues[75] found that pregnant women without symptoms of nausea and vomiting at the time of EGG recordings have normal 3-cpm myoelectrical activity. They also found that pregnant women with NVP had more unstable EGG activity compared with women after voluntary abortions and nonpregnant controls. Riezzo and colleagues speculated that this may be due to restoration of the normal gastric slow-wave pattern after abortion following normalization of estradiol and progesterone levels.

However, it is noteworthy that many studies have found no difference in gastric motility between pregnant and nonpregnant women. Using gastric scintigraphy, no significant differences in the liquid emptying rate were found in pregnant women before voluntary abortion, 6 weeks after abortion, and in nonpregnant control women.[76] Using dye dilution methods with phenol red, Davison and colleagues[77] found gastric emptying to be delayed in women during labor but not in the third trimester, as compared with nonpregnant controls. Similarly, studies using paracetamol showed no gastric emptying delay in the first, second, or third trimester.[78]

Alterations in gastric motility in pregnancy have been attributed to high levels of progesterone. Moreover, in late pregnancy, compression from an enlarged uterus may contribute to symptoms.

Meal composition may also serve a pathogenic role in NVP. Jednak and colleagues[79] demonstrated that protein-dominant meals were associated with decreased symptoms and corrected slow-wave dysrhythmias. Carbohydrate or fat-dominant meals had no effect on symptoms or slow-wave dysrhythmias.

Finally, small bowel transit time has been evaluated with regard to NVP pathogenesis. Using the lactulose hydrogen breath test, an indirect measure of small bowel transit time, Lawson and colleagues[80] found transit times to be prolonged in the second and third trimester compared with the first trimester, with the longest times found when progesterone levels were highest. Wald and colleagues[81] used similar techniques, and found transit time to be prolonged in the third trimester when progesterone and estrogen levels were high in comparison to the postpartum period. However, in both of these studies, delayed intestinal transit times did not correlate with NVP.

Psychosocial Factors

Early studies proposed that NVP may be a psychosomatic illness in which vomiting represents intrapsychic conflicts. Some have speculated that NVP is a manifestation of a pregnant woman's subconscious attempt to reject an unwanted pregnancy,[3] as studies have found that women with NVP in the first trimester are more likely to have unplanned or undesired pregnancies.[82]

HG has also been associated with psychological disturbances, namely neurotic tendencies, hysteria, rejection of femininity, and rejection of pregnancy, as well as depression and psychological stress related to poverty and marital conflicts.[39] Recent studies, however, have not found definite psychogenic causes of HG.[83,84] Some investigators, therefore, argue that sociocultural factors rather than scientific evidence have led to the labeling of HG as a psychologically based condition and that it is more likely that psychological disturbances such as depression are the result rather than the cause of HG.[85]

Thus although NVP and HG are likely not the result of a conversion disorder or other psychological disorder, it is well recognized that affected women have psychological responses that become intertwined with, and possibly exacerbate, their physical symptoms.

DIAGNOSIS AND CLINICAL FEATURES
History and Physical Examination

Despite popular use of the term "morning sickness," NVP persists throughout the day in the majority of affected women and has been found to be limited to the morning in less than 2% of women.[10] It often begins within weeks of missing menses and thus is caricatured across most cultures as the initial sign of pregnancy. Symptoms usually peak between 10 and 16 weeks' gestation and usually resolve after 20 weeks. Up to 10% of women, however, continue to be symptomatic beyond 22 weeks.[10]

Whereas dehydration and orthostasis can occur in women with HG, most women with NVP have normal vital signs and a benign physical examination. A careful abdominal examination, however, should be done to rule out peritonitis and other intraabdominal causes of nausea and vomiting.

Differential Diagnosis

Given the high prevalence of NVP, nausea and vomiting in the first trimester is usually attributable to NVP. However, if changes in bowel habits, abdominal pain, and bilious emesis are present, appropriate investigations should be conducted to exclude other causes. The differential diagnosis for NVP includes gastroesophageal reflux disease, peptic ulcer disease, small bowel obstruction, acute cholecystitis, cholelithiasis, and pancreatitis, as well as appendicitis, gastroenteritis, nephrolithiasis, pyelonephritis, and hepatitis (**Table 1**).[71]

Table 1
Differential diagnosis for nausea and vomiting in pregnancy

GI disorders	Metabolic disorders
Gastroenteritis	Hyperthyroidism
GERD	Addison's disease
Peptic ulcer disease	Diabetic complications
Intestinal obstruction	**Neurologic disorders**
Pancreatitis	Migraines
Appendicitis	CNS tumors
Hepatitis	Pseudotumor cerebri
Biliary disorders	Vestibular abnormalities
Genitourinary disorders	**Pregnancy-related disorders**
Nephrolithiasis	Preeclampsia/HELLP
Pyelonephritis	Acute fatty liver of pregnancy
Ovarian torsion	

Diagnostic and Laboratory Tests

Other than a pregnancy test, no specific laboratory studies are recommended for the diagnosis of NVP. Other tests, however, may be helpful in excluding other causes of nausea and vomiting. Leukocytosis should not be seen in NVP and may point to an infectious or inflammatory cause such as cholecystitis, urinary tract infections, or pancreatitis. Elevations in the aminotransferases could indicate chronic hepatitis but may also be the result of repetitive vomiting. An abnormal TSH could indicate hypothyroidism or hyperthyroidism, both of which can cause nausea and vomiting. Elevation in serum glucose could indicate diabetes, and may produce nausea and vomiting by decreasing antral contractility and precipitating gastric dysrhythmias.[86]

Radiographic imaging is generally not needed for the diagnosis of NVP. A pelvic ultrasonogram can be considered to document pregnancy and evaluate for conditions that increase the risk for NVP such as multiple gestation. Abdominal radiographs are generally not helpful, and although they pose low risk to the fetus are still relatively contradicted during the first trimester.

Upper endoscopy can be performed safely in pregnancy, and can be considered to rule out gastritis and peptic ulcer disease as causes of nausea and vomiting in pregnancy. In one large center, nausea and vomiting was the second most common indication for upper endoscopy in pregnancy after upper gastrointestinal bleeding.[87]

OUTCOME

Most studies have found NVP to be associated with a favorable outcome for the fetus. A meta-analysis of 11 studies by Weigel and Weigel[88] found a strong significant association between nausea and vomiting of pregnancy and decreased risk of miscarriage (common odds ratio = 0.36, 95% CI 0.32–0.42), and no consistent associations with perinatal mortality. Moreover, women without NVP have been found to deliver earlier than women with NVP.[89]

Adverse outcomes, however, have been reported in some studies, especially when NVP is deemed severe. Deuchar[90] found an increased risk for intrauterine growth retardation in women with severe NVP, but could not account for potential confounding by antiemetic medication use on fetal growth. Similarly, Zhou and colleagues[91] found an increased risk for low birth weight in women with severe NVP, likely due to the deleterious effects of nausea and vomiting on maternal nutrition.

In a prospective study of 16,398 women, no difference was found in congenital abnormalities between those with and without NVP.[92] In addition, a retrospective study showed a lower risk of congenital heart defects in infants born to women with early-onset of NVP requiring antiemetic use compared with women without nausea.[93]

It is not entirely clear how NVP protects the developing fetus; however, several theories have been described. Some have argued that nausea and vomiting allows the pregnant woman to avoid or expel foods that may be teratogenic or induce abortion. This notion may explain the close temporal relationship between the development of food aversions in pregnancy and the onset of nausea.[94] NVP may also lower energy intake and lower levels of anabolic hormones, insulin, and insulin growth factor, leading to a shunting of scarce nutrients to the placenta and fetus.[95]

Despite its favorable effects on the fetus, the psychosocial morbidity in pregnant women with NVP is substantial and perhaps underemphasized. In a study by Smith and colleagues[96] of 593 Australian women with NVP, most reported that their symptoms produced major negative impacts on employment, household duties, and parenting, with 96% of women reporting mild to moderate distress from nausea and 28% reporting moderate to severe distress. Similarly, a study by Mazzotta and colleagues[2] of Canadian women found more severe nausea and vomiting to be associated with more frequent feelings of depression, consideration of termination of pregnancy, adverse effects on women's relationships with their partners or their partners' everyday lives, and the perceived likelihood that NVP would harm their baby. Of note, women with mild symptoms also reported experiencing the same psychosocial problems, suggesting that the severity of nausea or vomiting does not adequately reflect the distress caused by NVP.

O'Brien and Naber[97] also showed significant psychosocial morbidity in women suffering from NVP, and found that affected women reported a decline in social commitments and impaired relationships with spouses and children. Women with severe symptoms also reported frequent tearfulness, irritability, increased sleep disturbances, and lowered mood. Using the Short-Form 36, Attard and colleagues[98] found that women with NVP had lower scores in physical functioning, physical role, bodily pain, vitality, social functioning, and emotional role as compared with healthy pregnant controls in early pregnancy and women with chronic depression. Mental health scores for the women with NVP were similar to those of the women with depression.

In addition to causing psychosocial morbidity, NVP also poses a significant financial burden. In 2002, the cost of severe NVP was estimated to be approximately $130 million based on hospital costs linked to an average of 39,000 hospital admissions. This figure is likely a gross underestimate, as it does not include the loss of productivity at home, physician fees, or cost of treatments.[99]

It has been estimated that 206 work hours are lost for each employed woman with NVP[2] and that NVP accounts for 28% of all sick leave during pregnancy before week 28.[18] Furthermore, work by Vallacott and colleagues[100] reveals that 50% of affected women believe their work efficiency to be significantly reduced.

HYPEREMESIS GRAVIDARUM

HG is a condition of severe nausea and vomiting during pregnancy leading to fluid, electrolyte, and acid-base imbalance, nutritional deficiency, and weight loss.[39] Some have defined it as the occurrence of greater than 3 episodes of vomiting per day accompanied by ketonuria and a weight loss of more than 3 kg or 5% of body weight.[61] HG is the most common reason for hospitalization in early pregnancy and is second only to preterm labor throughout the whole of pregnancy.[101] In the United

States more than 36,000 women are admitted to hospital each year because of HG, and the cost of care is estimated to be more than 250 million dollars annually for hospitalization alone.[102] Unlike NVP, which is associated with favorable fetal outcomes, HG poses significant health risks to mother and fetus.

Diagnosis and Clinical Features

HG presents in the first trimester of pregnancy, usually starting at 4 to 5 weeks' gestation. In addition to severe nausea and vomiting, 60% of women with HG also have excess salivation or ptyalism.[103] Patients may also complain of gastroesophageal reflux symptoms such as retrosternal discomfort and heartburn. A pregnancy-unique quantification of emesis and nausea (PUQE) score, calculated using the number of hours of nausea per day, number of episodes of emesis per day, and number of episodes of retching per day, can be used to track the severity of symptoms.[104]

Patients may present with signs of dehydration such as dry mucous membranes, tachycardia, poor skin turgor, and postural hypotension. Severely affected patients may also have muscle wasting and weakness and/or mental status changes.

Laboratory abnormalities in women with HG may include increased serum blood urea nitrogen, creatinine, and hematocrit, as well as ketonuria and increased urine specific gravity. In addition, electrolyte disturbances supporting a diagnosis of either hypochloremic metabolic alkalosis or metabolic acidosis with severe volume contraction may be found.[36] Pre-albumin (plasma transthyretin) levels may be low, reflecting poor protein nutrition status in the mother and possibly predicting lower fetal birth weights.[105] Vitamin and mineral deficiencies such as vitamin B1 (thiamine), iron, calcium, and folate are also possible.[71]

Liver function tests may be abnormal in up to 50% of hospitalized patients with HG.[106] Mild hyperbilirubinemia (bilirubin <4 mg/dL) and/or an increase in alkaline phosphatase to twice the upper limit of normal may be seen.[107] However, a moderate transaminitis is the most common liver function test abnormality, with alanine aminotransferase levels generally greater than aspartate aminotransferase levels. The transaminase elevation is usually 2 to 3 times the upper limit of normal; however, levels greater than 1000 U/mL have been reported.[108] The abnormal liver tests resolve promptly on resolution of the vomiting.

Serum amylase and lipase elevation are seen in 10% to 15% of women.[36] One study found elevated amylase levels in 24% of patients with HG.[109] This finding is believed to be due to excessive salivary gland production of amylase rather than pancreatic secretion, and a result rather than a cause of HG.[39]

TSH levels may be low in HG, due to cross-reaction between the α-subunit of hCG with the TSH receptor. In the majority of cases, this biochemical thyrotoxicosis is not clinically relevant because patients are euthyroid. Thyroid hormone levels generally normalize without treatment after delivery.

HG is a clinical diagnosis based on symptoms and the exclusion of other conditions. Like NVP, no specific testing is needed to diagnose HG; however, ultrasonography of the abdomen and pelvis may be helpful in excluding other causes such as gallbladder disease and hydatidiform mole, and in assessing for multiple gestations. The differential diagnosis includes NVP, acute thyroiditis, eating disorders, biliary tract disease, viral hepatitis, and gastroesophageal reflux disease.

Outcome

Unlike NVP, HG is associated with both adverse maternal and fetal outcomes. In a study of more than 150,000 singleton pregnancies, infants born to women with hyperemesis and low pregnancy weight gain (<7 kg) were more likely to be low birth weight, small for gestational age, born before 37 weeks of gestation, and have a 5-minute Apgar score of less than 7.[5]

Common maternal complications include weight loss, dehydration, micronutrient deficiency, and muscle weakness. More severe, albeit rare, complications include Mallory-Weiss tears, esophageal rupture, Wernicke encephalopathy with or without Korsakoff psychosis, central pontine myelinolysis due to rapid correction of severe hyponatremia, retinal hemorrhage, and spontaneous pneumomediastinum.[45] Vasospasm of the cerebral arteries due to increased sympathetic activity has also been reported.[110]

HG contributes to many psychological problems, and can result in termination of an otherwise wanted pregnancy and decreased likelihood to attempt a repeat pregnancy.[111] Pourshariff and colleagues[112] found that 15% of 808 women with HG had at least one termination because of their illness. Of interest, those women who terminated did not have more severe disease than women with HG who kept their pregnancy, but were twice as likely to perceive that their physician was uncaring or did not address the severity of their illness.

The long-term consequences of HG on mothers are unknown. Several studies show an increased risk of breast cancer.[113] There are also reports of increased rates of depression, posttraumatic stress disorder, and various neurologic disorders.[36]

Some studies have found no increased risk for adverse fetal outcomes in women with HG. Bashiri and colleagues,[6] for example, reported a lower incidence of spontaneous early pregnancy loss in women with HG compared with the general population, and found no differences in perinatal outcomes. However, other studies have found an association between HG and fetal growth retardation, preeclampsia, and infants small for gestational age.[114] In a retrospective study of 3068 women, HG was associated with earlier delivery and lower birth weight. These outcomes were most likely in women who had lost more than 5% of their prepregnancy body weight.[115] Similarly, Dodds and colleagues[5] found higher rates of low birth weight, preterm birth, and fetal death in women with HG who gained less than 7 kg overall during pregnancy. Multiple hospital admissions for HG appear to be another risk factor for lower neonatal birth weight.[103]

Various congenital malformations have been observed more in women with HG.[29] These conditions include Down syndrome, hip dysplasia, undescended testes, skeletal malformations, central nervous system defects, and skin abnormalities. Fetal coagulopathy and chondrodysplasia have been reported from vitamin K deficiency[116] with third-trimester fetal intracranial hemorrhage.[117] Several childhood cancers such as testicular cancer and leukemia have also been linked to maternal HG; however, data are conflicting.[36]

TREATMENT

The goal of treatment is to improve symptoms while minimizing risks to mother and fetus. To attain this goal, a multimodal approach tailored to each individual is usually needed. Treatment modalities range from simple dietary modifications to drug therapy and total parenteral nutrition. Severity of symptoms and maternal weight loss are useful in determining the aggressiveness of treatment. The PUQE score and the Hyperemesis Impact of Symptoms (HIS) Questionnaire can be considered to assess the severity of symptoms. The updated PUQE score evaluates symptoms over 24 hours[118] while the HIS takes into account psychosocial factors in addition to physical symptoms.[119]

Current studies demonstrate that management of NVP is suboptimal. One recent prospective study of 283 women with NVP during the first trimester found that only half were asked about the intensity and severity of their symptoms, and less than a quarter were asked if their symptoms interfered with their daily tasks and work. In this study by Lacasse and colleagues,[120] only 27% of women were offered an anti-emetic and an additional 14% were recommended a nonpharmacologic approach.

Nonpharmacologic Therapy

Dietary measures
The initial therapy for NVP and HG should include dietary changes. Affected women should avoid large meals and instead eat several small meals throughout the day that are bland and low in fat, as fatty foods may further delay gastric emptying. Eating protein more than carbohydrates and taking in more liquids than solids may also help nausea by improving the gastric dysrhythmias associated with NVP.[79] Small volumes of salty liquids such as electrolyte-replacement sport beverages are advisable, and if the smell of hot foods is noxious, cold foods should be prepared.[121]

Emotional support
Emotional support should always be offered by a medical professional. In addition, supportive psychotherapy, behavioral therapy, and hypnotherapy may be beneficial to women with severe symptoms and/or those in whom personality characteristics and/or marital or family conflict play a role.[58] The goal of psychotherapy is not to delve into the psychology that may be contributing to NVP but rather to encourage, explain, reassure, and allow the patient to express stress.[90]

Acupressure/acupuncture
Acupressure of the Chinese acupuncture point P6 (Neiguan) has been found to decrease nausea in patients with chemotherapy-induced nausea and postoperative nausea and vomiting, and may be helpful in treating HG. According to the principle of *Chi*, application of pressure to this point blocks abnormal energy slowly and relieves symptoms related to the pressure point.[12] Pressure may be placed manually or with elastic bands on the inside of the wrist. In addition, the ReliefBand, a battery-operated electrical nerve stimulator worn on the wrist, has recently been approved by the Food and Drug Administration (FDA) and can also be used to stimulate the P6 site.[122]

The evidence for acupressure is largely positive. One review of 7 trials indicated that acupressure of the Neiguan point could help symptoms of nausea.[123] A recent placebo-controlled study of 60 women with NVP found that the treatment group experienced relief from nausea the day after starting acupressure over the P6 site that lasted until the end of the observation period. In comparison, the group treated with acupressure over an insignificant site experienced initial symptom relief, but by day 6 symptoms had returned and were no different than the nontreated group.[124]

Although additional studies are needed, some experts believe this intervention should be offered because there are no known adverse side effects.[125]

Acupuncture has been less well studied, but one single-blind randomized, controlled trial with 593 women of less than 14 weeks' gestation showed that there was less nausea and dry retching in women treated weekly with acupuncture for 4 weeks as compared with controls.[126] However, it is possible that some women may have improved simply with advancing gestational age.[12]

Ginger
Ginger is the single nonpharmacologic intervention recommended by the American College of Obstetrics and Gynecology.[127] Ginger is believed to help improve NVP by stimulating gastrointestinal tract motility and stimulating the flow of saliva, bile,

and gastric secretions. One component of ginger has been shown to have similar activity to the 5-HT_3 antagonist, ondansetron. In addition, its extract has been found to inhibit the growth of some strains of *H pylori*.[128]

In a double-blind, randomized cross-over trial, 70% of women with HG treated with 250 mg of the powdered root of ginger 4 times daily preferred the period on ginger compared with the period on placebo.[129] Similarly, a second trial of 70 pregnant women at 17 weeks' gestation or less treated with either 250 mg of ginger 4 times a day or a placebo for 4 days found that women in the treatment group had significant improvement in nausea symptoms compared with women in the placebo group ($P<.001$).[130]

With regard to the safety of ginger in pregnancy,[130] a case-control study of 187 pregnant women found no increase in the rate of major malformations with first-trimester use.[131] A theoretical risk for bleeding, however, does exist, as ginger inhibits thromboxane synthetase and may inhibit platelet function. Thus, the concomitant use of anticoagulants with ginger is not advised.[132]

Pharmacologic Treatment

Pyridoxine-doxylamine

The combination of pyridoxine (vitamin B6) (pregnancy category A) and doxylamine (pregnancy category B), previously available as Bendectin, is the only medication that is specifically labeled for the treatment of NVP by the FDA. It remains available in Canada in a delayed-release tablet of 10 mg of pyridoxine and 10 mg of doxylamine under the trade name Diclectin.

Bendectin was taken off the market in 1983 in the United States following reports of congenital malformations with first-trimester use. Before its withdrawal, however, 30 million women had taken it over a nearly 25-year time span. Several small randomized controlled studies support its efficacy.[133] In addition, a meta-analysis that included 170,000 exposures found the pyridoxine-doxylamine combination to be safe and not to cause adverse effects in the fetus.[134] Other large studies have also shown no increase in congenital anomalies over the background rate.[135] Nevertheless, Bendectin remains off the market in the United States. Women can make their own preparation, however, by combining 10 mg of pyridoxine with half a tablet of Unisom, which is 25 mg of doxylamine.

Alternatively, pyridoxine can be taken on its own. Although no relationship has been found between pyridoxine levels and NVP, several studies have shown improvement in nausea scores in patients with severe nausea who take pyridoxine[136] and a reduction in the episodes of vomiting when compared with women taking placebo.[133] There is no definite evidence of vitamin B6 toxicity; however, in large doses pyridoxine has been linked to reversible peripheral neuropathy in nonpregnant adults.[12]

Antiemetics

The phenothiazines, chlorpromazine (Thorazine) and prochlorperazine (Compazine), are central and peripheral dopamine antagonists that have been shown to reduce symptoms in NVP and HG.[137] These agents are pregnancy category C.

A study of 12,764 pregnant women found a slightly increased risk of birth defects with phenothiazine use in the first trimester, particularly with chlorpromazine use; however, potential confounding factors such as alcohol use and treatment duration were not excluded.[138] Another study showed that infants of mothers who had taken chlorpromazine had extrapyramidal signs and jaundice; there was no significant impairment of postnatal development.[139]

Promethazine (Phenergan) was not found to have teratogenic effects in one study,[140] but increased congenital hip dislocation was seen in another study.[141]

Promotility agents

Metoclopramide (Reglan) is widely used for the treatment of NVP[142] and is graded as pregnancy category B. Metoclopramide is believed to improve symptoms by increasing LES pressure and increasing gastric transit. It also corrects gastric dysrhythmias by stimulating antral contractions and promoting antroduodenal contractions. A recent study found 10 mg of metoclopramide given every 8 hours to be as effective in reducing the number of vomiting episodes and increasing well-being in women with HG during their first hospitalization as 25 mg of promethazine given every 8 hours for 24 hours. The side effect profile was better in the metoclopramide-treated group, with less drowsiness, dizziness, and dystonia reported.[143]

With regard to safety, a study of 81,703 births between 1998 and 2007 in Israel wherein there was an exposure of metoclopramide in 4.2% of women found no increased risk of major congenital malformations, low birth weight, preterm delivery, or perinatal death with metoclopramide use.[144] Similarly, a Danish study of 309 pregnant women taking metoclopramide found no increased risk.[145]

Despite its efficacy, metoclopramide use is limited by its side-effect profile, which includes dystonia, restlessness, and somnolence. In 2009 the FDA added a black-box warning to metoclopramide because of the risk of tardive dyskinesia with chronic use.

Other prokinetics such as domperidone and erythromycin have not been studied in NVP.[71]

Antihistamines and anticholinergics

Antihistamines indirectly affect the vestibular system, decreasing stimulation of the vomiting center.[146] Randomized controlled trials of antihistamine use in NVP are limited; however, meclizine (Anitvert), dimenhydrinate (Dramamine), and diphenhydramine (Benadryl) have all been shown to control symptoms better than placebo.[137] These three agents are all pregnancy category B. In addition, pooled data from 7 trials between 1951 and 1975 found antihistamines to be effective.[147] A meta-analysis of more than 24 controlled studies with more than 200,000 pregnant women found that antihistamines (H1 blockers, in particular) given during the first trimester did not increase teratogenic risk.[148] Although meclizine had been previously thought to be teratogenic, studies now show it is safe to use during pregnancy.[149] Dimenhydrinate and diphenhydramine have conflicting results on safety.[71]

In one study of women undergoing elective cesarean delivery, transdermal scopolamine (pregnancy category C) was found to be more effective than placebo at decreasing nausea, vomiting, and retching due to epidural morphine analgesia.[150] However, scopolamine may produce sister-chromatid exchanges in healthy adult lymphocytes. This may lead to congenital malformations, including deformed limbs and trunks. Thus, first trimester use is not advised.[151]

Other agents

Ondansetron (Zofran) (pregnancy category B) is widely used for the treatment of postoperative and chemotherapy-induced nausea and vomiting, and is currently one of the most commonly prescribed antiemetics.[152] It is thought to work both centrally and peripherally by blocking serotonin receptors in the small bowel and medullary vomiting center.[146] Its safety in pregnancy was determined in a recent study, which showed no significant increase in the number of miscarriages, major malformations, or birth weight between infants exposed to ondansetron and unexposed controls.[153]

There has been one randomized controlled trial of ondansetron for the treatment of HG. In this small study of 30 women, no benefit of ondansetron, 10 mg given intravenously every 8 hours as needed, was found over promethazine, 50 mg given intravenously every 8 hours, in terms of nausea, weight gain, days of hospitalization, or total doses of medicine.[44] Promethazine, however, was found to cause more sedation. Nevertheless, case reports and widespread clinical experience do support the efficacy of ondansetron for the treatment of HG and its better tolerability over older antiemetics.[154,155]

Droperidol (pregnancy category C) is a dopamine antagonist that is an effective antiemetic for postoperative nausea and vomiting. A small study of women with HG found that the combination of continuous droperidol infusion and bolus intravenous diphenhydramine led to shorter hospitalizations and fewer readmissions compared with a historical control group that had received other forms of parenteral therapy. In addition, there were no significant differences in maternal or perinatal outcomes.[156] Of note, however, droperidol bears a black-box warning because it may cause QT prolongation and cardiac dysrhythmias.[71]

Oral and intravenous corticosteroids (pregnancy category C) have been used for refractory cases of HG, with variable results. Corticosteroids are believed to exert an antiemetic effect on the chemoreceptor trigger zone in the brainstem, and are also postulated to correct the "relative adrenal insufficiency" induced by HG in which the hypothalamic-pituitary-adrenal axis is unable to respond to the increased demands of cortisol during early pregnancy.

In a randomized controlled trial of 40 women with HG treated with methylprednisolone, 16 mg orally 3 times a day for 3 days followed by a 2-week tapering regimen, versus promethazine, 25 mg orally 3 times a day for 2 weeks, a lower rate of rehospitalization was found in the steroid-treated group.[157] Other studies have not shown a statistically significant benefit of corticosteroids. A randomized trial by Yost and colleagues[158] found no significant decrease in the number of visits to emergency departments or rehospitalizations with the addition of parenteral and oral methylprednisolone to a regimen of promethazine and metoclopramide.

There are no established guidelines for the use of corticosteroids for HG. A possible regimen that has been suggested, however, is 48 mg of methylprednisolone given orally or intravenously in 3 divided doses for 2 to 3 days. If no response is seen within 3 days, it is recommended that treatment be stopped, as response beyond 72 hours is unlikely.[146]

With regard to safety, a recent meta-analysis showed a slight increase in major malformations and a 3.4-fold increase in oral cleft in infants whose mothers took corticosteroids in the first trimester.[159]

There has been recent interest in acid-reducing medications for NVP, as one recent cohort study showed that women with NVP and heartburn and/or acid reflux had more severe nausea and vomiting than women without heartburn or acid reflux.[160] Furthermore, follow-up studies have shown that treatment of heartburn and/or reflux results in improved PUQE scores and quality-of-life scores.[161]

Antacids containing aluminum or calcium are first-line treatment during pregnancy for acid reflux and heartburn, and can be used to treat women with NVP. Magnesium-containing antacids are associated with nephrolithiasis, hypotonia, and respiratory distress in the fetus, and are not recommended during pregnancy. Bicarbonate-containing antacids can cause fetal metabolic acidosis and fluid overload, and are also not recommended.[162]

H2 blockers and proton-pump inhibitors can be used safely to treat acid reflux and/or heartburn in women with NVP.[163,164]

Pharmacologic therapies for NVP and HG are summarized in **Table 2**.

Table 2
Pharmacologic therapies for NVP and HG

Drug Name/Category	Pregnancy Category	Recommended Dose	Mechanism of Action	Efficacy in HG	Side Effects
Pyridoxine (136)	A	25 mg po q8 h	May treat underlying pyridoxine deficiency	+/-	Paresthesias, nausea, HA, fatigue
Diclectin (10 mg pyridoxine + 10 mg doxylamine) (133) *available only in Canada	A/B	2–4 tabs daily	Treats pyridoxine deficiency and H1 antagonist	+/-	Drowsiness
Antihistamines (147) • Dimenhydrinate • Diphenhydramine	B	25–50 mg po q4–8 h 50–100 mgpo q3–6 h	Peripheral H1 receptor antagonist	+	Drowsiness, dizziness, HA, fatigue
Phenothiazines (44) • Promethazine • Prochlorperazine	C	12.5–25 mg po q6–8 h 10 mg po q6–8 h	Central/peripheral dopamine antagonist	+	Drowsiness, decreased seizure threshold, akathisia
Metoclopramide (143)	B	10 mg po/IV q8 h	Central/peripheral dopamine antagonist	+	Dystonia, restlessness, somnolence *FDA black box warning: tardive dyskinesia
Ondansetron (154)	B	10 mg po/IV q8 h	Peripheral and central selective 5HT3 receptor antagonist	+/-	Constipation, diarrhea, HA, fatigue
Corticosteroids (157) • Methylprednisolone	C	16 mgpo q8hrx 3 d, then taper	May treat relative ACTH deficiency, inhibit central PG synthesis or decrease central 5-HT turnover	+/-	Hyperglycemia, possible increased risk of oral facial clefts with first trimester use
Droperidol (156)	C	0.25–2.5 mg iv loading with 1 mg iv/hour	Dopamine antagonist in chemoreceptor trigger zone	+/-	Drowsiness, dizziness; cardiac arrythmias, black box warning for QT prolongation
H2 blockers (137) • Ranitidine	B	150 mg po ql2 h or 50 mg IV q8 h	Peripheral H2 antagonist	Adjunct therapy	HA, drowsiness, dizziness, diarrhea or constipation
PPI • Lansoprazole • Esomeprazole	B	30 or 40 mg po/IV q24 h	Irreversible blocker of H+/K+ ATPase of parietal cell	Adjunct therapy	HA, nausea, diarrhea, fatigue

Citations are included in parentheses.
* N.B. Except for Diclectin, no drugs are FDA approved for the treatment of nausea and vomiting during pregnancy or HG. The expected benefits of treatment should outweigh the risk.

Nutritional Support

For women with intractable symptoms unresponsive to dietary modification and pharmacologic treatment and who are unable to maintain weight by oral intake, nutritional support may be required. In this population intravenous fluid therapy, enteral nutrition, or parenteral nutrition should be used to prevent fetal intrauterine growth restriction, maternal dehydration, and malnutrition.

The role of intravenous hydration is to increase volume and restore electrolytes. In hospitalized patients, normal saline or lactated Ringer solution can be infused rapidly if needed, and then later adjusted to match urine output. Intravenous thiamine should be administered before any dextrose-containing fluids to avoid Wernicke encephalopathy. Women requiring multiple hospitalizations may be considered for in-home intravenous hydration.[71]

Enteral tube feeding and total parenteral nutrition should be considered if intravenous therapy is not successful in reducing symptoms and there is still a caloric deficit. Studies on enteral feeding for HG, however, are limited. One small study of women with HG treated with enteral feeding using an 8F nasogastric tube reported symptom improvement within 24 hours of tube placement. After 8 days, patients were discharged with a mean of 43 additional days of outpatient enteral feeding, after which oral feeding was able to be resumed.[165]

In addition to nasogastric tubes, percutaneous endoscopic gastrostomy (PEG) tubes[166] have been used successfully to maintain nutrition in women with HG. Both of these modes of feeding are limited, however, by the risk of increased nausea and vomiting caused by intragastric feeding. Postpyloric feeding tubes, both nasojejunal[167,168] and PEG,[169] have been attempted to reduce this risk; however, dislodgment of the tubes[170] due to ongoing vomiting and retching and gastric coiling is a common complication. In addition, nasoenteric tubes, both nasogastric and nasojejunal, are poorly tolerated by many women for aesthetic reasons and because of physical discomfort. Recently, surgical jejunostomy has been described as an alternative mode of nutrition delivery to women with HG. In one small study, 5 women with HG underwent surgical jejunostomy in the second trimester. Isotonic tube feeds were administered to a goal caloric factor. Maternal weight gain occurred in 5 out of the 6 pregnancies, and all pregnancies ended in term deliveries. No major complications occurred, suggesting that jejunostomy may be a safe and effective mode of nutrition support in women with HG.[171]

For women unable to tolerate enteral feeding, parenteral nutrition should be considered. This therapy, however, is costly and is associated with significant maternal morbidity. Russo-Stieglitz and colleagues[172] reported a 9% complication rate for parenteral nutrition via peripherally inserted central catheters (PICC) in pregnancy and a 50% complication rate for centrally inserted catheters. Infection and thrombosis were the 2 most frequently occurring complications, and were hypothesized to result from pregnancy-associated hypercoagulability and immunologic suppression. Holmgren and colleagues[173] similarly showed a high rate of complications in women administered parenteral nutrition via PICC. In a study of 94 women with HG, 66.4% of those treated with parenteral nutrition via PICC required treatment for thromboembolism, infection, or both. Patients on parenteral nutrition also had higher rates of neonatal complications, including admission to the neonatal intensive care unit, small size for gestational age, termination of pregnancy from HG, and fetal loss, in comparison with women treated by enteral feeds. Thus, although it may be more tolerable to patients, parenteral nutrition should be reserved for selected patients with HG.

SUMMARY

NVP is an extremely common disorder in pregnancy that ranges in spectrum from mild to moderate nausea and vomiting to pathologic HG. Despite its prevalence, its pathogenesis is still largely unknown and consequently treatment is mainly symptomatic, ranging from dietary changes and oral pharmacologic treatment to hospitalization with intravenous fluid replacement and nutrition therapy.

Although most studies suggest that NVP is not harmful to the fetus, this condition is not benign in that it significantly reduces the quality of life of the pregnant woman and places a financial burden on the affected individual as well as the larger society. For women with HG, maternal and fetal morbidity may occur if the condition is unrecognized and not treated aggressively.

REFERENCES

1. O'Brien B, Zhou Q. Variables related to nausea and vomiting during pregnancy. Birth 1995;22:93–100.
2. Mazzotta P, Maltepe C, Navoiz Y, et al. Attitudes, management, and consequences of nausea and vomiting of pregnancy in the United States and Canada. Int J Gynaecol Obstet 2000;70:359–65.
3. Semmens JP. Female sexuality and life situations: an etiologic psycho-sociosexual profile of weight gain and nausea and vomiting of pregnancy. Obstet Gynecol 1971;38:555–63.
4. Lacasse A, Rey E, Ferreira E, et al. Epidemiology of nausea and vomiting of pregnancy: prevalence, severity, determinants, and the importance of race/ethnicity. BMC Pregnancy Childbirth 2009;9:26.
5. Dodds L, Fell DB, Joseph KS, et al. Outcome of pregnancies complicated by hyperemesis gravidarum. Obstet Gynecol 2006;107:285–92.
6. Bashiri A, Newmann L, Maymon E, et al. Hyperemesis gravidarum: epidemiologic features, complications, and outcome. Eur J Obstet Gynecol Reprod Biol 1995;63:135–8.
7. Blum R. Pregnancy, nausea, and vomiting: further explorations in theory. In: Blum RH, Heinrichs WL, editors. Nausea and vomiting. Overview, challenges, practical treatments and new perspectives. Philadelphia: Whurr Publishers; 2000. p. 246–68.
8. Klebanoff MA, Koslowe PA, Kaslow R, et al. Epidemiology of vomiting in early pregnancy. Obstet Gynecol 1985;66:612–6.
9. Brandes JM. First trimester nausea and vomiting as related to outcome of pregnancy. Obstet Gynecol 1967;30:427–31.
10. Lacroix R, Eason E, Melzack R. Nausea and vomiting during pregnancy: a prospective study of its frequency, intensity, and patterns of change. Am J Obstet Gynecol 2000;182:931–7.
11. Weigel RM, Weigel MM. The association of reproductive history, demographic factors, and alcohol and tobacco consumption with the risk of developing nausea and vomiting in early pregnancy. Am J Epidemiol 1988;127:562.
12. Davis M. Nausea and vomiting of pregnancy: an evidence-based review. J Perinat Neonatal Nurs 2004;18:312–28.
13. Corey LA, Berg K, Solaas MH, et al. The epidemiology of pregnancy complications and outcome in Norwegian twin population. Obstet Gynecol 1992;80:989–94.
14. Gadsby R, Barnie-Adshead A, Jagger C. Pregnancy nausea related to women's obstetric and personal histories. Gynecol Obstet Invest 1997;43:108–11.

15. Furneaux E, Langley-Evans A, Langley-Evans S. Nausea and vomiting of pregnancy; endocrine basis and contribution to pregnancy outcome. Obstet Gynecol Surv 2001;56:775–82.
16. Whitehead S, Holden W, Andrews P. Maternal susceptibility to nausea and vomiting of pregnancy: is the vestibular system involved? Am J Obstet Gynecol 2002;186:S204–9.
17. Heinrichs L. Linking olfaction with nausea and vomiting of pregnancy, recurrent abortion, hyperemesis gravidarum, and migraine headache. Am J Obstet Gynecol 2002;186:S215–9.
18. Kallen B, Lundberg G, Aberg A. Relationship between vitamin use, smoking, and nausea and vomiting of pregnancy. Acta Obstet Gynecol Scand 2003;82: 916–20.
19. Samisoe G, Crona N, Enk L, et al. Does position and size of corpus luteum have any effect on nausea and vomiting? Acta Obstet Gynecol Scand 1986;65:427–9.
20. Thorp JM, Watson WJ, Katz VL. Effect of corpus luteum position on hyperemesis gravidarum. A case report. J Reprod Med 1991;36:761–2.
21. Signorello L, Harlow B, Wang S, et al. Saturated fat intake and the risk of severe morning sickness. Epidemiology 1998;9:636–40.
22. Broussard CN, Richter JE. Nausea and vomiting of pregnancy. Gastroenterol Clin 1998;27:123–51.
23. Fejzo MS, Ingles SA, Wilson M, et al. High prevalence of severe nausea and vomiting of pregnancy and hyperemesis gravidarum among relatives of affected individuals. Eur J Obstet Gynecol Reprod Biol 2008;141:13–7.
24. Fell DB, Dodds L, Joseph KS, et al. Risk factors for hyperemesis gravidarum requiring hospital admission during pregnancy. Obstet Gynecol 2006;107:277–84.
25. Depue RH, Bernstsein L, Ross RK, et al. Hyperemesis gravidarum in relation to estradiol levels, pregnancy outcome and other maternal factors: sero-epidemiologic study. Am J Obstet Gynecol 1987;156:1137–41.
26. Cedergren M, Brynhildsen J, Josefesson A, et al. Hyperemesis gravidarum that requires hospitalization and the use of antiemetic drugs in relation to maternal body composition. Am J Obstet Gynecol 2008;198:412.e1–5.
27. Vikanes A, Grjibovski AM, Vangen S, et al. Maternal body composition, smoking, and hyperemesis gravidarum. Ann Epidemiol 2010;20:592–8.
28. Rochelson B, Vohra N, Darvishzadeh J, et al. Low prepregnancy ideal weight: height ratio in women with hyperemesis gravidarum. J Reprod Med 2003;48: 422–4.
29. Kallen B. Hyperemesis gravidarum during pregnancy and delivery outcome: a registry study. Eur J Obstet Gynecol Reprod Biol 1987;26:291.
30. Schiff M, Reed S, Daling J. The sex ratio of pregnancies complicated by hospitalization for hyperemesis gravidarum. BJOG 2004;111:27.
31. Schoeneck FJ. Gonadotropin hormone concentrations in hyperemesis gravidarum. Am J Obstet Gynecol 1943;43:308.
32. Masson GM, Anthony F, Chau E. Serum chorionic gonadotropin (hCG), schwangerschaftsprotein 1 (SP1), progesterone, and oestradiol levels in patients with nausea and vomiting in early pregnancy. Br J Obstet Gynaecol 1985;92:211–5.
33. Goodwin TM, Montoro M, Mestman JH, et al. The role of chorionic-gonadotropin in transient hyperthyroidism of hyperemesis gravidarum. J Clin Endocrinol Metab 1992;75:1333–7.
34. Soules MR, Hughs CL, Garcia JA, et al. Nausea and vomiting of pregnancy: role of human chorionic gonadotropin and 17-hydroxyprogesterone. Obstet Gynecol 1980;55:696.

35. Wenstrom KD, Owen J, Boots LR, et al. Elevated second-trimester human chorionic gonadotrophin levels in association with poor pregnancy outcome. Am J Obstet Gynecol 1994;171:1038–41.
36. Goodwin TM. Hyperemesis gravidarum. Obstet Gynecol Clin North Am 2008;35: 401–17.
37. Jordan V, Grebe SKG, Cooke PR, et al. Acidic isoforms of chorionic gonadotropin in European and Samoan women are associated with hyperemesis gravidarum and may be thyrotrophic. Clin Endocrinol 1999;50:619–27.
38. Goodwin T. Nausea and vomiting of pregnancy; an obstetric syndrome. Am J Obstet Gynecol 2002;186:S184–9.
39. Verberg MF, Gillott DJ, Al-Fardan N, et al. Hyperemesis gravidarum, a literature review. Hum Reprod Update 2005;11:527–39.
40. Walsh JW, Hasler WL, Nugent CE, et al. Progesterone and estrogen are potential mediators of gastric slow wave dysrhythmias in nausea of pregnancy. Am J Physiol 1996;270:506–14.
41. Sanders KM, Bauer AJ, Publicover NG. Regulation of gastric antral slow wave frequency by prostaglandins. In: Roman C, editor. Gastrointestinal motility. Lancaster (UK): MTP Press; 1983. p. 77–85.
42. North RA, Whitehead R, Larkins RG. Stimulation by human chorionic gonadotropin of prostaglandin synthesis by early human placental tissue. J Clin Endocrinol Metab 1991;73:60–70.
43. Borgeat A, Fathi M, Valiton A. Hyperemesis gravidarum: is serotonin implicated? Am J Obstet Gynecol 1997;176:476–7.
44. Sullivan CA, Johnson CA, Roach H, et al. A pilot study of intravenous ondansteron for hyperemesis gravidarum. Am J Obstet Gynecol 1996;174:1565–8.
45. Kuscu N, Koyuncu F. Hyperemesis gravidarum: current concepts and management. Postgrad Med J 2002;78:76–9.
46. Evans AJ, Li TC, Selby C, et al. Morning sickness and thyroid function. Br J Obstet Gynaecol 1986;93:520.
47. Goodwin TM, Hershmann JM. Hyperthyroidism due to inappropriate production of human chorionic gonadotropin. Clin Obstet Gynecol 1997;40:32–44.
48. Aka N, Atalay S, Sayharman S, et al. Leptin and leptin receptor levels in pregnant women with hyperemesis gravidarum. Aust N Z J Obstet Gynaecol 2006; 46:274–7.
49. Demir B, Erel CT, Haberal A. Adjusted leptin level (ALL) is a predictor for hyperemesis gravidarum. Eur J Obstet Gynecol Reprod Biol 2006;124:193–6.
50. Lee J, Lee K, Kim M, et al. The correlation of leptin and hCG (human chorionic gonadotrophin) levels in the serum between women with hyperemesis gravidarum and normal control. Fertil Steril 2003;80(Suppl 3):S251–2.
51. Unsel N, Benian A, Erel CT. Leptin levels in women with hyperemesis gravidarum. Int J Gynaecol Obstet 2004;84:162–3.
52. Sugito Y, Dekizawa A, Farina A, et al. Relationship between severity of HG and fetal DNA concentration in maternal plasma. Clin Chem 2003;49:1667–9.
53. Yoneyama Y, Suzuki S, Sawa R, et al. The T-helper 1/T-helper 2 balance in peripheral blood of women with hyperemesis gravidarum. Am J Obstet Gynecol 2002;187:1631–5.
54. Kaplan PB, Gucer F, Sayin NC, et al. Maternal serum cytokine levels in women with hyperemesis gravidarum in the first trimester of pregnancy. Fertil Steril 2003;1979:498–502.
55. Yoneyama Y, Shyunji S, Rinataro S, et al. Plasma adenosine concentrations increase in women with hyperemesis gravidarum. Clin Chim Acta 2004;342:99–103.

56. Kuscu NK, Yildirim Y, Koyuncu, et al. Interleukin-6 levels in hyperemesis gravidarum. Arch Gynecol Obstet 2003;269:13–5.
57. Leylek OA, Toyaksi M, Erselcan T, et al. Immunologic and biochemical factors in hyperemesis gravidarum with or without hyperthyroxinemia. Gynecol Obstet Invest 1999;47:229–34.
58. Hod M, Orvieto R, Kaplan B, et al. Hyperemesis gravidarum: a review. J Reprod Med 1994;39:605.
59. Frigo P, Lang C, Reisenberger K, et al. Hyperemesis gravidarum associated with Helicobacter pylori seropositivity. Obstet Gynecol 1998;91:615–7.
60. Bagis T, Gumurdulu Y, Kayaselcuk F, et al. Endoscopy in hyperemesis gravidarum and Helicobacter pylori infection. Int J Gynaecol Obstet 2002;79:105–9.
61. Golberg D, Szilagyi A, Graves L. Hyperemesis gravidarum and Helicobacter pylori infection: a systemic review. Obstet Gynecol 2007;110:695–703.
62. Sandven I, Abdelnoor M, Nesheim BI, et al. Helicobacter pylori infection and hyperemesis gravidarum: a systematic review and meta-analysis of case-control studies. Acta Obstet Gynecol Scand 2009;88:1190–200.
63. Kocak I, Akcan Y, Ustun C, et al. Helicobacter pylori seropositivity in patients with hyperemesis gravidarum. Int J Gynaecol Obstet 1999;66:251–4.
64. Lanciers S, Despinasse B, Mehta DI, et al. Increased susceptibility to Helicobacter pylori infection in pregnancy. Infect Dis Obstet Gynecol 1999;7:195–8.
65. Weyermann M, Brenner H, Adler G, et al. Helicobacter pylori infection and the occurrence and severity of gastrointestinal symptoms during pregnancy. Am J Obstet Gynecol 1989;2003:526–31.
66. Wu C-Y, Tseng J-J, Chou M-M, et al. Correlation between Helicobacter pylori infection and gastrointestinal symptoms in pregnancy. Adv Ther 2000;17:152–8.
67. Cutler A, Prasad V. Long-term followup for Helicobacter pylori serology after successful eradication. Am J Gastroenterol 1996;91:85–8.
68. Ali M, Khan A, Tiwari S, et al. Association between cag-pathogenicitiy island in Helicobacter pylori isolates from peptic ulcer, gastric carcinoma and non-ulcer dyspepsia subjects with histological changes. World J Gastroenterol 2005;11:6815–22.
69. Xia LB, Yang J, Li AM, et al. Relationship between hyperemesis gravidarum and H pylori seropositivity. Chin Med J 2004;117:301–2.
70. Nashaat EH, Mansour GM. Helicobacter pylori and hyperemesis gravidarum. Nat Sci 2010;8:22–6.
71. Koch KL, Frissora C. Nausea and vomiting during pregnancy. Gastroenterol Clin North Am 2003;32:201–34.
72. Brzana RJ, Koch KL. Intractable nausea presenting as gastroesophageal reflux disease. Ann Intern Med 1997;126:704–7.
73. Richter JE. Review article: the management of heartburn in pregnancy. Aliment Pharmacol Ther 2005;23:749–57.
74. Koch K, Stern RM, Vasey M, et al. Gastric dysrhythmias in nausea of pregnancy. Dig Dis Sci 1990;35:961–8.
75. Riezzo G, Pezzolla F, Darconza G, et al. Gastric myoelectrical activity in the first trimester of pregnancy: a cutaneous electrogastrographic study. Am J Gastroenterol 1992;87:702–7.
76. Schade RR, Pelekanose MJ, Tauze WN, et al. Gastric emptying during pregnancy [abstract]. Gastroenterol 1984;86:A1234.
77. Davison JS, Davison MC, Hay DM. Gastric emptying time in late pregnancy and labour. J Obstet Gynaecol Br Commonw 1970;77:37–41.

78. Macfie AG, Magides AD, Richmond MN, et al. Gastric emptying in pregnancy. Br J Anaesth 1991;67:54–7.
79. Jednak MA, Shadigian EM, Kim MS, et al. Protein meals reduced nausea and gastric slow waves dysrhythmic activity in first trimester pregnancy. Am J Physiol 1999;277:855–61.
80. Lawson M, Kern F, Everson GT. Gastrointestinal transit time in human pregnancy: prolongation in the second and third trimesters followed by postpartum normalization. Gastroenterol 1985;89:996.
81. Wald A, Van Thiel DH, Hoeschstetter L, et al. Effect of pregnancy on gastrointestinal transit. Dig Dis Sci 1982;27:1015.
82. Fitzgerald CM. Nausea and vomiting in pregnancy. Br J Med Psychol 1984;57:159.
83. Simpson SW, Goodwin TM, Robins SB, et al. Psychological factors and hyperemesis gravidarum. J Womens Health Gend Based Med 2001;10:471–7.
84. Munch S. Women's experiences with a pregnancy complication: causal explanations of hyperemesis gravidarum. Soc Work Health Care 2002;36:519–24.
85. Munch S. Chicken or the egg? The biological-psychological controversy surrounding hyperemesis gravidarum. Soc Sci Med 2002;55:1267–78.
86. Hasler WL, Soudah HC, Dulai G, et al. Mediation of hyperglycemia-evoked gastric slow waves dysrhythmias by endogenous prostaglandins. Gastroenterol 1995;108:727–36.
87. Cappell MS, Sidhom O, Colon V. A study at eight medical centers of the safety and clinical efficacy of esophagogastroduodenoscopy in 83 pregnancies with follow-up of fetal outcome. Am J Gastroenterol 1996;91:348.
88. Weigel RM, Weigel MM. Nausea and vomiting of early pregnancy and pregnancy outcome. A meta-analytical review. Br J Obstet Gynaecol 1989;96:1312–8.
89. Tierson FD, Olsen CL, Hook EG. Nausea and vomiting of pregnancy and association with pregnancy outcome. Am J Obstet Gynecol 1986;155:1017.
90. Deuchar N. Nausea and vomiting in pregnancy: a review of the problem with particular regard to psychological and social aspects. Br J Obstet Gynaecol 1995;120:6–8.
91. Zhou Q, O'Brien B, Relyea J. Severity of nausea and vomiting during pregnancy; what does it predict? Birth 1999;26:108–14.
92. Klebanoff M, Mills J. Is vomiting during pregnancy teratogenic? BMJ 1986;292:724–6.
93. Boneva RS, Moore CA, Potto L, et al. Nausea during pregnancy and congenital heart defects: population-based case-control study. Am J Epidemiol 1999;149:17–25.
94. Bayley T, Dye L, Jones S, et al. Food cravings and aversions during pregnancy: relationships with nausea and vomiting. Appetite 2002;38:45–51.
95. Huxley R. Nausea and vomiting in early pregnancy; its role in placental development. Obstet Gynecol 2000;95:779–82.
96. Smith C, Crowther C, Beilby J, et al. The impact of nausea and vomiting on women: a burden of early pregnancy. Aust N Z J Obstet Gynaecol 2000;4:397–401.
97. O'Brien B, Naber S. Nausea and vomiting during pregnancy; effects on the quality of women's lives. Birth 1992;19:138–43.
98. Attard C, Kohli M, Coleman S, et al. The burden of illness of severe nausea and vomiting of pregnancy in the United States. Am J Obstet Gynecol 2002;186:S220–7.
99. Miller F. Nausea and vomiting in pregnancy: the problem of perception—is it really a disease? Am J Obstet Gynecol 2002;186:S182–3.

100. Vallacott I, Cooke E, James C. Nausea and vomiting in early pregnancy. Int J Gynaecol Obstet 1988;27:7–62.
101. Gazmararian J, Peterson R, Jamieson D, et al. Hospitalization during pregnancy among managed care enrollees. Obstet Gynecol 2002;100:94–100.
102. Jiang HG, Elixhauser A, Nicholas J, et al. Care of women in US hospitals. Rockville (MD): Agency for Healthcare Research and Quality; 2000. 2002 HCUP Fact Book No. 3. AHRQ Pub No. 02–0044.
103. Godsey RK, Newman RB. Hyperemesis gravidarum: a comparison of single and multiple admissions. J Reprod Med 1991;36:287–90.
104. Koren G, Piwko C, Ahn E, et al. Validation studies of the Pregnancy Unique-Quantification of Emesis (PUQE) scores. J Obstet Gynaecol 2005;25:241–4.
105. Jain SK, Shah M, Ransonet L, et al. Maternal and neonatal plasma transthyretin (prealbumin) concentrations and birth weight of newborn infants. Biol Neonate 1995;68:10–4.
106. Wallstedt A, Riely CA, Shaver D, et al. Prevalence and characteristics of liver dysfunction in hyperemesis gravidarum. Clin Res 1990;38:970A.
107. Knox TA, Olans LB. Liver disease in pregnancy. N Engl J Med 1996;335: 569–76.
108. Conchillo JM, Pijnenborg JMA, Peeters P, et al. Liver enzyme elevation induced by hyperemesis gravidarum: aetiology, diagnosis and treatment. Neth J Med 2002;60:374–8.
109. Robertson C, Miller H. Hyperamylasemia in bulimia nervosa and hyperemesis gravidarum. Int J Eat Disord 1999;26:223–7.
110. Kanayama N, Khutan S, Belayet HM, et al. Vasospasms of cerebral arteries in hyperemesis gravidarum. Gynecol Obstet Invest 1998;46:139–41.
111. Trogstad L, Stoltenberg C, Magnus P, et al. Recurrence risk in hyperemesis gravidarum. BJOG 2005;112:1641–5.
112. Pourshariff B, Korst L, MacGibbon K, et al. Voluntary termination in a large cohort of women with hyperemesis gravidarum. Contraception 2007;76:451–5.
113. Erlandsson G, Lambe M, Cnattingius S, et al. Hyperemesis gravidarum and subsequent breast cancer risk. Br J Cancer 2002;87:974–6.
114. Zhang J, Cai W. Severe vomiting during pregnancy. Antenatal correlates and fetal outcomes. Epidemiology 1991;2:454.
115. Gross S, Librach C, Cecutti A. Maternal weight loss associate with hyperemesis gravidarum: a predictor of fetal outcome. Am J Obstet Gynecol 1989;160:906.
116. Brunetti-Pierri N, Hunter JV, Boerkoel CF. Gray matter heterotopias and brachytelephalangic chondrodysplasia punctata: a complication of hyperemesis gravidarum induced vitamin K deficiency? Am J Med Genet A 2007;154:200–4.
117. Eventov-Friedman S, Klinger G, Shinwell ES. Third trimester fetal intracranial hemorrhage owing to vitamin K deficiency associated with hyperemesis gravidarum. J Pediatr Hematol Oncol 2009;31:985–8.
118. Ebrahimi N, Maltepe C, Bournisssen FG, et al. Nausea and vomiting of pregnancy: using the 24-hour Pregnancy-Unique Quantification of Emesis (PUQE-24) scale. J Obstet Gynaecol Can 2009;31:803–7.
119. Power Z, Campbell M, Kilcoyne P, et al. The hyperemesis impact of symptoms questionnaire: development and validation of a clinical tool. Int J Nurs Stud 2010;47:67–77.
120. Lacasse A, Rey E, Ferreira E, et al. Determinants of early medical management of nausea and vomiting of pregnancy. Birth 2009;36:70–7.
121. Jueckstock JK, Kaestner R, Mylonas I. Managing hyperemesis gravidarum: a multimodal challenge. BMC Med 2010;8:46.

122. Rosen T, Veciana M, Miler H, et al. A randomized controlled trial of nerve stimulation for relief of nausea and vomiting in pregnancy. Obstet Gynecol 2003;102: 129–35.
123. Vickers AJ. Can acupuncture have specific effects on health? A systematic review of acupuncture antiemesis trials. J R Soc Med 1996;89:303–11.
124. Werntoft E, Dykes AK. Effect of acupressure on nausea and vomiting during pregnancy. A randomized, placebo-controlled pilot study. J Reprod Med 2001;46:835–9.
125. Quinlan PD, Hill DA. Nausea and vomiting of pregnancy. Am Fam Physician 2003;68:121–8.
126. Smith C, Crowther C, Beilby J. Acupuncture to treat nausea and vomiting in early pregnancy: a randomized controlled trial. Birth 2000;29:1–9.
127. American College of Obstreticians and Gynecologists. ACOG practice bulletin. Clinical management guidelines for obstetrician-gynecologists: nausea and vomiting of pregnancy. Obstet Gynecol 2004;103:803–11.
128. Mahady G, Pendland S, Yun G, et al. Ginger and the gingerols inhibits the growth of CagA+ strains of Helicobacter Pylori. Anticancer Res 2003;23: 3699–702.
129. Fischer-Rasmussen W, Kjaer S, Dahl C, et al. Ginger treatment of hyperemesis gravidarum. Eur J Obstet Gynecol Reprod Biol 1991;38:19–24.
130. Vutyavanich T, Kraisarin T, Ruangsri RA. Ginger for nausea and vomiting in pregnancy: a randomized, double-masked, placebo-controlled trial [abstract]. Obstet Gynecol 2001;97:577–82.
131. Portnoi G, Chang L, Karimi-Tabesh, et al. A prospective comparative study of the safety and effectiveness of ginger for the treatment of nausea and vomiting in pregnancy. Am J Obstet Gynecol 2003;189:1374–7.
132. Backon J. Ginger in preventing nausea and vomiting of pregnancy: a caveat due to its thromboxane synthetase activity and effect on testosterone binding. Eur J Obstet Gynecol Reprod Biol 1991;42:163–4.
133. Niebyl J, Goodwin T. Overview of nausea and vomiting of pregnancy with an emphasis on vitamins and ginger. Am J Obstet Gynecol 2002;186:S253–5.
134. McKeigue PM, Lamm SH, Linn S, et al. Bendectin and birth defects: a meta-analysis of the epidemiologic studies. Teratology 1994;50:881–4.
135. Einarson TR, Leeder JS, Koren G. Method of meta-analysis of epidemiological studies. Drug Intell Clin Pharm 1988;22:813–24.
136. Sahakian V, Rouse D, Spies S, et al. Vitamin B6 is effective therapy for nausea and vomiting of pregnancy: a randomized, double-blinded placebo-controlled study. Obstet Gynecol 1991;78:33.
137. Leathem A. Safety and efficacy of antiemetics used to treat nausea and vomiting in pregnancy. Clin Pharm 1986;5:660–8.
138. Rumeau-Rouquette C, Goujard J, Huel G. Possible teratogenic effect of phenothiazines in human beings. Teratology 1977;15:57–64.
139. Briggs G, Freeman R, Yaffe S, editors. Drugs in pregnancy and lactation: a reference guide to fetal and neonatal medicine. 4th edition. Baltimore (MD): Williams &Wilkins; 1994.
140. Witter FR, King TM, Blake D. The effects of chronic gastrointestinal medication on the fetus and neonate. Obstet Gynecol 1981;58:79.
141. Koussen M. Treatment of nausea and vomiting in pregnancy. Am Fam Physician 1993;48:1414.
142. Einarson A, Koren G, Bergman U. Nausea and vomiting of pregnancy: a comparative European study. Eur J Obstet Gynecol Reprod Biol 1998;76:1–3.

143. Tan PC, Khine PP, Vallikkannu N, et al. Promethazine compared with metoclopramide for hyperemesis gravidarum: a randomized controlled trial. Am J Obstet Gynecol 2010;115:975–81.
144. Matok I, Gorodischer R, Koren G, et al. The safety of metoclopramide use in the first trimester of pregnancy. N Engl J Med 2009;360:2528–35.
145. Sorensen HT, Nielsen GL, Christensen K, et al. Birth outcome following maternal use of metoclopramide: the Euromap study group. Br J Clin Pharmacol 2000;49: 264–8.
146. Badell ML, Ramin SM, Smith JA. Treatment options for nausea and vomiting of pregnancy. Pharmacotherapy 2006;26:1273–87.
147. Mazzotta P, Magee LA. A risk-benefit assessment of pharmacological and non-pharmacological treatments for nausea and vomiting of pregnancy. Drugs 2000; 59:781–800.
148. Seto A, Einarson T, Koren G. Pregnancy outcomes following first trimester exposure to antihistamines: a meta-analysis. Am J Perinatol 1997;14:119–24.
149. Miklovich L, Van den Berg BJ. An evaluation of the teratogenicity of certain antinauseant drugs. Am J Obstet Gynecol 1976;125:244–8.
150. Kotelko DM, Rottman RL, Wright WC, et al. Transdermal scopolamine decreases nausea and vomiting following cesarean section in patients receiving epidural morphine. Anesthesiology 1989;71:675.
151. Yu JF, Yang YS, Wang WY, et al. Mutagenicity and teratogenicity of chlorpromazine and scopolamine. Chin Med J 1988;101:339.
152. Rubenstein EB, Slusher BS, Rojas C, et al. New approaches to chemotherapy-induced nausea and vomiting: from neuropharmacology to clinical investigations. Cancer J 2006;12:341–7.
153. Einarson A, Malatepe C, Navioz Y. The safety of ondansetron for nausea and vomiting of pregnancy: a prospective comparative study. Br J Obstet Gynaecol 2004;111:940–3.
154. Tincello DJ, Johnstone MJ. Treatment of hyperemesis gravidarum with the 5-HT3 antagonist ondansetron (Zofran). Postgrad Med J 1996;72:688–9.
155. Siu SS, Yip SK, Cheung CW. Treatment of intractable hyperemesis gravidarum by ondansetron. Eur J Obstet Gynecol Reprod Biol 2002;105:73–4.
156. Nageotte MP, Briggs GG, Towers CV, et al. Droperidol and diphenhydramine in the management of hyperemesis gravidarum. Am J Obstet Gynecol 1996;174: 1801–5.
157. Safari HR, Alsulyman OM, Gherman RB, et al. Experience with oral methylprednisolone in the treatment of refractory hyperemesis gravidarum. Am J Obstet Gynecol 1998;178:1054–8.
158. Yost NP, McIntire DD, Wians FH, et al. A randomized, placebo-controlled trial of corticosteroids for hyperemesis due to pregnancy. Obstet Gynecol 2003;102: 1250–4.
159. Park-Wyllie L, Mazzotta P, Pastuszak A, et al. Birth defects after maternal exposure to corticosteroids: prospective cohort study and meta-analysis of epidemiological studies. Teratology 2000;62:385–92.
160. Gill SK, Maltepe C, Mastali K, et al. The effect of acid-reducing pharmacotherapy on the severity of nausea and vomiting of pregnancy. Obstet Gynecol Int 2009;2009:585269.
161. Gill SK, Maltepe C, Koren G. The effect of heartburn and acid reflux on the severity of nausea and vomiting of pregnancy. Can J Gastroenterol 2008;23:270–2.
162. Mahadevan U. Gastrointestinal medications in pregnancy. Best Pract Res Clin Gastroenterol 2007;21:849–77.

163. Gill SK, O'Brien L, Koren G. The safety of histamine 2 (H2) blockers in pregnancy: a meta-analysis. Dig Dis Sci 2009;54:1835–8.
164. Gill SK, O'Brien L, Einarson TR, et al. The safety of proton pump inhibitors (PPIs) in pregnancy: a meta-analysis. Am J Gastroenterol 2009;104:1541–5.
165. Hsu JJ, Clark-Glena R, Nelson DK, et al. Nasogastric enteral feeding in the management of hyperemesis gravidarum. Obstet Gynecol 1996;88:343–6.
166. Godil A, Chen YK. Percutaneous endoscopic gastrostomy for nutrition support in pregnancy associated hyperemesis gravidarum and anorexia nervosa. JPEN J Parenter Enteral Nutr 1998;22:238–41.
167. Vaisman N, Kaider R, Levin I, et al. Nasojejunal feeding in hyperemesis gravidarum—a preliminary study. Clin Nutr 2004;23:53–7.
168. Pearce CB, Collett J, Goggin PM, et al. Enteral nutrition by nasojejunal tube in hyperemesis gravidarum. Clin Nutr 2001;20:461–4.
169. Serrano P, Velloso A, Garcia-Luna PP, et al. Enteral nutrition by percutaneous endoscopic gastrojejunostomy in severe hyperemesis gravidarum: a report of two cases. Clin Nutr 1998;17:135–9.
170. Barclay BA. Experience with enteral nutrition in the treatment of hyperemesis gravidarum. Nutr Clin Pract 1990;5:153–5.
171. Saha S, Loranger D, Pricolo V, et al. Feeding jejunostomy for the treatment of severe hyperemesis gravidarum: a case series. JPEN J Parenter Enteral Nutr 2009;33:529–34.
172. Russo-Stieglitz KE, Levine AB, Wagner BA, et al. Pregnancy outcome in patients requiring parenteral nutrition. J Matern Fetal Med 1999;8:164–7.
173. Holmgren C, Aagaard-Tillery KM, Silver RM, et al. Hyperemesis in pregnancy: an evaluation of treatment strategies with maternal and neonatal outcomes. Am J Obstet Gynecol 2008;198:56, e1–4.

Liver Disease in Pregnancy

Ayaz Matin, MD, David A. Sass, MD, AGAF*

KEYWORDS

- Pregnancy • HELLP • Hyperemesis gravidarum
- Acute fatty liver • Intrahepatic cholestasis • Pruritus

This article briefly discusses gestational physiologic changes and thereafter reviews liver diseases during pregnancy, which are divided into 3 main categories. The first category includes conditions that are unique to pregnancy and generally resolve with the termination of pregnancy. These include hyperemesis gravidarum (HG); intrahepatic cholestasis of pregnancy (ICP); hemolysis, elevated liver enzymes, and low platelet count occurring in association with preeclampsia (HELLP) syndrome; and acute fatty liver of pregnancy (AFLP) (**Table 1**). The second category includes liver diseases that are not unique to the pregnant population but occur commonly or are severely affected by pregnancy. These include Budd-Chiari syndrome, acute intermittent porphyria, choledochal cysts, hepatic adenomas, splenic artery aneurysm, and hepatitis E. The third category includes diseases that occur coincidentally with pregnancy and in patients with underlying chronic liver disease, with cirrhosis, or after liver transplant who become pregnant.

PHYSIOLOGIC CHANGES AND DIAGNOSTIC TESTING IN PREGNANCY

Pregnancy is a state of altered, albeit normal, physiology. During pregnancy, the synthetic and metabolic functions of the liver are affected by the increased serum estrogen and progesterone levels.[1] Knowledge of the changes associated with normal pregnancy is essential for the interpretation of liver test values and the management of liver diseases during pregnancy.

Pregnancy is associated with many normal physiologic changes that can mimic chronic liver disease. Physical findings can include spider angiomata and palmar erythema, which can disappear after delivery. It is presumed that hyperestrogenemia during pregnancy is responsible for these changes. The plasma volume increases steadily between weeks 6 and 36 of gestation by about 50%. The red cell volume

Funding support: None.
Financial disclosures: Both authors have no financial disclosures and conflicts of interest.
Division of Gastroenterology and Hepatology, Drexel University College of Medicine, 12th Floor New College Building, 245 North 15th Street, Suite 12324, Philadelphia, PA 19102, USA
* Corresponding author.
E-mail address: dsass@drexelmed.edu

Gastroenterol Clin N Am 40 (2011) 335–353
doi:10.1016/j.gtc.2011.03.010
0889-8553/11/$ – see front matter © 2011 Elsevier Inc. All rights reserved.

Table 1
Liver diseases unique to pregnancy

Diagnosis	Onset (trimester)	Typical Features	Treatment	Prevalence (%)
HG	First	Nausea, vomiting, dehydration, electrolyte abnormalities	Supportive	0.3–1.0
Preeclampsia/ Eclampsia	Second and/or third	Hypertension, edema, proteinuria	Supportive, prompt delivery	5–7
HELLP	70% midsecond to midthird, 30% postpartum	Hemolysis, thrombocytopenia	Supportive, prompt delivery	0.2–0.6
AFLP	Third	Liver failure, coagulopathy, encephalopathy, hypoglycemia, DIC	Supportive, prompt delivery	0.005–0.010
ICP	Third	Pruritus, mild jaundice, elevated serum bile acid levels	UDCA, delivery after fetal maturity	0.1–0.3
Liver hematoma/ rupture	Third to postpartum	RUQ pain, preeclampsia, hypotension, shock	Surgery	1 (in patients with HELLP syndrome)

Abbreviations: DIC, disseminated intravascular coagulation; RUQ, right upper quadrant; UDCA, ursodeoxycholic acid.

also increases, but the increase is not as much, leading to hemodilution and a lower hematocrit caused by increased total blood volume. Cardiac output increases until the second trimester, then decreases and normalizes near term. Absolute hepatic blood flow remains unchanged, but the percentage of cardiac output to the liver decreases. The blood pressure during pregnancy is usually lower than normal, and an increase in level may suggest preeclampsia or eclampsia.

Serum albumin levels decrease because of hemodilution and decreased synthesis, but serum cholesterol and triglyceride concentrations increase markedly because of increased synthesis. The serum alkaline phosphatase levels increase late in pregnancy, mainly during the third trimester as a result of production of the placental isoenzyme and an increase in the bone isoenzyme.[2] The serum values of alanine aminotransferase (ALT) and aspartate aminotransferase (AST) are usually within normal limits.[2] Serum γ-glutamyl transpeptidase (GGT) activity decreases slightly during late pregnancy. The total and free bilirubin concentrations are lower in the pregnant population than in nonpregnant controls during all 3 trimesters, as are the concentrations of conjugated bilirubin during the second and third trimesters. The fasting serum total bile acid (TBA) concentrations usually remain within normal limits. Hence, elevated levels of ALT, AST, serum bilirubin, and fasting TBA should be considered pathologic, as they are in nonpregnant women, and further evaluation should be considered.

The differential diagnosis for elevated liver function tests and abdominal pain in a pregnant patient is extensive. To reach the diagnosis, physicians need to make sure that all the diagnostic tests used are safe for the mother and the fetus. Diagnostic imaging, such as ultrasonography, is considered safe during pregnancy, and no adverse effects have been noted in children from birth up to 8 years of age because of in utero exposure. Magnetic resonance imaging (MRI) is also considered safe. However, gadolinium should be avoided especially in the first trimester because it crosses the placenta and its effects on the fetus are not known. Computed tomography (CT) or radiography should be avoided because radiation poses a big risk to the fetus. However, CT scans expose the fetus to less than 1 rad of radiation and can be used if strongly indicated. Exposure to more than 5 rad during the first 14 days after fertilization can lead to intrauterine death, and exposure to more than 15 rad during the remainder of the pregnancy may cause congenital anomalies, growth restriction, and intellectual disability.[3,4]

A liver biopsy is rarely necessary for the diagnosis of liver disease during pregnancy unless the diagnosis is in question and if establishing the diagnosis will change the management course. In the absence of coagulopathy, a percutaneous liver biopsy can be safely performed under ultrasound guidance. If the patient is coagulopathic, a transjugular liver biopsy can be performed.

LIVER DISEASES UNIQUE TO PREGNANCY
HG

Nausea and vomiting are not uncommon during pregnancy, with symptoms ranging from mild morning sickness to severe disease requiring hospitalization. Morning sickness is a common occurrence, occurring in 50% to 90% of all pregnant women, and is almost an accepted physiologic phenomenon of pregnancy. On the other hand, HG can significantly affect a pregnant woman's quality of life.[5] This topic is discussed in another article by Saha and colleagues elsewhere in this issue and so is only briefly addressed here.

HG is an idiopathic syndrome of severe intolerable nausea and vomiting in the first trimester of pregnancy, usually before 10 weeks of gestation, occurring in approximately 0.3% of pregnancies.[6,7] Objectively, HG is defined as persisting vomiting accompanied by weight loss exceeding 5% of prepregnancy body weight and ketonuria unrelated to other causes.[8] The pathophysiology is poorly understood but immunologic, hormonal, and psychological factors are thought to play a role.[6] The risk factors for HG are noted in **Box 1**.

Approximately 50% of women are hospitalized with HG.[9] Half of these patients have liver dysfunction with minimal to several fold elevation in aminotransferase levels, mild unconjugated hyperbilirubinemia (up to 4 mg/dL), or pruritus. The true incidence of abnormal liver function tests in HG is difficult to predict because the incidence is related to the severity of symptoms.[7] The hepatic dysfunction is thought to be related to dehydration, malnutrition, and electrolyte abnormalities.[10] There may be elevation in amylase levels, likely from a salivary source and not pancreatic.[9,11] Symptoms usually resolve at 14 to 18 weeks of gestation; however, they may continue until the third trimester in 15% to 20% or even until delivery in 5% of patients.[12]

The diagnosis is usually made on clinical grounds. It remains a diagnosis of exclusion after other pathologic conditions, such as gastrointestinal disorders (gastroenteritis, viral hepatitis, pancreatitis, cholelithiasis, peptic ulcer disease), genitourinary tract disorders, metabolic disturbances (diabetes, porphyria), neurologic diseases (migraine, tumor, vestibular lesions), drug toxicity, and psychological problems, have been ruled out.[12] Rarely, a liver biopsy need to be performed only to exclude other more serious diseases. The hepatic histologic appearance is generally normal or shows bland cholestasis, mild fatty change, or no abnormality.[6,7]

> **Box 1**
> **Risk factors for developing HG**
>
> Young age
> Obesity
> Nulliparity
> Tobacco use
> Hyperthyroidism
> Psychiatric illnesses
> Molar pregnancy
> Preexisting diabetes
> Multiple pregnancies
> Abnormal gastric motility during pregnancy
> Specific nutrient deficiencies
> Alterations in lipid levels
> Changes in autonomic nervous system

Treatment is symptomatic, focuses on alleviating vomiting, and includes bowel rest and intravenous fluids. Antiemetics, such as metoclopramide, promethazine, ondansetron, or droperidol, have been reported to be safe and useful in the treatment; however, no medications are currently approved by the US Food and Drug Administration (FDA).[11,13–15] Dietary management generally consists of frequent high-carbohydrate, low-fat, small meals. Fluids are better tolerated if they are cold, clear, and carbonated and if taken in small amounts between meals. Thiamine supplementation should be given to patients with prolonged vomiting to prevent Wernicke encephalopathy. Patients who are not able to maintain their weight because of excessive vomiting may need enteral feeding.[16]

HG may rarely lead to serious complications, including Wernicke encephalopathy, renal damage, retinal hemorrhage, immunosuppression, pneumomediastinum, and spontaneous esophageal rupture. Mild hyperthyroidism may be associated with HG likely because of the high serum concentrations of human chorionic gonadotrophin, which increases thyroid-stimulating activity in pregnant women. With adequate supportive treatment, the pregnancy outcome is favorable.[17]

ICP

ICP is characterized by pruritus and elevated serum bile acid levels, which occur in the second and third trimester of pregnancy. The disorder resolves after delivery but often recurs in subsequent pregnancies. ICP was initially described in the Scandinavian countries, and the incidence in the region is 1% to 2%. However, the incidence varies significantly, and there are clear ethnic and racial differences. In the United States, the population prevalence varies from 0.3% to 5.6% in a primarily Latin population in Los Angeles.[18,19] The highest incidence is found in Chile and Bolivia with rates ranging from 4% to 22%.[20] The cause for the disorder is unknown; however, genetic, hormonal, and environmental factors may play a role.[21]

The association with ethnic background supports the presence of a genetic component.[6,7] Some women have defects in the *ABCB 4* (adenosine triphosphate–binding cassette subfamily B member 4) gene, which codes for the multidrug-resistance

P-glycoprotein 3 (MDR 3). MDR 3 is a hepatocellular phospholipid transporter, transporting phospholipids across the canalicular membrane, and mutations may result in loss of function and increased bile acid levels as a secondary effect. At least 10 different MDR 3 mutations have been identified in ICP, and MDR 3 mutations may account for 15% of cases of ICP.[22-25] Some genes encoding other canalicular transport proteins or their regulator may also play a role in the pathogenesis of ICP.[26] Sex hormones have known cholestatic effects and are thought to play a role in causing ICP. There is increased hormonal activity in the third trimester and in twin pregnancies, which may lead to ICP because it is more common in these situations. Estrogens and progesterones can impair the function of bile transporters (such as MDR 3), saturating the hepatic transport systems, in some genetically predisposed women.[27] Progesterone treatment in pregnant women for the prevention of premature labor can lead to symptoms of ICP, and it is recommended that progesterone be avoided in patients with a history of ICP or stopped immediately if the patients develop symptoms of cholestasis while on progesterone therapy.[28]

A new hypothesis for the pathogenesis of ICP was proposed in a recent study. It was found that patients with ICP had increased intestinal permeability, and it has been hypothesized that a leaky gut can increase the intestinal absorption of endotoxins and contribute to the pathogenesis of the disease.[29] Environmental factors are certainly thought to play a role because of the climatic and geographic variability. Selenium deficiency has also been implicated in a study from Chile where the increased levels of selenium over the years especially during the summers has led to a decrease in the incidence of ICP.[30]

The disease is manifested by pruritus, at times severe and intractable, in the third trimester; however, symptoms as early as the first trimester have been noted. The pruritus is usually generalized, starting peripherally and spreading centrally, but it may be present more on the palms and soles and gets more intense at night. There is no clear rash, but there may be excoriations on various areas because of scratching. Jaundice is fairly uncommon, occurring in less than 15% of patients with ICP. Jaundice usually occurs 2 to 4 weeks after the onset of pruritus, and if it precedes pruritus, other causes of liver disease should be investigated. Patients may also develop diarrhea or steatorrhea.

Fasting levels of TBAs, particularly conjugated bile acids and especially cholic acid, are elevated.[31,32] These increased levels may be the first or only laboratory abnormality seen and are the most sensitive and specific markers of the disease.[33] There is mild, predominantly conjugated hyperbilirubinemia. Transaminase levels are usually 2 to 10 fold above normal levels (in 20%–60% of cases with pruritus), serum alkaline phosphatase level is modestly elevated (not specific because of production of the placental isoenzyme), and GGT level is normal.[28,34] Liver biopsy is usually not necessary and if done, shows bland cholestasis with minimal or no inflammation. Bile plugs in hepatocytes and canaliculi predominate in zone 3, and the portal tracts are unaffected.[7,35] Ultrasonographically, the liver appears normal and the biliary ducts are not dilated.

The treatment of ICP is focused on reducing the debilitating symptoms, improving biochemical test results, and preventing maternal and fetal complications. There is no associated maternal mortality; however, there may be significant fetal morbidity and mortality.[28,36] The risks for the fetus include fetal prematurity, meconium-stained amniotic fluid, intrauterine demise, and increased risk of fetal respiratory distress syndrome. The rate of fetal demise ranges from 1% to 3% but can be as high as 5%.[28] There is no ideal method for fetal surveillance, and even though biophysical profile testing and nonstress tests are recommended by some physicians, their role in predicting the risk of fetal demise is very limited. It has been suggested that fetal complications increase with increasing serum bile acid levels, with significant complications arising when the levels are more than 40 μmol/L.[33] However, this method is very impractical because of delay in reported results. The delivery of the fetus leads to resolution of symptoms but may not be feasible until fetal lung maturity is established.

Ursodeoxycholic acid (UDCA) has shown efficacy in the treatment of ICP in multiple trials, improving the symptoms, bile flow, and biochemical test results. There are no significant adverse maternal or fetal effects reported; however, the effect of UDCA in reducing fetal complications is unknown.[33,37–39] UDCA seems to restore the transport capabilities of the placenta, which are affected in ICP, and it also helps normalize the maternal serum bile acid concentration to that of a healthy pregnant woman.[40] A study compared UDCA dose of 8 to 10 mg/kg/d in divided doses versus cholestyramine. Pruritus and biochemical studies significantly improved with UDCA compared with cholestyramine, and the babies were delivered closer to term. There were no adverse effects noted.[39] With all the supporting data, UDCA is considered to be a first-line therapy for ICP.[38,41–43] The dosage is not clearly defined but the usual dose is 10 to 15 mg/kg/d in divided doses. However, even when used in higher doses, UDCA is completely safe for the fetus.[39]

Other drugs that are used include antihistamines, such as hydroxyzine; cholestyramine; and S-adenosylmethionine (SAMe). Cholestyramine works by decreasing ileal absorption of bile salts and increasing fecal elimination. Cholestyramine has not shown benefit over UDCA in clinical trials and may lead to significant steatorrhea. If cholestyramine is used, vitamin K should be administered along with it because it can lead to exacerbation of vitamin K deficiency, leading to postpartum bleeding. Antihistamines may aggravate respiratory difficulties in preterm babies. SAMe is a glutathione precursor and when used alone has not shown benefit but if combined with UDCA, may have an additive effect.[44] Cholestasis can lead to deficiency of fat-soluble vitamins; hence, vitamin K should be given to all patients with jaundice to decrease postpartum bleeding.

Cholestasis recurs in 60% to 70% of the patients, and affected women are also at an increased risk of having gallstones. It is prudent to check patients for underlying liver disease.[45] Liver function tests should also be checked a few months after delivery to confirm normalization. Use of oral contraceptives is associated with a small risk of recurrence of pruritus; however, low-dose estrogen contraception can be used safely after liver function tests have normalized.

AFLP

AFLP is a sudden catastrophic illness characterized by microvesicular steatosis associated with mitochondrial dysfunction. When described in 1940, AFLP was thought to be universally fatal, but now with early diagnosis and prompt delivery, the prognosis has significantly improved, with maternal mortality being a rarity.[46] AFLP occurs in approximately 1 out of 10,000 pregnancies and is a disease of the third trimester; however, there are patients presenting in the late second trimester or who are diagnosed after delivery.[47–49] Approximately half of the patients are nulliparous, with an increased incidence in twin pregnancies and preeclamptic patients.[47–50] There is no ethnic, geographic, or age distribution.[7]

There is a strong association with defects in the mitochondrial beta-oxidation pathway, particularly in the long-chain 3-hydroxyacyl-CoA dehydrogenase (LCHAD). The LCHAD, 1 of the 4 enzymes responsible for long-chain fatty acid oxidation (FAO) in the liver, is part of a larger enzyme complex on the mitochondrial inner membrane called mitochondrial trifunctional protein. Defects in the LCHAD lead to accumulation of long-chain 3-hydroxyacyl metabolites produced by the fetus or placenta. These metabolites are hepatotoxic and can lead to liver disease. The most common mutations are Glu474Gln and G1548C.[48,51] The risk of developing AFLP in mothers of infants with LCHAD homozygosity is very high. There is also increased risk of developing HELLP syndrome in mothers of babies with LCHAD mutations. This strong association supports the need to screen for this defect in the fetuses of mothers with AFLP. Testing for the known genetic variants of LCHAD is available and should be performed in affected women, their infants, and fathers.[12] However, LCHAD deficiencies may not be the only defects leading to AFLP, and other defects in the mitochondrial beta-oxidation pathway may play a role, including short- and medium-chain fatty acid defects.[50] Factors such as carnitine deficiency or other dietary factors may also play a role.[48]

The diagnosis of AFLP is made by a combination of clinical presentation, laboratory findings, and imaging. Presentation of AFLP may range from asymptomatic elevation in aminotransferases to fulminant hepatic failure. Patients usually have 1 or 2 weeks of nonspecific symptoms, such as anorexia, nausea and vomiting, headache, and right upper quadrant pain. The patients may develop progressive jaundice with the bilirubin level usually being less than 5 mg/dL, but pruritus is rare. Aminotransferases vary from near normal to 1000s, with the majority being in the 300 to 500 range. If the levels are very high, other diagnoses, such as hepatic ischemia and viral hepatitis, should also be entertained. Other laboratory studies may show a normochromic normocytic anemia, leukocytosis, normal to low platelet levels, coagulopathy with or without disseminated intravascular coagulation (DIC), metabolic acidosis, renal dysfunction, hypoglycemia, high ammonia levels, and biochemical pancreatitis with elevated amylase and lipase.[50] As the disease progresses, patients appear ill with worsening jaundice and development of complications such as hypertension, edema, ascites, polyuria and polydipsia caused by transient diabetes insipidus, oliguric renal failure, gastrointestinal bleeding, intra-abdominal bleeding, and hepatic encephalopathy.[7,49,52,53]

Definitive diagnosis is made histologically; however, it is not always required because doing a biopsy may prove hazardous in a pregnant patient. If done, the biopsy shows microvesicular fatty infiltration predominantly in zone 3 within hepatocytes. The fat droplets surround centrally located nuclei, giving the cytoplasm a foamy appearance. There is lobular disarray, and there might be mild inflammation with cholestasis. The frozen section can be stained with oil red O stain or can be viewed under electron microscopy, which shows evidence of cytoplasmic fat and can be helpful if the fat is not obvious on regular hematoxylin-eosin staining.

Differential diagnosis includes acute viral hepatitis, especially hepatitis E; herpes simplex virus disease; drug-induced hepatitis; HELLP syndrome; and biliary tract disorders. Features of AFLP may overlap with HELLP syndrome, making the distinction between the two very difficult at times. But in AFLP, the degree of hepatic impairment is much more significant. Even though AFLP can culminate in severe disease, early recognition and diagnosis with immediate delivery of the fetus and aggressive supportive care has increased both maternal and fetal survival, with fetal mortality being less than 15%.[47,51]

Patients generally improve clinically and biochemically shortly after delivery; however, there may be cases with transient worsening followed by definitive improvement.[49] There are no reports of improvement before delivery. The method of delivery is dependent on obstetric assessment. Vaginal delivery can be attempted in a stable patient if it can be achieved in a rapid controlled fashion within 24 hours. Vaginal delivery decreases the incidence of major intra-abdominal bleeding caused by coagulopathy. However, in most cases, a cesarean section is the mode of delivery. Supportive care is of the utmost importance, especially in severe cases or when the diagnosis was delayed. Mechanical ventilation, blood products to correct coagulopathy, glucose infusion, dialysis, parenteral nutrition, or even surgery to treat bleeding may be required.[47] Lactulose therapy can be used for hepatic encephalopathy associated with elevated ammonia levels. Occasionally, liver transplant may be required.[54]

Patients typically recover without any clinical sequelae, even after severe liver disease. The disease recurs in approximately 25% of pregnancies, even though there might be negative testing for LCHAD deficiencies. Patients need counseling regarding risks, and if they decide to proceed with another pregnancy, they should be closely followed up at a tertiary referral center by a high-risk obstetrician.[47,51]

Preeclampsia and HELLP Syndrome

Preeclampsia is a triad of hypertension, edema, and proteinuria seen in the third trimester of 5% to 7% of pregnancies. Liver involvement is not common but when present signifies severe disease. The mechanism of injury involves vasospasm and precipitation of fibrin in the liver. Histologically, there is periportal hemorrhage, ischemic lesions, and microvesicular fat deposition. Clinically, the patients may have nausea, vomiting, and right upper quadrant abdominal pain. Liver enzyme levels may be elevated 10- to 20-fold, and this elevation reflects the development of HELLP syndrome. In the most severe cases, it may progress to subcapsular hemorrhage or hepatic rupture. Prompt delivery is indicated to avoid progressing to eclampsia and hepatic complications as mentioned earlier.

HELLP syndrome is characterized by microangiopathic hemolytic anemia, elevated liver enzyme levels, and low platelet counts. This syndrome complicates 2% to 12% of cases with severe preeclampsia and about 0.2% to 0.6% of all pregnancies.[55–57] Although preeclampsia may lead to development of HELLP syndrome, there are patients without hypertension and proteinuria but with defining criteria of HELLP syndrome, leading many experts to believe that it is a separate entity.[57,58] Most women present antepartum, usually in the third trimester, with most cases being diagnosed in the 28 to 36 weeks of gestation.[57,59] Up to 30% of women may present in the postpartum period, ranging from 48 hours after delivery to as long as 7 days after childbirth.[10]

The precipitating injury is not known. There is some overlap with AFLP and FAO defects; however, this association is not well established. Although families with FAO deficiencies have an increased incidence of HELLP, the babies born to women with HELLP do not necessarily have an increased risk of having FAO deficiencies.[48,60] HELLP is a disease of abnormal hepatic endothelial reactivity or disruption. Initially, abnormal trophoblastic implantation may lead to reduced tissue perfusion and endothelial dysfunction, which leads to platelet activation and aggregation along with activation of the complement and coagulation cascades, increased vascular tone, and alteration of the thromboxane to prostacyclin ratio.[9] The endothelial injury results in microangiopathic hemolytic anemia with schistocytes seen on peripheral smear. The liver enzymes are elevated because of periportal hepatic necrosis.

It is difficult to clinically distinguish HELLP from preeclampsia. Most women have right upper quadrant abdominal pain and tenderness, nausea and vomiting, malaise, headache, edema, and weight gain. Most patients have hypertension and proteinuria; however, 15% of patients can have absence of either one or both even with severe HELLP syndrome. Jaundice is only seen in 5% of patients. HELLP is more common in older, white, multiparous women but can occur in any parity and age.

Diagnosis is made by changes in complete blood cell count, peripheral smear, and transaminase levels. Patients have anemia with schistocytes on peripheral smear, elevated lactate dehydrogenase level (more than 600 IU/L), and platelet count usually less than 100,000 cells/μL. The transaminase levels are elevated, with the AST levels being at least 70 IU/L.[7,57,61] Patients who fulfill all 3 criteria usually have severe disease and are considered to have "true" HELLP syndrome, whereas some patients may only have "partial" HELLP. These include patients with "ELLP," in which hemolysis is absent; "EL," in which severe preeclampsia is present; or "HEL," in which platelet counts are normal.[7] Patients may also develop DIC.

Radiological imaging is considered when complications are suspected because of pain radiating to the shoulder or neck. CT or MRI scans can show subcapsular hematomas, intraparenchymal hemorrhage, or infarction or hepatic rupture. These findings usually correlate with platelet counts less than 20,000 but not with liver dysfunction.[6] Liver biopsy is rarely necessary and can be dangerous because of coagulopathy. However, if biopsy is done, it shows periportal hemorrhage and fibrin deposition.[62] Certain other conditions can have a similar presentation as HELLP. In particular, some features of AFLP may overlap with those of HELLP, but in AFLP, the degree of hepatic impairment is much more significant.[9] Thrombocytopenia can be caused by gestational thrombocytopenia, immune thrombocytopenia or thrombotic thrombocytopenia (TTP), and hemolytic uremic syndrome (HUS).[63,64] These conditions do not have elevated liver enzyme levels, and HELLP lacks the neurologic and renal manifestations found in patients with TTP and HUS.[64]

Delivery is the only definitive therapy because there can be rapid progressive maternal deterioration. Mortality is as high as 3%, and serious morbidity can include DIC, abruption placenta, acute renal failure, pulmonary edema, subcapsular liver hematoma, and retinal detachment.[57] Pregnant women with HELLP should be hospitalized immediately for antepartum stabilization and transferred to a tertiary referral center if needed. A limited-view hepatic CT scan should also be obtained in deteriorating or critical patients to rule out hepatic complications. Temporizing measures, such as magnesium sulfate for seizure prophylaxis, and vasodilators (labetalol; hydralazine; nifedipine; or, in severe cases, sodium nitroprusside) should be administered and may improve fetal and neonatal as well as maternal outcomes.[12,65] If there are no obstetric complications or DIC and if the pregnancy is at term, well-established labor should be allowed to proceed. However, most patients require caesarean section. Usually, there is resolution of HELLP after delivery with platelet levels normalizing in 5 days; however, some patients may develop persistent thrombocytopenia or hemolysis or may have complications of HELLP. In these situations, more aggressive therapy is indicated, including plasmapheresis, plasma volume expansion, antithrombotic agents, steroids, plasma exchange with fresh frozen plasma, or dialysis.

There may be an indication to proceed with liver transplant in rare situations, such as persistent bleeding from a hematoma or hepatic rupture or liver failure from extensive necrosis.[66] Hepatic hemorrhage without rupture is managed conservatively with close hemodynamic monitoring, correction of coagulopathy, and immediate intervention for any maternal deterioration or expansion of hematoma on hepatic imaging. Any stressful situation, such as abdominal palpation, unnecessary transportation, convulsions, or emesis, should be avoided.[6] Rarely, hepatic hemorrhage may lead to hepatic rupture. Hepatic hemorrhage is associated with severe thrombocytopenia and occurs primarily in the right lobe, occurring just before or after delivery. Diagnosis is made on finding intraperitoneal blood during emergency caesarean section or by imaging. Operative management includes packing; drainage; hepatic artery ligation; resection; angiographic embolization; or, rarely, transplant.[67–71]

Perinatal mortality is high (7%–20%) because of prematurity, dysmaturity due to placental insufficiency, or the consequences of severe maternal complications. If the maternal condition is stable and the pregnancy is not at term, options include conservative management until fetal lung maturity is achieved or corticosteroids to help achieve fetal lung maturity. However, the longer the conservative management, the higher the risk of deterioration with resultant increase in fetal loss. Despite lacking randomized trials, the National Institutes of Health Consensus Development Panel recommends using corticosteroids for fetal lung maturity at less than 34 weeks gestation and consequently improving perinatal outcome. Using steroids may also improve the maternal platelets.[72] High-dose intravenous dexamethasone is preferable to intramuscular betamethasone for 24 to 48 hours, with delivery thereafter.[73,74] Surviving babies have the same outcome as other babies of similar gestational age. Subsequent pregnancies carry a high risk of complications and recurrence occurs in 2% to 6%. No long-term effects have been noted.[12]

LIVER DISEASES SEVERELY AFFECTED BY PREGNANCY

Certain liver diseases that may occur coincidentally with the pregnancy are severely affected by it and can be significant in determining maternal and fetal outcomes. These disorders need to be considered when evaluating a patient with abdominal symptoms and abnormal liver function tests or radiographic studies. **Table 2** summarizes these liver disorders.

LIVER DISEASE COINCIDENTAL TO PREGNANCY
Hepatitis A

The incidence of acute hepatitis A in pregnant women is comparable to that in the nonpregnant population.[82] The clinical presentation and course is also similar except for increased pruritus due to increased estrogen. In most endemic areas, many women are immune to the virus because of exposure in earlier years. However, if there is no immunity, both the inactivated vaccine and postexposure prophylaxis are safe in pregnancy.[83]

Hepatitis B and D

Hepatitis B virus (HBV) infection is a common health problem in many countries. Acute HBV complicates 1 to 2 per 1000 pregnancies, and chronic HBV infection is seen in 1% of pregnancies in North America.[83] Pregnant patients are routinely offered screening tests for HBV. If the test for hepatitis B surface antigen (HBsAg) gives positive results, the infection is confirmed with test for hepatitis B e antigen (HBeAg). In addition to complications during pregnancy from chronic hepatitis, there is a significant risk of perinatal transmission. Almost all infections occur around the time of delivery. The highest rates of transmission are in HBeAg-positive mothers. Infections acquired through childbirth tend to confer as high as 90% chronicity when compared with 5% when acquired in adulthood. Since 1991 it has been recommended to check the hepatitis B status of a pregnant woman using HBsAg. If a pregnant woman is HBsAg negative, vaccination against HBV is recommended for the infant. However, if the mother is HBsAg positive, it is recommended that the infant receives HBV immunoglobulin as well. The combination of active and passive immunizations is very effective, reducing the carrier state of infants born to HBeAg/HBsAg-positive mothers to almost zero. Delivery by caesarean section is not safer, and with proper immunoprophylaxis, breastfeeding has been shown to be safe.[84] Failures of immunoprophylaxis can occur in women with very high viral loads. To prevent these failures, lamivudine has been

Table 2
Disorders severely affected by pregnancy

Disorder	Mechanisms of Effect of Pregnancy	Clinical Presentation	Diagnosis	Therapy
Hepatitis E	Particularly severe during pregnancy, especially third trimester. Possibly related to immunologic changes during pregnancy[75–77]	Malaise, anorexia, nausea, vomiting, abdominal pain, and jaundice	IgM antibody to hepatitis E, PCR analysis of blood or feces for hepatitis E	Supportive therapy for acute infection. May require liver transplant
Hepatic adenoma	Increased growth of adenoma because of hyperestrogenemia	Nausea, vomiting, and RUQ pain	Abdominal US	Size<5 cm, observe; size≥5 cm or symptomatic or intralesional hemorrhage, surgery[78]
Budd-Chiari syndrome	Thrombosis promoted by increased gestational serum levels of estrogen and decrease in AT III levels	RUQ pain, hepatomegaly, and ascites	Doppler abdominal US, hepatic venography, or magnetic resonance angiography	Selective thrombolytic therapy, surgical shunt, or TIPS; anticoagulation with heparin because warfarin is contraindicated during pregnancy[79,80]
Splenic artery aneurysm	Can rupture during pregnancy because of compression by gravid uterus	Abdominal pain, pulsatile left upper quadrant mass, and abdominal bruit in patient with portal hypertension	Abdominal Doppler US	Surgical removal or angiographic occlusion[81]
AIP	Symptoms worsened by hyperestrogenemia	Abdominal pain, vomiting, constipation, paresthesias in extremities, mental status changes, tachycardia, and ileus	Increased urinary porphobilinogen, and δ-aminolevulinic acid	Discontinue precipitating drugs, avoid prolonged fasting, and administer hematin and glucose to prevent attacks
Choledochal cysts	Cyst compression by gravid uterus can lead to cyst rupture or cholangitis	Abdominal pain, jaundice, and abdominal mass	Abdominal US, may require cholangiography	Frequently requires surgery: cystectomy and cholecystectomy, with either Roux-en-Y hepaticojejunostomy or choledochojejunostomy

Abbreviations: AIP, acute intermittent porphyria; AT III, antithrombin III; RUQ, right upper quadrant; TIPS, transjugular intrahepatic portosystemic shunt; US, ultrasonography.

Data from Cappell MS. Hepatic disorders severely affected by pregnancy: medical and obstetric management. Med Clin North Am 2008;92:739–60.

used in the third trimester in HBeAg-positive patients with high viral loads. Lamivudine (a category C drug) has been shown to decrease perinatal transmission with no clear evidence of harmful effects to the fetus.[59,85–87] Alternatively, one may use tenofovir or telbivudine (both category B drugs) in the third trimester to prevent perinatal transmission. It is recommended that such individuals be enrolled in the antiretroviral pregnancy registry to monitor for the safety of these agents (http://www.apregistry.com).

Coinfection may occur with hepatitis D virus (delta virus) and lead to a more severe infection, with a rapid course and higher risk of progression to chronic infection and cirrhosis.[83]

Hepatitis C

The prevalence of hepatitis C virus (HCV) in pregnant women is comparable to that in the general population. Vertical transmission seems to be the most common route of HCV infection.[88] The viral levels fluctuate during pregnancy, and it is recommended to check them during the third trimester. Chronic infection is not associated with a higher risk to the pregnancy and its outcome.[89] Transmission to the fetus is increased if there is active infection with detectable HCV RNA. The viral load and not the genotype confer a higher risk of transmission. There is passive passage of maternal anti-HCV antibodies to the fetus via the placenta, and detection of anti-HCV antibodies in newborns does not mean the presence of active infection. However, if there is presence of HCV RNA in infants 3 to 6 months of age or persistence of anti-HCV antibodies beyond 18 months, it can be concluded that the infant has had transmission of infection. Long-term sequelae in children with chronic infection acquired by vertical transmission are not well studied.[90,91] Coinfection with human immunodeficiency virus (HIV) significantly increases the risk of transmission, and antiretroviral treatment of HIV during pregnancy decreases the rate of HCV transmission to levels of women who do not have HIV.[92] Amniocentesis in women infected with hepatitis C does not seem to significantly increase the risk of vertical transmission, but women should be counseled that very few studies have properly addressed this possibility.[93] The mode of delivery does not affect transmission rates. Even though the HCV virus can be detected in breast milk, breast-feeding is considered to be safe.

Treatment of chronic hepatitis C in pregnancy is currently not recommended. Although interferon does not seem to have an adverse effect on the embryo or fetus, there are limited data on its use and potential harmful effects to the fetus are not known.[94] Ribavirin is teratogenic in multiple animal species, and its use during pregnancy is contraindicated. Screening is recommended in high-risk women.

Autoimmune Hepatitis

Autoimmune hepatitis (AIH) is a chronic liver disease that may progress to cirrhosis. AIH occurs in young women and may predispose to infertility. With adequate immunosuppression and regression of disease, normal menstruation can be achieved with a chance of conception. There is variability reported in disease activity during pregnancy, with some reports of increase in disease activity, whereas others report improvement in the course of the disease, with frequent exacerbation in the postpartum period.[95,96] The improvement is speculated to be because of immunotolerance induced by pregnancy. Prednisone is considered to be safe and is recommended to be continued at a low dose during pregnancy.[95] Azathioprine is also considered to be safe and has been used in various conditions during pregnancy with good results.[96] Because the disease often exacerbates in the postpartum period, immunosuppression should be continued or even elevated during that time.[97]

Primary Biliary Cirrhosis and Primary Sclerosing Cholangitis

Primary biliary cirrhosis (PBC) and primary sclerosing cholangitis (PSC) are both chronic cholestatic conditions leading to destruction of the bile ducts. There are limited data on the natural course of pregnancy in both these diseases because most young women with these conditions are usually infertile. If pregnancy occurs, patients may experience increased pruritus and elevation of cholestatic liver enzyme levels, which should prompt evaluation for biliary strictures and choledocholithiasis by ultrasonography. There is no definitive treatment of either PBC or PSC during pregnancy, but UDCA is recommended and has been shown to be safe during pregnancy.[98,99]

Cirrhosis in Pregnancy

Some women may exhibit signs of liver disease during pregnancy because of preexisting chronic liver disease. The severity of these hepatic disorders may affect the ability to conceive and maintain a healthy pregnancy. Cirrhotic patients, with portal hypertension in particular, have a very high risk of complications during pregnancy. However, cirrhosis is not a contraindication for pregnancy.

Portal pressures increase throughout pregnancy and more so in patients with preexisting portal hypertension. Complications, such as hepatic encephalopathy; hepatic failure; jaundice; malnutrition; splenic artery aneurysms; and, in particular, variceal bleeding, can seriously affect the mortality and morbidity of the pregnant patient.[100,101] Variceal bleeding may complicate 20% to 25% of pregnancies in cirrhotic patients.[6] All pregnant patients with cirrhosis should be screened for varices in their second trimester and started on β-blockers if present. Patients with large varices may also undergo prophylactic variceal band ligation. Endoscopic management is used in cases of active variceal hemorrhage. The use of vasopressin is contraindicated because it is teratogenic; however, the safety of octreotide has not been well studied.[102] Even though there are no data to date suggesting the risk of vaginal delivery in patients with varices, caesarean section is recommended to prevent excessive straining.[103] Hepatic encephalopathy is treated similar to that in the nonpregnant patient. Lactulose is a pregnancy category B drug and should be used over rifaximin, a category C drug.

Pregnancy and Liver Transplant

Amenorrhea and infertility are common in women with end-stage liver disease, affecting up to 50% of patients. In premenopausal women, a return to normal reproductive function is expected after liver transplant. In fact, more than 80% of women have a normal menstrual cycle in the first year after transplant, and restoration of menstrual bleeding may occur as early as 2 months posttransplant.[104,105] This restoration to normal condition allows for the opportunity of pregnancy, which, if handled with rigorous hepatological and obstetric follow-up, leads to success in most cases. Although there are no clear guidelines regarding the interval of conception from liver transplant, it is prudent to wait at least a year before conception, and counseling about family planning should be offered to all patients. Immunosuppressive therapy should be continued; however, the effects of most immunosuppressive agents on the fetus have not been well studied. Tacrolimus (FK506), cyclosporine, mycophenolate mofetil, sirolimus, and prednisone are all FDA category C drugs.

Liver transplant is associated with a considerable risk to the fetus, with a significant increase in fetal and neonatal complications and mortality, particularly prematurity and low birth weight. However, about 70% of live-born babies do well without congenital anomalies or neonatal complications.[106–108] Maternal complications are also common, including hypertension, preeclampsia, and infections associated with immunosuppression.[106,108] These complications are rarely fatal. The rate of graft rejection is also not affected by pregnancy.[107]

SUMMARY

Although relatively uncommon, hepatic disorders during pregnancy are clinically important because of their potentially severe effects on both the mother and the fetus. These disorders are often complex and clinically challenging, and a rapid diagnosis differentiating between liver diseases related and unrelated to pregnancy is required to render appropriate therapeutic interventions effective. The spectrum of disease ranges from subtle alterations in liver biochemical profile to fulminant hepatic failure. Patients presenting with severe liver dysfunction during pregnancy should be managed by experienced physicians in specialized centers. Research has improved our understanding of pregnancy-related liver disease pathogenesis, which has translated into improved maternal and fetal outcomes.

REFERENCES

1. Van Thiel DH, Gavaler JS. Pregnancy-associated sex steroids and their effects on the liver. Semin Liver Dis 1987;7(1):1–7.
2. Valenzuela GJ, Munson LA, Tarbaux NM, et al. Time-dependent changes in bone, placental, intestinal, and hepatic alkaline phosphatase activities in serum during human pregnancy. Clin Chem 1987;33(10):1801–6.
3. De Santis M, Cesari E, Nobili E, et al. Radiation effects on development. Birth Defects Res C Embryo Today 2007;81(3):177–82.
4. De Santis M, Di Gianantonio E, Straface G, et al. Ionizing radiations in pregnancy and teratogenesis: a review of literature. Reprod Toxicol 2005;20(3): 323–9.
5. Lacasse A, Rey E, Ferreira E, et al. Nausea and vomiting of pregnancy: what about quality of life? BJOG 2008;115(12):1484–93.
6. Hay JE. Liver disease in pregnancy. Hepatology 2008;47(3):1067–76.
7. Su GL. Pregnancy and liver disease. Curr Gastroenterol Rep 2008;10(1):15–21.
8. Goodwin TM. Hyperemesis gravidarum. Clin Obstet Gynecol 1998;41(3): 597–605.
9. Benjaminov FS, Heathcote J. Liver disease in pregnancy. Am J Gastroenterol 2004;99(12):2479–88.
10. Cappell MS. Hepatic disorders severely affected by pregnancy: medical and obstetric management. Med Clin North Am 2008;92(4):739–60, vii–viii.
11. Riely CA. Liver disease in the pregnant patient. American College of Gastroenterology. Am J Gastroenterol 1999;94(7):1728–32.
12. Kupcinskas L, Kondrackiene J. Liver diseases unique to pregnancy. Medicina (Kaunas) 2008;44(5):337–45.
13. Seto A, Einarson T, Koren G. Pregnancy outcome following first trimester exposure to antihistamines: meta-analysis. Am J Perinatol 1997;14(3):119–24.
14. Johnson C, Roach H, Morrison J, et al. A pilot study of intravenous ondansetron for hyperemesis gravidarum. Am J Obstet Gynecol 1996;174(5):1565–8.
15. Asrat T, Briggs G, Towers C, et al. Droperidol and diphenhydramine in the management of hyperemesis gravidarum. Am J Obstet Gynecol 1996;174(6): 1801–6.

16. Jewell D, Young G. Interventions for nausea and vomiting in early pregnancy. Cochrane Database Syst Rev 2003;4:CD000145.

17. Dodds L, Fell DB, Joseph KS, et al. Outcomes of pregnancies complicated by hyperemesis gravidarum. Obstet Gynecol 2006;107(2 Pt 1):285–92.

18. Laifer SA, Stiller RJ, Siddiqui DS, et al. Ursodeoxycholic acid for the treatment of intrahepatic cholestasis of pregnancy. J Matern Fetal Med 2001;10(2):131–5.

19. Lee RH, Goodwin TM, Greenspoon J, et al. The prevalence of intrahepatic cholestasis of pregnancy in a primarily Latina Los Angeles population. J Perinatol 2006;26(9):527–32.

20. Reyes H, Gonzalez MC, Ribalta J, et al. Prevalence of intrahepatic cholestasis of pregnancy in Chile. Ann Intern Med 1978;88(4):487–93.

21. Arrese M, Macias RI, Briz O, et al. Molecular pathogenesis of intrahepatic cholestasis of pregnancy. Expert Rev Mol Med 2008;10:e9.

22. Dixon PH, Weerasekera N, Linton KJ, et al. Heterozygous MDR3 missense mutation associated with intrahepatic cholestasis of pregnancy: evidence for a defect in protein trafficking. Hum Mol Genet 2000;9(8):1209–17.

23. Schneider G, Paus TC, Kullak-Ublick GA, et al. Linkage between a new splicing site mutation in the MDR3 alias ABCB4 gene and intrahepatic cholestasis of pregnancy. Hepatology 2007;45(1):150–8.

24. Keitel V, Vogt C, Haussinger D, et al. Combined mutations of canalicular transporter proteins cause severe intrahepatic cholestasis of pregnancy. Gastroenterology 2006;131(2):624–9.

25. Floreani A, Carderi I, Paternoster D, et al. Intrahepatic cholestasis of pregnancy: three novel MDR3 gene mutations. Aliment Pharmacol Ther 2006;23(11):1649–53.

26. Sookoian S, Castano G, Burgueno A, et al. Association of the multidrug-resistance-associated protein gene (ABCC2) variants with intrahepatic cholestasis of pregnancy. J Hepatol 2008;48(1):125–32.

27. Beuers U, Pusl T. Intrahepatic cholestasis of pregnancy—a heterogeneous group of pregnancy-related disorders? Hepatology 2006;43(4):647–9.

28. Bacq Y, Sapey T, Brechot MC, et al. Intrahepatic cholestasis of pregnancy: a French prospective study. Hepatology 1997;26(2):358–64.

29. Reyes H, Zapata R, Hernandez I, et al. Is a leaky gut involved in the pathogenesis of intrahepatic cholestasis of pregnancy? Hepatology 2006;43(4):715–22.

30. Reyes H, Baez ME, Gonzalez MC, et al. Selenium, zinc and copper plasma levels in intrahepatic cholestasis of pregnancy, in normal pregnancies and in healthy individuals, in Chile. J Hepatol 2000;32(4):542–9.

31. Mullally BA, Hansen WF. Intrahepatic cholestasis of pregnancy: review of the literature. Obstet Gynecol Surv 2002;57(1):47–52.

32. Heikkinen J. Serum bile acids in the early diagnosis of intrahepatic cholestasis of pregnancy. Obstet Gynecol 1983;61(5):581–7.

33. Glantz A, Marschall HU, Mattsson LA. Intrahepatic cholestasis of pregnancy: relationships between bile acid levels and fetal complication rates. Hepatology 2004;40(2):467–74.

34. Bacq Y, Zarka O, Brechot JF, et al. Liver function tests in normal pregnancy: a prospective study of 103 pregnant women and 103 matched controls. Hepatology 1996;23(5):1030–4.

35. Rolfes DB, Ishak KG. Liver disease in pregnancy. Histopathology 1986;10(6):555–70.

36. Rioseco AJ, Ivankovic MB, Manzur A, et al. Intrahepatic cholestasis of pregnancy: a retrospective case-control study of perinatal outcome. Am J Obstet Gynecol 1994;170(3):890–5.

37. Meng LJ, Reyes H, Axelson M, et al. Progesterone metabolites and bile acids in serum of patients with intrahepatic cholestasis of pregnancy: effect of ursodeoxycholic acid therapy. Hepatology 1997;26(6):1573–9.
38. Palma J, Reyes H, Ribalta J, et al. Ursodeoxycholic acid in the treatment of cholestasis of pregnancy: a randomized, double-blind study controlled with placebo. J Hepatol 1997;27(6):1022–8.
39. Kondrackiene J, Beuers U, Kupcinskas L. Efficacy and safety of ursodeoxycholic acid versus cholestyramine in intrahepatic cholestasis of pregnancy. Gastroenterology 2005;129(3):894–901.
40. Brites D, Rodrigues CM, Oliveira N, et al. Correction of maternal serum bile acid profile during ursodeoxycholic acid therapy in cholestasis of pregnancy. J Hepatol 1998;28(1):91–8.
41. Pusl T, Beuers U. Intrahepatic cholestasis of pregnancy. Orphanet J Rare Dis 2007;2:26.
42. Glantz A, Marschall HU, Lammert F, et al. Intrahepatic cholestasis of pregnancy: a randomized controlled trial comparing dexamethasone and ursodeoxycholic acid. Hepatology 2005;42(6):1399–405.
43. Zapata R, Sandoval L, Palma J, et al. Ursodeoxycholic acid in the treatment of intrahepatic cholestasis of pregnancy. A 12-year experience. Liver Int 2005; 25(3):548–54.
44. Binder T, Salaj P, Zima T, et al. Randomized prospective comparative study of ursodeoxycholic acid and S-adenosyl-L-methionine in the treatment of intrahepatic cholestasis of pregnancy. J Perinat Med 2006;34(5):383–91.
45. Ropponen A, Sund R, Riikonen S, et al. Intrahepatic cholestasis of pregnancy as an indicator of liver and biliary diseases: a population-based study. Hepatology 2006;43(4):723–8.
46. Bacq Y, Riely CA. Acute fatty liver of pregnancy: the hepatologist's view. Gastro-enterologist 1993;1(4):257–64.
47. Castro MA, Fassett MJ, Reynolds TB, et al. Reversible peripartum liver failure: a new perspective on the diagnosis, treatment, and cause of acute fatty liver of pregnancy, based on 28 consecutive cases. Am J Obstet Gynecol 1999; 181(2):389–95.
48. Ibdah JA. Acute fatty liver of pregnancy: an update on pathogenesis and clinical implications. World J Gastroenterol 2006;12(46):7397–404.
49. Monga M, Katz AR. Acute fatty liver in the second trimester. Obstet Gynecol 1999;93(5 Pt 2):811–3.
50. Browning MF, Levy HL, Wilkins-Haug LE, et al. Fetal fatty acid oxidation defects and maternal liver disease in pregnancy. Obstet Gynecol 2006;107(1):115–20.
51. Ibdah JA, Bennett MJ, Rinaldo P, et al. A fetal fatty-acid oxidation disorder as a cause of liver disease in pregnant women. N Engl J Med 1999;340(22):1723–31.
52. Pereira SP, O'Donohue J, Wendon J, et al. Maternal and perinatal outcome in severe pregnancy-related liver disease. Hepatology 1997;26(5):1258–62.
53. Cammu H, Velkeniers B, Charels K, et al. Idiopathic acute fatty liver of pregnancy associated with transient diabetes insipidus. Case report. Br J Obstet Gynaecol 1987;94(2):173–8.
54. Knight M, Nelson-Piercy C, Kurinczuk JJ, et al. A prospective national study of acute fatty liver of pregnancy in the UK. Gut 2008;57(7):951–6.
55. Baxter JK, Weinstein L. HELLP syndrome: the state of the art. Obstet Gynecol Surv 2004;59(12):838–45.
56. Barton JR, Sibai BM. Diagnosis and management of hemolysis, elevated liver enzymes, and low platelets syndrome. Clin Perinatol 2004;31(4):807–33, vii.

57. Sibai BM, Ramadan MK, Usta I, et al. Maternal morbidity and mortality in 442 pregnancies with hemolysis, elevated liver enzymes, and low platelets (HELLP syndrome). Am J Obstet Gynecol 1993;169(4):1000–6.

58. Reubinoff BE, Schenker JG. HELLP syndrome—a syndrome of hemolysis, elevated liver enzymes and low platelet count–complicating preeclampsia-eclampsia. Int J Gynaecol Obstet 1991;36(2):95–102.

59. del Canho R, Grosheide PM, Mazel JA, et al. Ten-year neonatal hepatitis B vaccination program, The Netherlands, 1982–1992: protective efficacy and long-term immunogenicity. Vaccine 1997;15(15):1624–30.

60. Sibai BM. Imitators of severe preeclampsia. Obstet Gynecol 2007;109(4): 956–66.

61. Sibai BM, Taslimi MM, el-Nazer A, et al. Maternal-perinatal outcome associated with the syndrome of hemolysis, elevated liver enzymes, and low platelets in severe preeclampsia-eclampsia. Am J Obstet Gynecol 1986;155(3):501–9.

62. Barton JR, Riely CA, Adamec TA, et al. Hepatic histopathologic condition does not correlate with laboratory abnormalities in HELLP syndrome (hemolysis, elevated liver enzymes, and low platelet count). Am J Obstet Gynecol 1992; 167(6):1538–43.

63. Shehata N, Burrows R, Kelton JG. Gestational thrombocytopenia. Clin Obstet Gynecol 1999;42(2):327–34.

64. Saphier CJ, Repke JT. Hemolysis, elevated liver enzymes, and low platelets (HELLP) syndrome: a review of diagnosis and management. Semin Perinatol 1998;22(2):118–33.

65. Visser W, Wallenburg HC. Temporising management of severe pre-eclampsia with and without the HELLP syndrome. Br J Obstet Gynaecol 1995;102(2):111–7.

66. Shames BD, Fernandez LA, Sollinger HW, et al. Liver transplantation for HELLP syndrome. Liver Transpl 2005;11(2):224–8.

67. Stevenson JT, Graham DJ. Hepatic hemorrhage and the HELLP syndrome: a surgeon's perspective. Am Surg 1995;61(9):756–60.

68. Hunter SK, Martin M, Benda JA, et al. Liver transplant after massive spontaneous hepatic rupture in pregnancy complicated by preeclampsia. Obstet Gynecol 1995;85(5 Pt 2):819–22.

69. Henny CP, Lim AE, Brummelkamp WH, et al. A review of the importance of acute multidisciplinary treatment following spontaneous rupture of the liver capsule during pregnancy. Surg Gynecol Obstet 1983;156(5):593–8.

70. Barton JR, Sibai BM. Hepatic imaging in HELLP syndrome (hemolysis, elevated liver enzymes, and low platelet count). Am J Obstet Gynecol 1996;174(6): 1820–5 [discussion: 1825–7].

71. Gyang AN, Srivastava G, Asaad K. Liver capsule rupture in eclampsia: treatment with hepatic artery embolisation. Arch Gynecol Obstet 2006;274(6): 377–9.

72. Tompkins MJ, Thiagarajah S. HELLP (hemolysis, elevated liver enzymes, and low platelet count) syndrome: the benefit of corticosteroids. Am J Obstet Gynecol 1999;181(2):304–9.

73. Martin JN Jr, Perry KG Jr, Blake PG, et al. Better maternal outcomes are achieved with dexamethasone therapy for postpartum HELLP (hemolysis, elevated liver enzymes, and thrombocytopenia) syndrome. Am J Obstet Gynecol 1997;177(5):1011–7.

74. Isler CM, Barrilleaux PS, Magann EF, et al. A prospective, randomized trial comparing the efficacy of dexamethasone and betamethasone for the treatment of antepartum HELLP (hemolysis, elevated liver enzymes, and low platelet

count) syndrome. Am J Obstet Gynecol 2001;184(7):1332–7 [discussion: 1337–9].

75. Khuroo MS, Kamili S, Jameel S. Vertical transmission of hepatitis E virus. Lancet 1995;345(8956):1025–6.
76. Kane MA, Bradley DW, Shrestha SM, et al. Epidemic non-A, non-B hepatitis in Nepal. Recovery of a possible etiologic agent and transmission studies in marmosets. JAMA 1984;252(22):3140–5.
77. Kumar RM, Uduman S, Rana S, et al. Sero-prevalence and mother-to-infant transmission of hepatitis E virus among pregnant women in the United Arab Emirates. Eur J Obstet Gynecol Reprod Biol 2001;100(1):9–15.
78. Terkivatan T, de Wilt JH, de Man RA, et al. Management of hepatocellular adenoma during pregnancy. Liver 2000;20(2):186–7.
79. Singh V, Sinha SK, Nain CK, et al. Budd-Chiari syndrome: our experience of 71 patients. J Gastroenterol Hepatol 2000;15(5):550–4.
80. Slakey DP, Klein AS, Venbrux AC, et al. Budd-Chiari syndrome: current management options. Ann Surg 2001;233(4):522–7.
81. He MX, Zheng JM, Zhang SH, et al. Rupture of splenic artery aneurysm in pregnancy: a review of the literature and report of two cases. Am J Forensic Med Pathol 2010;31(1):92–4.
82. Rustgi VK, Hoofnagle JH. Viral hepatitis during pregnancy. Semin Liver Dis 1987;7(1):40–6.
83. Magriples U. Hepatitis in pregnancy. Semin Perinatol 1998;22(2):112–7.
84. Hill JB, Sheffield JS, Kim MJ, et al. Risk of hepatitis B transmission in breast-fed infants of chronic hepatitis B carriers. Obstet Gynecol 2002;99(6):1049–52.
85. Shi Z, Yang Y, Ma L, et al. Lamivudine in late pregnancy to interrupt in utero transmission of hepatitis B virus: a systematic review and meta-analysis. Obstet Gynecol 2010;116(1):147–59.
86. van Zonneveld M, van Nunen AB, Niesters HG, et al. Lamivudine treatment during pregnancy to prevent perinatal transmission of hepatitis B virus infection. J Viral Hepat 2003;10(4):294–7.
87. Su GG, Pan KH, Zhao NF, et al. Efficacy and safety of lamivudine treatment for chronic hepatitis B in pregnancy. World J Gastroenterol 2004;10(6):910–2.
88. Bortolotti F, Resti M, Giacchino R, et al. Changing epidemiologic pattern of chronic hepatitis C virus infection in Italian children. J Pediatr 1998;133(3): 378–81.
89. Jabeen T, Cannon B, Hogan J, et al. Pregnancy and pregnancy outcome in hepatitis C type 1b. QJM 2000;93(9):597–601.
90. Ceci O, Margiotta M, Marello F, et al. High rate of spontaneous viral clearance in a cohort of vertically infected hepatitis C virus infants: what lies behind? J Hepatol 2001;35(5):687–8.
91. Ketzinel-Gilad M, Colodner SL, Hadary R, et al. Transient transmission of hepatitis C virus from mothers to newborns. Eur J Clin Microbiol Infect Dis 2000;19(4): 267–74.
92. Conte D, Fraquelli M, Prati D, et al. Prevalence and clinical course of chronic hepatitis C virus (HCV) infection and rate of HCV vertical transmission in a cohort of 15,250 pregnant women. Hepatology 2000;31(3):751–5.
93. Davies G, Wilson RD, Desilets V, et al. Amniocentesis and women with hepatitis B, hepatitis C, or human immunodeficiency virus. J Obstet Gynaecol Can 2003; 25(2):145–52.
94. Ozaslan E, Yilmaz R, Simsek H, et al. Interferon therapy for acute hepatitis C during pregnancy. Ann Pharmacother 2002;36(11):1715–8.

95. Candia L, Marquez J, Espinoza LR. Autoimmune hepatitis and pregnancy: a rheumatologist's dilemma. Semin Arthritis Rheum 2005;35(1):49–56.
96. Heneghan MA, Norris SM, O'Grady JG, et al. Management and outcome of pregnancy in autoimmune hepatitis. Gut 2001;48(1):97–102.
97. Buchel E, Van Steenbergen W, Nevens F, et al. Improvement of autoimmune hepatitis during pregnancy followed by flare-up after delivery. Am J Gastroenterol 2002;97(12):3160–5.
98. Poupon R, Chretien Y, Chazouilleres O, et al. Pregnancy in women with urso-deoxycholic acid-treated primary biliary cirrhosis. J Hepatol 2005;42(3):418–9.
99. Gossard AA, Lindor KD. Pregnancy in a patient with primary sclerosing cholangitis. J Clin Gastroenterol 2002;35(4):353–5.
100. Sandhu BS, Sanyal AJ. Pregnancy and liver disease. Gastroenterol Clin North Am 2003;32(1):407–36, ix.
101. Cheng YS. Pregnancy in liver cirrhosis and/or portal hypertension. Am J Obstet Gynecol 1977;128(7):812–22.
102. Russell MA, Craigo SD. Cirrhosis and portal hypertension in pregnancy. Semin Perinatol 1998;22(2):156–65.
103. Britton RC. Pregnancy and esophageal varices. Am J Surg 1982;143(4):421–5.
104. Riely CA. Contraception and pregnancy after liver transplantation. Liver Transpl 2001;7(11 Suppl 1):S74–6.
105. Cundy TF, O'Grady JG, Williams R. Recovery of menstruation and pregnancy after liver transplantation. Gut 1990;31(3):337–8.
106. Armenti VT, Herrine SK, Radomski JS, et al. Pregnancy after liver transplantation. Liver Transpl 2000;6(6):671–85.
107. Armenti VT, Radomski JS, Moritz MJ, et al. Report from the National Transplantation Pregnancy Registry (NTPR): outcomes of pregnancy after transplantation. Clin Transpl 2005;69–83.
108. Christopher V, Al-Chalabi T, Richardson PD, et al. Pregnancy outcome after liver transplantation: a single-center experience of 71 pregnancies in 45 recipients. Liver Transpl 2006;12(7):1138–43.

Hepatitis B in Pregnancy: Challenges and Treatment

Silvia Degli Esposti, MD[a,b,*], Dhvani Shah, BA[a]

KEYWORDS

- Hepatitis B • Pregnancy • Antiretroviral therapy
- Vertical transmission

DISEASE BURDEN

An estimated 350 million people, 5% of the world's population, are chronically infected with the hepatitis B virus (HBV); of those, 70% live in the western Pacific area.[1] Despite global adoption of hepatitis B immunization programs over the past 2 decades, chronic HBV infection and its complications, cirrhosis and hepatocellular carcinoma, remain significant medical and financial burdens to the health care system. The prevalence of HBV infection varies greatly among countries. In high endemic areas such as China, most of Africa, and South America, more than 10% of the population is infected.

In the United States, an estimated 1.4 million individuals are infected with HBV.[1,2] Between 2000 and 2003, HBV infection was responsible for 2000 to 4000 deaths. Chronic HBV prevalence is the highest among immigrants from high endemic countries, people who have human immunodeficiency virus (HIV), injecting drug users, men who have sex with men, and household contacts of people with chronic HBV infection.

MODE OF INFECTION

HBV has two primary modes of transmission: from infected mother to newborn during delivery (vertical transmission) and from an infected sexual or household contact (horizontal transmission). Unlike adult-acquired HBV infection, in which the risk of chronic infection is only 5% to 10%, perinatally acquired infection carries an 85% to 95% risk of chronic infection, with a 25% to 30% lifetime risk of a serious complication or fatal liver disease.[3]

The authors have nothing to disclose.
[a] The Alpert Medical School, Department of Medicine, 97 Waterman Street, Providence, RI 02912, USA
[b] Department of Medicine, Center for Women's Gastrointestinal Services, Women & Infants Hospital of Rhode Island, 101 Dudley Street, Providence, RI 02905, USA
* Corresponding author. Department of Medicine, Center for Women's Gastrointestinal Services, Women & Infants Hospital of Rhode Island, 101 Dudley Street, Providence, RI 02905.
E-mail address: Silvia_Degli_Esposti@Brown.edu

Gastroenterol Clin N Am 40 (2011) 355–372
doi:10.1016/j.gtc.2011.03.005
0889-8553/11/$ – see front matter © 2011 Elsevier Inc. All rights reserved.

gastro.theclinics.com

In the United States, the incidence of new HBV infection has fallen 82% since the implementation of universal vaccination at birth in the early 1990s.[4] Today, new infections occur mainly among unvaccinated adults. In the United States, vertical transmission is responsible for a very small fraction of new HBV infections; and of the 43,000 new infections in the United States each year, only 1000 are estimated to occur in children.[5] Worldwide, however, 50% of chronically infected individuals acquired their infection perinatally or in early childhood, much of which is attributed to high rates of hepatitis B e-antigen (HBeAg)–positive infections in women of childbearing age.

PREVENTION STRATEGIES

Vaccination at birth has been a successful strategy adopted by the United States and the rest of the world to prevent HBV infection. Immunization of the adult population has also been encouraged by some countries but has been deemed too costly. The vaccine is reserved for adults at high risk of acquiring the infection. Currently, 175 countries, or 91% of all nations, have a child immunization program. The modality and success of implementing a vaccination program vary greatly and depend on the country's available resources.

The United States began an infant vaccination program in 1991, and a catch-up vaccination program in 1999 for every individual younger than 19 years of age. In 2010, the Institute of Medicine (IOM) released a document describing future strategies to control and prevent HBV infection in the United States.[1] Recommendations include an enhanced immunization schedule at birth, public education in collaboration with community-based programs, and targeted vaccination of high-risk adults.

PREVENTION OF PERINATAL TRANSMISSION: CURRENT RECOMMENDATIONS
Universal HBV Prenatal Screening

The prevalence of chronic HBV infection in pregnant women in the United States varies by race and ethnicity, with Asian women having the highest rate of infection (6%). An estimated 24,000 HBV-infected women give birth in the United States each year.[6]

In the United States, routine universal prenatal screening for HBV identifies women who are positive for the hepatitis B surface antigen (HBsAg) before they give birth. This practice achieves two goals: newborns receive the appropriate postexposure prophylaxis, and infected mothers receive appropriate medical care during and after pregnancy. The delivery hospital functions as a safety net where all women of unknown status (lack of evidence of HBV testing) are required to be tested on admission. This program has been successful, with 97% of all pregnant women currently tested before childbirth.[7] Universal screening of pregnant women is not practiced in every country. Many European countries, for example, still practice screening models driven by risk factors.[5]

The hepatitis B vaccine is considered safe during pregnancy with no adverse reactions reported in the literature. Women who test negative for HBsAg and are at risk of acquiring HBV infection should be immunized during pregnancy. Proof of absent immunity (defined as absence of the antibody to hepatitis B surface antigen [HBsAb-negative]) is not required before vaccination. Women considered to be at greatest risk are those with multiple sexual partners (more than two in the last 6 months), those who have been evaluated or treated for sexually transmitted diseases, recent or current injecting drug users, and those who have an HBsAg-positive sexual partner.[8]

Although several individuals infected with HBV will test negative for the HBsAg, the virus is detectable in the blood and therefore DNA testing will show positive results. These individuals have a very low viral load and are called occult infected. The prevalence of occult HBV infection in the pregnant population and its contribution to childhood HBV infection are unknown. Case reports have suggested that occult HBV infection in pregnancy might be a significant problem in populations with a high prevalence of HBV.[9]

Perinatal Hepatitis B Prevention Program

The American Congress of Obstetricians and Gynecologists (ACOG), the Centers for Disease Control and Prevention (CDC), and the IOM support the referral of all HBV-positive mothers to the state's Perinatal Hepatitis B Prevention Program and to subspecialists for counseling and medical treatment. The Perinatal Hepatitis B Prevention Program is a state-run, CDC-funded program with the goal of implementing current perinatal immunoprophylaxis recommendations throughout the United States. Pregnant women infected with HBV are identified early in pregnancy through prenatal testing and referred to case managers in the Perinatal Hepatitis B Prevention Program. Case managers provide counseling and encourage appropriate testing and vaccination of household contacts. They also coordinate appropriate vaccination and testing of the infant and medical treatment for the mother during pregnancy and postpartum.

Infant Immunoprophylaxis

Current CDC guidelines stipulate that infants of women who are HBsAg-positive or whose status is unknown at delivery should receive both hepatitis B hyperimmune gamma globulin (HBIG) and hepatitis B vaccine within 12 hours of birth, preferably in the delivery room. This initial vaccine administration should be followed by at least two more injections of hepatitis B vaccine within the first 6 months of life. After completion of the vaccine series, testing for the antibody against HBsAg (anti-HBsAb) and for HBsAg should be performed at 9 to 18 months of age. HBsAg-negative infants with HBsAb levels greater than 10 mIU/mL are considered protected and no further medical management is required. Those with HBsAb levels less than 10 mIU/mL are not protected and should be revaccinated with a second three-dose series followed by retesting 1 to 2 months after the final dose. Passive immunoprophylaxis with HBIG at birth followed by at least 3 doses of hepatitis B vaccine provides approximately 95% protection from perinatal infection, whereas the vaccine alone is approximately 75% protective.

Report Card

Although immunoprophylaxis guidelines are important for decreasing the transmission of perinatal HBV, they must be endorsed properly. A study conducted in 2006 reviewed infant and maternal records in a representative sample of 242 delivery hospitals in the 50 states, Washington DC, and Puerto Rico. The records of 4762 mothers and 4786 infants were reviewed. Among infants born to the 18 HBsAg-positive women with documented prenatal test results, 62.1% received both hepatitis B vaccine and HBIG within 12 hours. However, 13.7% were unvaccinated and 19.7% did not receive HBIG before discharge. Among infants born to the 320 women with unknown HBsAg status, only 52.4% were vaccinated within 12 hours of birth and 20.1% were unvaccinated before discharge. These findings indicate significant inconsistency in hospital policies and practices to achieve prevention of vertical transmission of HBV.[10,11]

VERTICAL TRANSMISSION

The risk of perinatal infection for infants born to HBeAg-positive mothers in the absence of prophylaxis is as high as 70% to 90% by the age of 6 months; and approximately 90% of these children will remain chronically infected. HBeAg-negative mothers carry a 10% to 40% transmission risk, and 40% to 70% of infants who become infected remain chronically infected.[1] The likelihood of acquiring HBV infection through vertical transmission is probably linked to the viral replication status of the mother rather than to e-antigen status. E-antigen–negative mothers with a high viral load are at great risk for transmitting the virus to their infant.[12]

Active and passive postexposure prophylaxis of the newborn with HBIG and hepatitis B vaccine is known to be safe and effective and dramatically reduces the risk of HBV transmission.[13,14] This strategy has been acknowledged as the most effective intervention to contain HBV infection. Unfortunately, administration of HBIG is costly and not all countries have the resources to support this intervention, resulting in a wide variety of immunization protocols around the world.

Mode of Transmission From Mother to Infant

The vertical transmission of HBV from mother to infant occurs in the perinatal period. During delivery, maternal secretions in the birth canal come in contact with the infant's mucosal membranes. In the immediate postpartum period, transmission results from close contact between mother and baby. Of infants born to HBeAg-positive mothers who are uninfected at birth, 34% will acquire the infection in the next 6 months. A small number of infants will be infected in utero. In a study performed in the Republic of China,[15] 3.7% of babies tested HBsAg-positive at birth from in utero infection. Zhang and colleagues[16] showed the ability of the virus to translocate through the placenta from the mother to the fetal trophoblast. This finding suggests a direct transplacental route of infection. Factors that cause transplacental infection remain unknown, but high maternal viral load and preterm labor are predisposing factors.[15,17]

Special Circumstances

Breastfeeding is not contraindicated for HBV-positive mothers. Several studies found no difference in rates of infection between breast fed and formula fed babies.[18] The American Academy of Pediatrics supports breastfeeding as long as the infant has received HBIG and hepatitis B vaccine as recommended.

Experts consider amniocentesis to be relatively safe. Current data, however, are limited to few observations.[19] Given the small number of cases reported, it should be performed only if absolutely necessary.

Assisted reproduction can be safely achieved for discordant couples in which one partner is HBV-infected and the other is not. Sperm preparation techniques greatly decrease the viral load, minimizing the chances of cross-infection.[20]

Immunoprophylaxis Failure

Despite enormous strides in preventing perinatal HBV infection, vertical transmission remains a significant route of virus acquisition worldwide. Recent statistics show that only 36% of all newborns received the HBV vaccine at birth in the 87 countries in which chronic HBV is endemic (affecting ≥8% of the total population).[21] The lack of a universal and consistent global policy to prevent vertical transmission, and barriers to the implementation of an immunization protocol in the poorest countries, account for most infected infants worldwide.

Even in countries in which proper immunization is practiced, as many as 9% of infants whose mothers are HBsAg-positive will become infected with HBV.[1] Another 1% to 2% of properly vaccinated infants are unable to develop sufficient amounts of HBsAb to afford long-lasting immunity. Although immunoprophylaxis failure is known to exist, the magnitude of the problem is difficult to estimate. The rate of reported immunization failure varies greatly among countries because of different immunization schedules, modes of vaccine delivery, and compliance with completing the vaccination series.

Asian countries such as China and Korea have reported immunoprophylaxis failure as high as 25% in HBeAg-positive mothers,[22] and in 10% to 20% of all infants born to HBV-infected mothers. More recent Chinese data[23] reported a much lower rate. In a Canadian retrospective review of data from pregnant women, 1485 HBV-positive women were identified, with an immunization failure rate of 2.1%.[24] In an Australian study, 2% of all HBsAg-positive mothers gave birth to children who were HBV-positive.[25] Given the variability of practices during delivery and prophylaxis protocols around the world, data obtained in foreign countries should be interpreted with caution.

Current data on immunization failure in the United States is lacking because not all infants born to HBsAg-positive mothers have the mandatory testing at 9 months of age. A study by Andre and Zuckerman[26] reported that vertical transmission despite immunoprophylaxis (true immunization failure) is estimated to be approximately 5%. The CDC estimated that in the United States in 2007, 800 infants were infected perinatally (John Ward, MD, personal communication, 2010).[27] Elimination of vertical transmission was identified as one of the strategic goals by the IOM in an effort to eliminate HBV infection. Determining the rate of true immunization failure in the United States is the first step toward achieving this goal. The effectiveness of the more stringent immunization protocol suggested by the IOM in 2010 must be evaluated before additional interventions are formulated.

Causes of Immunoprophylaxis Failure

Examination of the causes of vertical transmission should help identify the causes of immunoprophylaxis failure. Failure to identify infected mothers and inadequate newborn prophylaxis contribute significantly to vertical transmission.[11] In the Australian study discussed previously, of the four children (2%) infected vertically, one was improperly immunized.[25] Delay of the second dose of vaccine may also contribute to the rate of immunoprophylaxis failure.[27] Only documented peripartum transmission despite adherence to an adequate immunization protocol should be considered true immunization failure. Because this is a rare event, establishing the risk factors associated with immunization failure would help identify populations to target for intervention.

True immunoprophylaxis failure has been linked to high maternal viral load. The viral load range of concern has not been defined because viral load can change over several logs during pregnancy and HBV DNA is not routinely tested during pregnancy in the United States.

Available data suggest that the measure of HBV DNA associated with immunization failure is approximately 10^8 copies/mL. The recent study in Australia[25] examined 313 HBsAg-positive pregnant women from 2002 to 2008, and found that 47 were HBeAg-positive and had HBV DNA viral loads greater than 10^8 copies/mL. Subsequent testing showed that 4 of the 47 infants born were HBsAg-positive and HBsAb-negative. All 4 infants received the HBV vaccination series, and 3 of these received HBIG at birth. No perinatal transmission of HBV occurred in any newborns of mothers with viral loads less than 10^8 copies/mL. Thus, this study suggests that HBeAg positivity and high maternal viral load correlate with perinatal transmission. Transplacental infection might also play an important role in the transmission of HBV.

Polymorphism of maternal cytokine involved in the immune response to HBV, particularly tumor necrosis factor, interferon-γ, or interleukin-10, has also been linked to immunization failure. This polymorphism may also correlate with other factors, including intrauterine infection and high viremia.[28] Other risk factors related to pregnancy outcome, such as preterm labor, premature rupture of membranes, and a complicated delivery, need further study. Cesarean section does not seem to protect against vertical transmission and immunization failure, although data are still controversial.

Minimizing the Immunization Failure

Programs encouraging proper immunoprophylaxis remain the most effective way to reduce vertical transmission worldwide. Countries such as China, where vertical transmission contributes significantly to the overall burden of disease, have implemented several strategies. For example, despite the lack of evidence that these strategies reduce vertical transmission, the rate of caesarian section and bottle feeding among HBsAg-positive Chinese mothers is 95%.

One approach to prevent perinatal HBV transmission is maternal administration of HBIG during pregnancy; several studies show varying results. Different doses and routes of HBIG were administered with different outcomes used to determine neonatal infection, including HBV DNA in cord blood or HBsAg present in infants at 6 months of age. Three of the four studies documented a beneficial effect of HIBG, whereas one study reported no obvious difference.[29,30] One study examined the effect of maternal HBIG treatment on newborn vaccination and found that maternal HBIG treatment was associated with higher HBsAb rates than in infants of both HBeAg-positive and HBeAg-negative women not treated with HBIG.[31]

ANTIRETROVIRAL THERAPY AND VERTICAL TRANSMISSION

Because the risk of vertical transmission despite immunoprophylaxis is higher for mothers with high viremia, a sensible strategy to interrupt perinatal infection is to reduce the mother's viral load with antiretroviral drugs before delivery. Antiretroviral nucleo(t)side analogs are a category of drug with direct antiviral action. They are used extensively to treat HBV- and HIV-infected individuals. In HIV-infected pregnant women, administration of nucleo(t)side analog therapy helped reduce the perinatal HIV transmission rate from 25% to 30% to less than 2%.[32]

Chinese physicians have published several reports of successful use of lamivudine in the third trimester for the sole purpose of interrupting vertical transmission of HBV.[33] Based on these reports, some experts advocate for this strategy and suggest antiretroviral therapy (ART) for all pregnant women with high HBV viremia in the United States. However, this practice remains controversial; the need and efficacy of ART to prevent immunization failure in the American population have not been proven. Studies available to support the use of ART in pregnancy are few and their scientific merit is questionable. To date, only one randomized trial and one case series have been published in the western literature.

A meta-analysis summarizing trials published in foreign languages is also available, but the studies included are of poor quality. The first report was published in 2003[34] from a European group in which eight pregnant women who were highly viremic (1.2×10^9 copies/mL) were treated with 150 mg of lamivudine daily from gestational week 34 until delivery. The infants received both active and passive immunization at birth. Within 6 to 40 days, the HBV DNA levels declined at least 1 log in five of the eight women. Although four of the infants were HBsAg-positive at birth, all but one were negative by 12 months of age (12.5%). The rate of HBV infection in a group of 24 historical controls was 28%. Xu and colleagues[33] published the first randomized trial in 2009, enrolling 115 women who were HBsAg-positive with high viral loads; 59 women were controls and 56 were treated with 100 mg of lamivudine beginning in the third trimester and until 4 weeks postpartum. Despite a 50% decrease in vertical transmission in the treated group, these data were invalid given the high drop-out rate in the control group.

More recently, a randomized controlled trial with telbivudine was presented at the 2010 American Association for the Study of Liver Diseases (AASLD) meeting in Boston, Massachusetts.[23] In this trial, 190 Asian mothers with high viral loads were recruited in an open-label prospective study. The study group received 600 mg daily of telbivudine from gestational weeks 20 to 32 through 4 weeks postpartum. The rate of vertical transmission was 2.1% in the treated group and 13.4% in the untreated women. If these data can be confirmed, this will be the first trial proving efficacy. However, other considerations must be weighed before recommending late-trimester ART, such as the effect of ART on the mother, the likelihood of flares as ART is discontinued postpartum, and the potential risks, albeit small, of generating drug resistance. Furthermore, lamivudine is no longer used as a first-line drug and newer, more efficacious agents should be considered. Thus, the AASLD 2007 consensus statement concluded that more data were needed before treatment with ART to block vertical transmission could be recommended.

CHRONIC HEPATITIS B: ASSESSMENT AND MONITORING DURING PREGNANCY

As a result of universal screening for HBV, pregnancy often coincides with the initial diagnosis in many HBV-infected women. Thus, pregnancy is a time of challenge for the mother, but also an opportunity to deliver appropriate medical care to thousands of infected women. The ACOG, AASLD, and CDC guidelines suggest that HBsAg-positive mothers be referred for further medical evaluation and not deferred post-partum. Although most patients will do well in pregnancy, a small percentage have significant liver disease that requires close monitoring and therapeutic intervention. Complications such as cholestasis, flare of underlying hepatitis, and hepatic failure[35,36] have been described in pregnancy. In addition, more patients are becoming pregnant while on ART, which presents unique challenges. Fig. 1 presents the algorithm used to guide clinical care in the authors' facility.

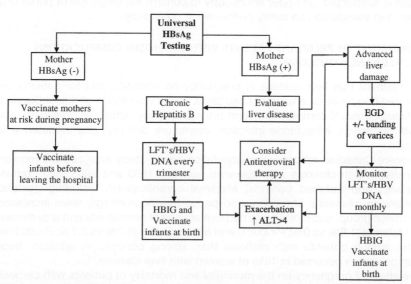

Fig. 1. Management of hepatitis B–positive mothers during pregnancy. Arrows indicate the next step in clinical care.

Assessment of Liver Disease in Pregnancy

During pregnancy the liver undergoes metabolic, immunologic, and hemodynamic changes, which unmask, modulate, or worsen underlying liver disease. Women with advanced chronic liver disease, regardless of origin, have decreased fertility as a result of anovulatory cycles and amenorrhea. In recent years, the availability of reproductive technologies and advanced support measures have changed the attitude toward liver disease in pregnancy. With appropriate care, women with chronic liver disease and cirrhosis carry successful pregnancies to term.

Evaluation of Liver Disease

Physiologic changes in pregnancy make the evaluation of liver damage difficult. Common biochemical tests including albumin, total protein, hematocrit, and alkaline phosphatase, are physiologically altered. Physical signs of liver disease are also common in pregnancy, particularly in the third trimester, such as palmar erythema, spider angiomas, and leg edema. Fatigue and abdominal pain are also common in both conditions. Liver biopsy remains the definitive test to evaluate liver damage, but it is considered too invasive by many patients. When it is critical to establish a firm diagnosis, the risk of liver biopsy is justified and does not carry any greater risk than in the nonpregnant population.

Noninvasive markers of liver fibrosis could be very useful but have not yet been validated in pregnancy. For example, aspartate aminotransferase (AST) level and platelets are not influenced by pregnancy, and the AST-to-platelet ratio index is a good predictor of significant fibrosis in many liver diseases. More sensitive techniques, such as transient elastography fibroscan and other algorithms combining less commonly ordered blood tests, might add sensitivity to the diagnosis.

In most cases, the presumptive diagnosis and subsequent medical management is based on clinical information, such as duration of disease and past evaluations, combined with blood tests (AST, platelets), HBeAg status, viral load, and noninvasive imaging (right upper quadrant ultrasound with Doppler study). When advanced liver disease is suspected, an upper endoscopy to confirm the diagnosis of portal hypertension and varices can be safely performed in pregnancy.

MANAGEMENT OF PREGNANT PATIENTS WITH CIRRHOSIS: COMPLICATIONS AND PREGNANCY OUTCOME

It is important that liver disease in pregnancy be identified and for patients to be monitored frequently by a team of specialists. These women are at risk of developing significant perinatal complications and poor pregnancy outcomes, including uterine growth restriction, intrauterine infection, premature delivery, and intrauterine fetal demise.

A recent Canadian retrospective population-based study analyzed the records of 339 patients with cirrhosis who delivered between 1993 and 2005, and compared them with age-matched controls. Maternal complications, including gestational hypertension, placental abruption, and peripartum hemorrhage, were increased in the cirrhotic group, and their infants had higher rates of prematurity and growth restriction. Maternal (1.8% vs 0%; $P<.0001$) and fetal mortality (5.2% vs 2.1%; $P<.001$) were greater among patients with cirrhosis than among controls. In addition, hepatic decompensation occurred in 15% of women with liver disease.[37]

The effect of pregnancy on the morbidity and mortality of patients with cirrhosis is controversial. As suggested by many case reports, pregnancy may accelerate the disease process, leading to decompensation. Variceal bleeding occurs more often in the third trimester and during labor from increased intra-abdominal pressure and volume expansion. Other reported complications include thromboembolic complications, Budd-Chiari syndrome, worsening of cholestasis, and acute decompensation with ascites. To avert variceal bleeding in pregnancy, an upper endoscopy and obliteration of varices in the second trimester is recommended, and is preferable to the use of nonselective ß-blockers, which have been linked to toxicity in pregnancy.[38] An elective operative delivery should be considered for patients who did not have obliteration of their varices. Correction of coagulopathy and prevention of bacterial peritonitis in cases of cesarean delivery are also recommended.

When complications occur, management is similar to that for nonpregnant patients. An emergency endoscopic treatment of a variceal bleed can be safely performed in pregnancy with banding, sclerotherapy, or glue injection.[39] However, during the variceal bleed, the use of octreotide is not recommended given the possible uterine ischemia associated with this drug.

CHRONIC HBV IN PREGNANCY

As with many diseases in pregnancy, little is known about chronic HBV infection and how it affects gestation and pregnancy outcome. To date, studies addressing these questions are limited and available information is mostly from endemic countries in Asia.

Effect of Chronic HBV on Pregnancy

It was generally accepted that acute or chronic HBV infection did not affect gestation or pregnancy outcome. Recent reports, although conflicting, challenge this belief. In a large study by Wong and colleagues,[40] no differences were seen in gestational age at delivery, birth weight, incidence of prematurity, neonatal jaundice, congenital anomalies, or perinatal mortality when comparing HBsAg-positive women with noninfected controls. Conversely, the analysis of 186,619 deliveries in a population-based study in Israel found that HBV infection was an independent risk factor for poor pregnancy outcome.[41] Two additional studies in Hong Kong noted that maternal HBV infection is associated with increased inflammation, as indicated by elevated ferritin levels and higher incidence of gestational diabetes and antepartum hemorrhage.[42] These studies provide some insight into the effect of chronic HBV on pregnancy; however, whether data gathered from the homogenous Asian population are applicable to Western society is unclear.

Effect of Pregnancy on Chronic HBV

Limited data are available about the effect of pregnancy on chronic HBV infection in the absence of severe liver damage. A normal pregnancy is associated with high levels of adrenal corticosteroid and modulation of cytokines involved in the immune response, both of which can result in an increased viremia. Often, these changes lead to clinically insignificant fluctuations in liver function tests. However, case reports exist of hepatic exacerbation and hepatic decompensation, and even fulminant hepatic failure.[43] In one study, no significant differences in HBV viremia were noted during pregnancy, but alanine aminotransferase (ALT) levels tended to increase late in pregnancy and postpartum.[44] In another retrospective study[35] evaluating 29 pregnant women with chronic HBV infection in California, adverse events were reported in 7 women, 4 women developed liver failure, and 9 required ART initiation during pregnancy. Maternal age seemed to be the only predictor of increased risk of negative maternal outcomes.

Other studies point to the postpartum period as the vulnerable time for exacerbations, when the immune system is reconstituted. Ter Borg and colleagues[45] followed a group of 38 HBV-positive mothers. A postpartum flare (defined as a fourfold elevation of ALT) was described in 17 of these women. In a Japanese study of 269 pregnant women with chronic HBV infection, overt liver dysfunction was observed within the first month postpartum in 43% of mothers who were HBeAg-positive. Exacerbations of underlying liver disease can lead to HBV seroconversion, with rates of 12% to 17% reported.[46] More studies are needed to better understand the natural history of HBV in pregnancy. Given the available data, HBsAg-positive mothers should be monitored closely in pregnancy for decompensation and followed up carefully in the postpartum period.

Treatment of HBV in pregnancy

Although a full evaluation of the symptoms of HBV is recommended in pregnancy, the initiation of therapy is often delayed until after delivery. Liver function tests and viral DNA fluctuate during gestation and in the postpartum period. Thus, the decision to treat with ART should be postponed until the biochemical profile has stabilized.

For patients presenting with advanced disease and those with an acute exacerbation or liver failure, the benefits of treating the mother supersede any concern about the theoretical possibility of harming the fetus with toxic drugs. The effectiveness of ART during acute exacerbations has been reported in pregnant and nonpregnant women, such as in the successful treatment of acute liver failure in pregnancy.[43]

ANTIRETROVIRAL THERAPY IN PREGNANCY
"Safe" Drugs in Pregnancy

Some general considerations guide clinicians in prescribing medications in pregnancy. Definitive pregnancy safety data are not available for many drugs because gathering data requires large, long and costly trials. Trials must be large enough to evidentiate events that occur infrequently. They have to be long because, although birth defects linked to teratogenesis are seen at birth, long-term adverse effects on neurologic development, childhood behavior, and impaired organ function may not be identified for several years. Very few drugs have been studied this extensively. Therefore, no drug can be described as completely safe in pregnancy. Often an alternative medication can be considered, and as part of the decision to treat, the clinician should prescribe the drug for which more safety data are available.[47]

Teratogenesis and Birth Defects

The safety of a drug refers to its teratogenetic effect/potential to cause birth defects. The most critical period for the development of the embryo occurs in the first trimester. Most birth defects are caused by exposure of the embryo to a medication during organogenesis in the first 4 to 14 weeks of gestation. Therefore, initiation of new therapy is often delayed until after the first trimester. **Fig. 2** summarizes the most common birth defects and susceptible gestational ages.

The teratogenic potential of a drug is reported by the U.S. Food and Drug Administration (FDA) and by birth defect registries available to consumers and health care providers. The FDA issues a category for each drug at approval for general use, but these data are infrequently updated. These categories reflect a summary of data on teratogenicity in animals and, for a few drugs, human data are also included.

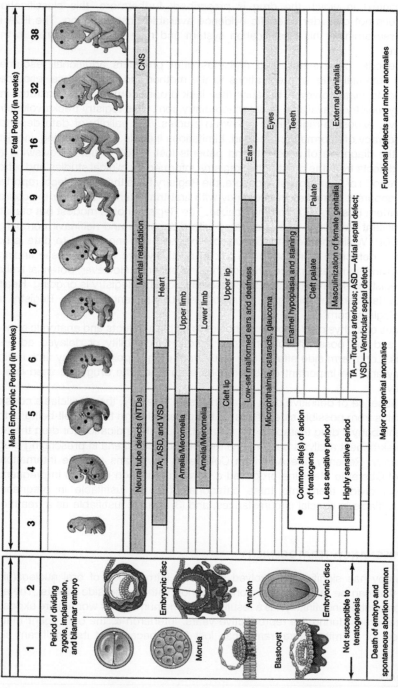

Fig. 2. The developing fetus. (*From* Moore K. The developing human: clinically oriented embryology. Philadelphia: WB Saunders; 2003. p. 173; with permission.)

Experts in the field of obstetric medicine have questioned the validity of this classification. It is often misinterpreted as a grading system and does not reflect the clinical context in which the drug is prescribed; furthermore, this classification system does not consider scientific evidence available postmarketing. The FDA is currently reexamining this classification system and may abolish it entirely in the near future.

Case reports, case series, and registries offer providers additional resources regarding potential risks of medications to the mother and fetus. These resources are subject to bias, however, because they lack proper controls. One antiretroviral pregnancy registry is available at www.apregistry.com. This registry tracks voluntary prospective, exposure-registration follow-up studies. The validity of data depends on the accuracy of information reported. Limitations include underreporting, inability to verify the diagnosis of a defect, and patients lost to follow-up. In reviewing all reported defects from the prospective registry, informed by clinical studies and retrospective reports of antiretroviral exposure, the Registry finds that the defects reported show no apparent increases in frequency with first trimester versus later exposures and no pattern to suggest a common cause. The Registry notes modest but statistically significant elevations of overall rates with didanosine and nelfinavir compared with MACDP. While the Registry population exposed and monitored to date is not sufficient to detect an increase in the risk of relatively rare defects, these findings should provide some assurance when counseling patients. However, potential limitations of registries such as this should be recognized. The Registry is ongoing. Health care providers are encouraged to report eligible patients to the Registry at www.APRegistry.com.

The focus of a physician's concern should be on birth defects and anatomic abnormalities, and the possibility of long-term functional disability or delayed adverse outcomes. Long-term side effects can result from drug exposure at any time during pregnancy and are important considerations even when the drug was used late in pregnancy.

In the absence of definitive data regarding "safe" therapy, the physician's consideration shifts from possible side effects, to the potential harm to the well-being of the mother and baby if drug therapy is not initiated. Thus, the indication for drug therapy and the risk/benefit analysis become the most important criteria in prescribing drugs in pregnancy. Recently, the American College of Physicians and the International Society of Obstetric Medicine proposed a new classification of drugs in pregnancy that would divide them into three categories: (1) use justifiable in pregnancy, (2) use justifiable in special circumstances, and (3) use not justifiable as a treatment option.

ART IN PREGNANCY: TERATOGENICITY

HBV therapy has significantly evolved since the introduction of oral nucleos(t)ide analogs that can be taken for a prolonged period with limited side effects. Therapy is often prescribed indefinitely. As a result, increasing numbers of women are exposed to antiviral drugs during the reproductive years. Interferon-α, the only agent that is prescribed for a limited time frame, has lost favor because of its significant side effects.

ART Agents

Lamivudine, telbivudine, adefovir, tenofovir, entecavir, and emtricitabine have received indication for HBV infection treatment and are collectively referred to as

ART drugs. They have been assigned category B or C by the FDA based on animal exposure data. They freely distribute through the placenta and the fetal compartment. The concentration in the amniotic fluid varies depending on the compound and patient's gestational age. Lamivudine reaches a higher concentration in the amniotic compartment than in the mother's serum.[48] Both lamivudine and tenofovir have been found to be excreted in breast milk.[49]

Studies addressing the safety of ART in pregnancy in HBV-infected patients are not available. In seven published studies, pregnant patients were exposed to lamivudine and telbivudine, respectively, in the third trimester with no birth defects reported.[23,25,33] These data must be interpreted with caution however, given the late exposure in pregnancy well beyond the period of organogenesis, the small number of patients, and concern about the quality of some of these studies. Most safety data are obtained from the ART registry (updated as of July, 2010). Although none of the antiretroviral drugs showed increased birth defects above the national average, only the number of patients exposed in the first trimester to lamivudine is substantial. Moreover, most data collected in the ART registry are from the HIV-infected population, in whom lamivudine, tenofovir, and emtricitabine are used in combination with other agents. Whether these data are completely applicable to monoinfected HBV patients is unclear. Currently, the registry is collecting data on HBV-infected patients on monotherapy with antiretroviral drugs.

The safety of interferon-α in pregnancy has not been established and women are required to practice an effective method of birth control while on therapy. No birth defects were seen in the offspring of pregnant women who were exposed to interferon-α during treatment for melanoma.[50] However, neurotoxicity has been described when interferon-α is used in children younger than 3 years. The FDA category and ART registry data as of July 2010 are summarized in **Table 1.**

Table 1
Birth defects associated with antiviral exposure

Antiviral Agent	FDA Pregnancy Category	Live Births Earliest Exposure	Prevalence Birth Defects (95% CI)
Telbivudine	B	6 first trimester	0
		8 second trimester	0
Entecavir	C	20 first trimester	1
		2 second trimester	0
Lamivudine	C	3754 first trimester	3.0% (CI, 2.5%, 3.6%)
		6080 second trimester	2.7% (CI, 2.3%, 3.2%)
Tenofovir	B	981 first trimester	2.5 (CI, 1.6%, 3.7%)
		584 second trimester	2.2 (CI, 1.2%, 3.8%)
Adefovir	C	39 first trimester	0
		0 second trimester	0

Prevalence of birth defects by trimester of earliest exposure for antiviral agents in any ART combination. Any regimen, combinations or monotherapy, monoinfected, or coinfected.

Data from Antiretroviral Pregnancy Registry Steering Committee. Antiretroviral Pregnancy Registry International Interim Report for 1 January 1989 through 31 July 2010. Wilmington, NC: Registry Coordinating Center; 2010. Available at http://www.apregistry.com/forms/interim_report.pdf. Accessed April 1, 2011.

Safety of ART Late in Pregnancy

Toxicity and functional abnormalities associated with the use of ART in animal studies and nonpregnant patients have raised concern regarding ART use in pregnancy. Mitochondrial damage, lactic acidosis, and acute fatty liver are described as potential side effects. Lactic acidosis is a serious and occasionally fatal complication of all antiretroviral drugs. It is characterized by muscular cramps, fatigue, and accumulation of lactic acid in the blood.[51] This side effect is particularly disconcerting in pregnancy because acidosis is not tolerated by the fetus and can lead to fetal death even if the mother recovers. Routine assessment of lactic acid in pregnant patients on ART therapy is not recommended because asymptomatic and clinically insignificant elevations have been described in HIV-positive pregnant women.

ART therapy, particularly lamivudine, has been associated with mitochondrial toxicity in the newborns of mothers exposed to ART.[52] The current limited literature on HBV-infected pregnant patients taking ART have reported no occurrences of fatty liver or lactic acidosis in the newborn or mother. Concern still remains, however, because of the pregnant patient's susceptibility to develop acute fatty liver.

Tenofovir causes a remodeling of bone and osteoporosis in nonpregnant patients.[53] In Macaca mulatta (rhesus monkeys), bone abnormalities occurred in the offspring of exposed monkeys.[54] Kidney impairment has also been reported as a complication of ART, but no data are available in pregnancy.

Breastfeeding

Breastfeeding is discouraged in all mothers exposed to ART. Lamivudine and tenofovir are known to be excreted in the breast milk, but no adverse results have been reported.[49] The recommendation not to breastfeed might be reflective of the protocol recommendations for HIV-positive mothers. The safety of breastfeeding in HBV-positive women must be further evaluated.

No increased birth defects with ART have been reported above the background incidence, nor has toxicity been reported in the clinical use of ART in patients with HBV. Lamivudine has been used the longest in pregnancy and, therefore, has accumulated more safety data than the newer drugs. Currently, much more effective drugs are available that are a better therapeutic choice. The use of a less-effective therapy must be balanced with concerns regarding potential toxicity. The most recent AASLD consensus stated that no recommendations could be made regarding HBV therapy in pregnancy, given the paucity of data. Some considerations pertinent to the use of ART in specific clinical scenarios are discussed in the following sections.

TREATMENT WITH ART IN THE CLINICAL SCENARIO

Drug toxicity must be interpreted in the clinical context because the risk/benefit analysis depends on multiple factors, including the duration of therapy, gestational age, and indication.

Initiation of ART During the Reproductive Years

The prevalence of HBV infection is highest among immigrants from endemic areas where it is often acquired in infancy or childhood. By the time these women reach the reproductive years, they have been infected for many years. ART for these women can contain liver damage and prevent hepatocellular carcinoma.

Therapy that clearly benefits the mother should not be withdrawn or delayed because of pregnancy. Fertility spans 35 years of a woman's life and can include multiple pregnancies. Delaying therapy could result in serious maternal harm.

Because the patient will be on the drug throughout the pregnancy, current ART options should be considered based on safety data regarding teratogenicity and toxicity.

Tenofovir or entecavir are most commonly used as first-line therapy because they combine the best antiviral efficacy with a minimal chance of developing viral strains resistant to therapy. More patients on tenofovir are reported on the ART registry, but potential bone toxicity makes tenofovir less appealing for long-term use in women. Lamivudine, which has the largest safety profile, is no longer used because it is prone to fostering the emergence of mutant viruses that are cross-resistant to other therapy. Interferon therapy is an appealing choice because it is a time-limited therapy, whereas oral agents, once started, often must be continued indefinitely.

Patients Trying to Conceive: Stop, Switch, or Continue ART?

A patient who conceives while on ART will often have her first prenatal appointment after gestational week 4 to 14, which is the most critical period of organogenesis, risking the possibility that the teratogenetic effect of the drug has already occurred. Discontinuation or change of therapy after the fact does not seem to be a logical strategy. Moreover, discontinuation of ART can cause dangerous exacerbations leading to hepatic failure.[55]

Although tenofovir has been shown to cause bone abnormalities in offspring of animals, no one agent has been seen to be less toxic than another in the latter half of pregnancy. Changing therapy might cause new side effects.

Initiation of ART During Gestation

Patients with chronic HBV who develop liver failure or are at risk of decompensating in pregnancy, both in the setting of a flare or severe underlying disease, should be treated. Theoretical toxicity concern should not detract from initiating therapy that is potentially life-saving for both mother and fetus. The choice of drug should be guided by clinical considerations similar to those for nonpregnant patients. The ideal drug is one with a strong and fast antiviral effect.

Initiating therapy in the third trimester to avoid immunization failure and vertical transmission is controversial. Not enough evidence supports the need and efficacy of therapy to make a recommendation at this point; and expert opinions have been divided. A quick and effective suppression of viral load is desirable. Lamivudine has been used the most for this purpose, although a recent abstract reported the use of telbivudine instead. Because the drug is started in the third trimester, toxicity rather than teratogenicity is a concern.

SUMMARY

HBV during pregnancy presents unique management challenges. Varying aspects of care must be considered, including the effects of HBV on maternal and fetal health, effects of pregnancy on the course of HBV infection, treatment of HBV during and after pregnancy, and prevention of perinatal infection. Acute infection in pregnant women is often similar to that of the general population; however, the risk of perinatal transmission increases later in gestation. For those with chronic HBV infection, the course of disease is usually unchanged during pregnancy. However, flares have been reported shortly after delivery. Women with high viremia have an increased likelihood of perinatal transmission and may contribute to the failure rate of current immunoprophylaxis strategies. ART has not been associated with increased risk of birth defects or toxicity, but despite studies designed to elucidate the drug efficacy and safety in affected individuals and the developing fetus, recommendations are inconclusive. Clinicians and patients must make individualized decisions after carefully evaluating the risks and benefits summarized in this article.

REFERENCES

1. Institute of Medicine (IOM). Hepatitis and liver cancer: a national strategy for prevention and control of hepatitis B and C. Washington, DC: The National Academies Press; 2010.
2. Goldstein ST, Zhou F, Hadler SC, et al. A mathematical model to estimate global hepatitis B disease burden and vaccination impact. Int J Epidemiol 2005;34: 1329–39.
3. McMahon BJ, Alvard WL, Hall DB, et al. Acute hepatitis B virus infection: relation of age to the clinical expression of disease and subsequent development of the carrier state. J Infect Dis 1985;151:599–603.
4. Centers for Disease Control and Prevention (CDC). Summary of notifiable diseases, United States, 2008. MMWR Morb Mortal Wkly Rep 2008;57:1–94.
5. Alter MJ. Epidemiology of hepatitis B in Europe and worldwide. J Hepatol 2003; 39(Suppl 1):S64–9.
6. Euler GL, Wooten KG, Baughman AL, et al. Hepatitis B surface antigen prevalence among pregnant women in urban areas: implications for testing, reporting and preventing perinatal transmission. Pediatrics 2003;111:1192–7.
7. Schrag SJ, Arnold KE, Mohle-Boetani JC, et al. Prenatal screening for infectious diseases and opportunities for prevention. Obstet Gynecol 2003;102: 753–60.
8. American College of Obstetricians and Gynecologists. American Congress of Obstetricians and Gynecologists (ACOG) Practice Bulletin No. 86. Viral hepatitis in pregnancy. Obstet Gynecol 2007;110:941–56.
9. Kim SM, Lee KS, Park CJ, et al. Prevalence of occult HBV infection among subjects with normal serum ALT levels in Korea. J Infect 2007;54:185–91.
10. Willis BT, Wortley P, Wang SA, et al. Gaps in hospital policies and practices to prevent perinatal transmission of HBV. Pediatrics 2010;125:704–11.
11. Anderson TA, Wexler DL. States report hundreds of medical errors in perinatal hepatitis B prevention. St Paul (MN): Immunization Action Coalition; 2005.
12. Burk RD, Hwang LY, Ho GY, et al. Outcome of perinatal hepatitis B virus exposure is dependent on maternal virus load. J Infect Dis 1994;170:1418–23.
13. Beasley RP, Hwang LY, Lin CC, et al. Hepatitis B immune globulin (HBIG) efficacy in the interruption of perinatal transmission of hepatitis B virus carrier state. Initial report of a randomized double-blind placebo-controlled trial. Lancet 1981; 2(8243):388–93.
14. Lee C, Gong Y, Brok J, et al. Effect of hepatitis B immunization in newborn infants of mothers positive for hepatitis surface antigen: systematic review and meta-analysis. BMJ 2006;332:328–36.
15. Xu DZ, Yan YP, Choi BC, et al. Risk factors and mechanism of transplacental transmission of hepatitis B virus: a case-control study. J Med Virol 2002;67(1): 20–6.
16. Zhang SL, Yue YF, Bai GQ, et al. Mechanism of intrauterine infection of hepatitis B virus. World J Gastroenterol 2004;10(3):437–8.
17. Bai H, Zhang L, Ma L, et al. Relationship of hepatitis B infection of placental barrier and hepatitis B virus intra-uterine transmission mechanism. World J Gastroenterol 2007;13(26):3625–30.

18. Hill JB, Sheffield JS, Kim MJ, et al. Risk of hepatitis B transmission in breast-fed infants of chronic hepatitis B carriers. Obstet Gynecol 2002;99:1049–52.
19. Alexander JM, Ramus R, Jackson G, et al. Risk of hepatitis B transmission after amniocentesis in chronic hepatitis B carriers. Infect Dis Obstet Gynecol 1999;7: 283–6.
20. Englert Y, Lesage B, Van Vooren JP, et al. Medically assisted reproduction in the presence of chronic viral diseases. Hum Reprod Update 2004;10(20):149–62.
21. CDC. Implementation of newborn hepatitis B vaccination-worldwide. MMWR Morb Mortal Wkly Rep 2008;57(46):1249–52.
22. Wang JS, Chen H, Zhu QR. Transformation of hepatitis B serologic markers in babies born to hepatitis B surface antigen positive mothers. World J Gastroenterol 2005;11(23):3582–5.
23. Han G, Zhao W, Cao M, et al. A prospective and open-label study for the efficacy and safety of telbivudine (ldt) in pregnancy for the prevention of perinatal transmission of hepatitis B virus (HBV) to the infants. Hepatology 2010;52(4): 427A.
24. Plitt SS, Somily AM, Singh AE. Outcomes from a Canadian public health prenatal screening program for hepatitis B: 1997–2004. Can J Public Health 2007;98(3): 194–7.
25. Wiseman E, Fraser MA, Holden S, et al. Perinatal transmission of hepatitis B virus: an Australian experience. Med J Aust 2009;190:489–92.
26. Andre FE, Zuckerman AJ. Review: protective efficacy of hepatitis B vaccines in neonates. J Med Virol 1994;44:144–51.
27. Tharmaphornpilas P, Rasdjarmrearnsook AO, Plianpanich S, et al. Increased risk of developing chronic HBV infection in infants born to chronically HBV infected mothers as a result of delayed second dose of hepatitis B vaccination. Vaccine 2009;27(44):6110–5.
28. Zhu QR, Ge YL, Gu SQ, et al. Relationship between cytokines gene polymorphism and susceptibility to hepatitis B virus intrauterine infection. Chin Med J 2005;118(19):1604–9.
29. Li XM, Shi MF, Yang YB, et al. Effect of hepatitis B immunoglobulin on interruption of HBV intrauterine infection. World J Gastroenterol 2004;10:3215–7.
30. Xu Q, Xiao L, Lu XB, et al. A randomized controlled clinical trial: interruption of intrauterine transmission of hepatitis B virus infection with HBIG. World J Gastroenterol 2006;12:3434–7.
31. Xiao XM, Li AZ, Zhu YK, et al. Prevention of vertical hepatitis B transmission by hepatitis B immunoglobulin in the third trimester of pregnancy. Int J Gynaecol Obstet 2007;96:167–70.
32. Connor EM, Sperling RS, Geiber R, et al. Reduction of maternal-infant transmission of human immunodeficiency virus type 1 with zidovudine treatment. N Engl J Med 1994;331(18):1173–80.
33. Xu WM, Cui YT, Wang L, et al. Lamivudine in late pregnancy to prevent perinatal transmission of hepatitis B virus infection: a multicentre, randomized, double-blind, placebo-controlled study. J Viral Hepat 2009;16(2):94–103.
34. Van Zonneveld M, van Nunen AB, Niesters HG, et al. Lamivudine treatment during pregnancy to prevent perinatal transmission of hepatitis B virus infection. J Viral Hepat 2003;10:294–7.
35. Nguyen G, Garcia RT, Nguyen N, et al. Clinical course of hepatitis B virus infection during pregnancy. Aliment Pharmacol Ther 2009;29:755–64.
36. Potthoff A, Rifai K, Wedemeyer H, et al. Successful treatment of fulminant hepatitis B during pregnancy. Gastroenterol 2009;47(7):667–70.

37. Shaheen AA, Myers RP. The outcomes of pregnancy in patients with cirrhosis: a population-based study. Liver Int 2010;30(2):275–83.
38. Sandhu BS, Sanyal AJ. Pregnancy and liver disease. Gastroenterol Clin North Am 2003;32:407–36.
39. Iwase H, Morise K, Kawase T, et al. Endoscopic injection sclerotherapy for esophageal varices during pregnancy. J Clin Gastroenterol 1994;18:80–3.
40. Wong S, Chan LY, Yu V, et al. Hepatitis B carrier and perinatal outcome in singleton pregnancy. Am J Perinatol 1999;16(9):485–8.
41. Safir A, Levy A, Sikuler E, et al. Maternal hepatitis B virus or hepatitis C virus carrier status as an independent risk factor for adverse perinatal outcome. Liver Int 2010;30(5):765–70.
42. Lao TT, Tse KY, Chan LY, et al. HBsAg carrier status and the association between gestational diabetes with increased serum ferritin concentration in Chinese women. Diabetes Care 2003;26(11):3011–6.
43. Hung JH, Chu CJ, Sung PL, et al. Lamivudine therapy in the treatment of chronic hepatitis B with acute exacerbation during pregnancy. J Chin Med Assoc 2008; 71(3):155–8.
44. Tan HH, Lui HF, Chow WC. Chronic hepatitis B virus (HBV) infection in pregnancy. Hepatol Int 2008;2:370–5.
45. Ter Borg MJ, Leemans WF, de Man RA, et al. Exacerbation of chronic hepatitis B infection after delivery. J Viral Hepat 2008;15:37–41.
46. Lin HH, Wu WY, Kao JH, et al. Hepatitis B post-partum e antigen clearance in hepatitis B carrier mothers: correlation with viral characteristics. J Gastroenterol Hepatol 2006;21(3):605–9.
47. Powrie RO. Principles for drug prescribing in pregnancy. In: Rosene-Montella K, Keely E, Barbour LA, Lee R, editors. Medical care of the pregnant patient. 2nd ed. Philadelphia: American College of Physicians Press; 2008. p. 18–25.
48. Bennetto-Hood C, Bryson YJ, Stek A, et al. Zidovudine, lamivudine, and nelfinavir concentrations in amniotic fluid and maternal serum. HIV Clin Trials 2009;10(1): 41–7.
49. Van Rompay KK, Hamilton M, Kearney B, et al. Pharmacokinetics of tenofovir in breast milk of lactating rhesus macaques. Antimicrob Agents Chemother 2005; 49(5):2093–4.
50. Sakata H, Karamitsos J, Kundaria B, et al. Case report of interferon alfa therapy for multiple myeloma during pregnancy. Am J Obstet Gynecol 1995;172(1): 217–9.
51. Cohen SM, Levy RM, Jovanovich JF, et al. Fatal lactic acidosis associated with the use of combination oral medications to treat reactivation of hepatitis B. J Clin Gastroenterol 2009;43(10):1008–10.
52. Shah I. Lactic acidosis in HIV-exposed infants with perinatal exposure to antiretroviral therapy. Ann Trop Paediatr 2009;29(4):257–61.
53. Woodward CL, Hall AM, Williams IG, et al. Tenofovir-associated renal and bone toxicity. HIV Med 2009;10(8):482–7.
54. Van Rompay KK, Durand-Gasselin L, Brignolo LL, et al. Chronic administration of tenofovir to rhesus macaques from infancy through adulthood and pregnancy: summary of pharmacokinetics and biological and virological effects. Antimicrob Agents Chemother 2008;52(9):3144–60.
55. Núñez M, Soriano V. Hepatotoxicity of antiretrovirals: incidence, mechanisms and management. Drug Saf 2005;28(1):53–66.

Primary Biliary Cirrhosis

Bhavik M. Bhandari, MD[a],*, Hasan Bayat, BS[b],
Kenneth D. Rothstein, MD[a]

KEYWORDS

• Primary biliary cirrhosis • Ursodeoxycholic acid • Liver failure

Primary biliary cirrhosis is a chronic autoimmune inflammatory disease of the liver with a striking female preponderance. It has an insidious onset and typically affects middle-aged women. The disease manifests gradually with symptoms of fatigue, pruritis, and increased alkaline phosphatase levels on laboratory evaluation. The hallmark of the disease is the circulating antimitochondrial antibody (AMA), found in up to 95% of patients.[1,2] Histology is characterized by inflammation of the bile ducts, destruction of cholangiocytes, and subsequent cholestasis, progressing to biliary cirrhosis.[2,3] The standard treatment of primary biliary cirrhosis (PBC) is ursodeoxycholic acid (UDCA), which improves survival, but the disease can still lead to cirrhosis and liver failure over decades.[4,5]

HISTORICAL TIMELINE

The description of diseases similar to PBC extends back to 1851, when Addison and Gull[6] reported a skin condition with a clinical relation to liver affection. Similar cases appeared in the literature until 1949, when Dauphinee and Sinclair[7] coined the term PBC to distinguish the disease from obstructive biliary jaundice. In the 1950s, Ahrens and colleagues[8] along with Sherlock[9] reported the clinical spectrum of jaundice, pruritus, osteoporosis, xanthomas, portal hypertension, and liver failure.

In 1965 the hallmark of the disease, the AMA, was discovered via immunofluorescence by Walker and colleagues.[1] Evaluation of this serum marker led to the recognition of a familial component in PBC.[10] Immunofluorescence detection of AMA remains the most sensitive and specific marker for diagnosis of PBC.

The histologic continuum of PBC was first described in 1965 by Rubin and colleagues.[11] Over time, genetic and environmental factors were considered to play an independent role in the development of PBC, with reports of case clustering.[12,13] The association of PBC with other autoimmune conditions also led to the investigation

[a] Division of Gastroenterology & Hepatology, Drexel University College of Medicine, 219 North Broad Street, Fifth Floor, Philadelphia, PA 19107, USA
[b] Drexel University College of Medicine, Philadelphia, PA, USA
* Corresponding author.
E-mail address: bhandabh@gmail.com

of genetic polymorphisms, which may cause immune dysregulation, but the precise cause of PBC remains a mystery.[14]

EPIDEMIOLOGY

PBC is a disease that is rare but universally present. It is most prevalent in Northern European countries (England and Scotland) and the Northern United States (Minnesota).[2,15] In a recent systematic review by Prince and James,[16] the prevalence of the disease ranged from 7 to 400 cases per million. Although it is a geographically variable disease, evidence suggests that both the prevalence and incidence are rising. The identification of geographic clusters of PBC has also raised the question of whether genetic and environmental factors are dominant factors in disease development.[17]

CAUSE

It is believed that PBC results when an individual with a susceptible genetic makeup encounters a superimposed environmental trigger that, in combination with other factors, leads to dysregulation of the immune system and an attack on target tissues within the liver. The genetic predisposition is shown by the high concordance rate among monozygotic twins, which is 63%.[18] In this same study, dizygotic twins had a concordance rate of 0%, showing the complexity of genetic friability in patients who are susceptible. Approximately 6% of patients with PBC have a first-degree relative who suffers from PBC. The prevalence is nearly 100 times higher of developing PBC than in the general population if a first-degree relative suffers from the disease.[16] There is a high female/male disease incidence ratio, which suggests a significant role for X chromosome defects in PBC. The increased risk of having PBC with genetic polymorphism of the vitamin D receptor is also of note.[19] Allelic variations in the major histocompatibility complex along with innate and adaptive immunity have also been shown to increase genetic susceptibility for PBC.

Several etiologic environmental risk factors have been evaluated. One of the most widely studied environmental factors is a past history of infection. In an interview-based study, female patients with PBC had a history of increased number of genitourinary infections when compared with women without the disease.[20] These findings were statistically significant, and PBC developing as a result of such infections is theorized under the mechanism of molecular mimicry. Infectious agents that have been studied in conjunction with PBC are *Chlamydia pneumoniae*, *Escherichia coli*, mouse mammary tumor virus, human betaretrovirus and *Novosphingobium aromaticivorans*.[2,17,21,22]

Smoking consistently has been found to be a risk factor in the development of this disease and may also play a role in accelerating its progression.[23] Toxin exposure by compounds such as halogenated hydrocarbons is also considered a potential risk factor for the development of PBC. Animal studies have shown that exposure to halogenated hydrocarbons can induce antimitochondrial antibodies but whether these lead to the development of liver disease is unclear.[24] The role of the use of cosmetics, frequency of pregnancy, and hormone replacement therapy in contributing to disease development is unclear.[25]

GENDER IN PBC

The ratio of women to men who have PBC is disproportionately 9:1.[2] This ratio suggests the importance of gender in the development of PBC. This finding is supported by evidence that women with PBC have a significantly enhanced monosomy X frequency in peripheral white blood cells compared with age-matched healthy women and that the X chromosome loss is preferential. Recent data suggest that the role played by the X chromosome in immune function may be the critical factor.[26] Studying the nature of autoimmunity that develops as a result of acquiring such monosomy is an important area of research.

The role of sex hormones is also a consideration in the cause of PBC. The higher prevalence of autoimmune conditions in women is believed to be secondary to the effect of sex hormones on the differentiation of immune responses. A recent study has shown pregnancy to be a precipitating factor associated with the development of PBC.[27]

When comparing the presentation of PBC in men and women, studies have shown few, if any, differences.[28] One study found that pruritus, and hyperpigmentation related to pruritus, was seen more frequently in women, most notably postmenopausal patients. Women were also found to have Sjögren syndrome more commonly than men.[29]

PATHOPHYSIOLOGY

Even although a definitive cause for PBC has not been explained, a multihit hypothesis leading to autoimmunity and subsequent disease is postulated. Although not yet clearly defined, genetic susceptibility is critical overall, and depends particularly on multiple inherited deficits in immune tolerance. Regardless of cause, the common pathway for injury is the hallmark of the disease and the development of antimitochondrial antibodies. Amongst the multiple antimitochondrial antigens, the so-called M2 antibody was shown to be the most specifically associated with PBC. These M2 antibodies target the 2-oxo-acid dehydrogenase complexes located on the inner mitochondrial membranes, and predominantly include the E2 binding protein components of the pyruvate dehydrogenase complex (PDC-E2).[30] Recent evidence showed that CD4+ and CD8+ T cells reactive against PDC-E2 are found in higher titers in the livers of patients with PBC.[31] The overexpression of PDC-E2 in biliary epithelial cells may also play a role in the recruitment of T cells to the liver.[32]

The sequence of events in the initiation of PBC may begin with initiation by an autoantigenic stimulus provided either by a bacterial mimic of PDC-E2 or from a native mitochondrial antigen from apoptotic cells. This sequence of events in turn activates antigen-presenting cells, which present immunogenic peptides to autoreactive CD4+ T lymphocytes. These cells subsequently activate CD8+ cytotoxic T lymphocytes and B lymphocytes, which produce AMA. Regulatory T lymphocytes that normally restrain activated T cells are deficient in PBC, thus further augmenting T-cell proliferation and AMA production. Effector mechanisms converge on the target cell, the biliary epithelial cell, which can be damaged by injurious cytokines, direct cytotoxicity, or transcytosis of immunogenic peptides. A toxic effect might also be supplied by activated eosinophils and the release of eosinophil major basic protein. Biliary epithelial cells then undergo apoptosis and in doing so contribute immunogenic mitochondrial PDC-E2 antigen to sustain a self-perpetuating autoimmunization process. Destruction of biliary epithelial cells and bile ducts leads to chronic cholestasis and liver injury.[33]

A patient with a susceptible genetic makeup undergoes an environmental insult, which then triggers AMA production. This production in turn leads to cholangiocyte apoptosis, inflammation, and cholestasis. Through a continued cycle of insult and injury, there is fibrosis, ductopenia, cirrhosis, and ultimately, liver failure.

CLINICAL PRESENTATION

The typical patient is a woman between the ages of 40 and 60 years who undergoes an investigation for PBC as a result of increased liver enzymes such as alkaline phosphatase and γ-glutamyl transpeptidase found on routine blood work. With progressively earlier diagnosis of PBC as a result of health maintenance blood work, most patients (nearly 60%) are diagnosed in the asymptomatic phase.[2] Symptomatic patients generally present at a younger age, perhaps because of either a different clinical course or because their symptoms prompt an earlier clinical investigation. Early manifestations of the disease include symptoms of fatigue and pruritis followed by complications as a result of a long-standing history and progression of the disease such as osteoporosis, vitamin deficiencies, hyperlipidemia, and cirrhosis. These manifestations are discussed in further detail later.

In most asymptomatic patients afflicted with PBC, the physical examination is normal. A few patients may have hepatomegaly (4%–52%), splenomegaly (6%–24%), and abdominal pain in the right upper quadrant.[34] Jaundice is seen in only 3% to 8% of patients at the time of diagnosis, and is a marker for advanced disease and poor prognosis.[3] Routine blood work may reveal increased alkaline phosphatase and γ-glutamyl transpeptidase levels. In addition, hypercholesterolemia with an increase in low-density lipoprotein cholesterol is found in nearly 20% of patients with PBC.[5] If the bilirubin is greater than 3 mg/L, patients are likely to have advanced fibrosis and less likely to respond to medical treatment and require liver transplantation. An ultrasound of the abdomen is of paramount importance to evaluate the liver parenchyma and biliary tree. The typical cholestatic liver profile can also be seen in biliary obstruction. Identification of antimitochondrial antibodies by indirect immunofluorescence and immunoblotting, and/or investigation by liver biopsy, leads to the eventual diagnosis of PBC.[35]

Fatigue

A major symptom affecting the quality of life of patients with PBC is fatigue. A large percentage of patients with PBC, ranging from 40% to 80%, reported experiencing fatigue.[36] Assessing a subjective finding such as fatigue can be difficult, but tools such as the Fatigue Impact Scale (FIS) have traditionally been used to make such an assessment in patients with PBC.[37] The FIS was developed with the intention of quantifying the effects of fatigue on quality of life in patients with any illness. For an assessment tool specific for patients with PBC, the PBC-40 has been developed.[38] The PBC-40 is a questionnaire that addresses concerns that relate most to patients with PBC.

Despite being a common finding, the presence or severity of fatigue does not correlate with the severity of the liver disease.[39] Nearly half of the patients who had fatigue described it as the worst symptom of their disease.[37] Given the near normal life expectancy in patients undergoing medical management of PBC it is important to address the problems with the highest effect to improve their quality of life.

Pruritus

Another common symptom experienced by patients with PBC is pruritus. Up to 80% of patients reported having pruritus when seeking medical evaluation. Similarly to fatigue, pruritus does not correlate with the extent of liver disease.[35] Complications that may arise secondary to untreated pruritus include sleep deprivation, fatigue, and even suicidal ideation.[40] Many treatments are available to counteract the morbidity from pruritus, which results in significant improvement in the quality of life in these patients.

Osteoporosis

Osteoporosis in a well-known complication of PBC, with most significant studies reporting a prevalence of approximately 35%.[41] Osteoporosis is also associated with the postmenopausal state, and because many patients with PBC are postmenopausal, it may be difficult to determine the exact cause. A recent study of women with PBC and age-matched controls showed that osteoporosis was more prevalent in women with PBC. The same study concluded that age and severity of disease were the main risk factors for developing osteoporosis.[42] Whether or not osteoporosis in women with PBC translates into more frequent fractures is also an area of debate. A population-based cohort study showed that women with PBC who developed osteoporosis had an increase in both relative and absolute risk of fracture when compared with the general population.[43]

In order to diagnose osteoporosis, bone mineral density scans should be performed.[44] In patients with normal scans, the study should be repeated in 2 to 3 years, or every year if they have other risk factors for osteoporosis.[45] Serologic studies to complete the workup include calcium, phosphorus, parathyroid hormone, and 25-hydroxyvitamin D.[41]

Vitamin Deficiencies

Fat-soluble vitamin deficiencies (vitamins A, D, E, and K) are of concern in patients with PBC. Their prevalence is variable and largely attributable to malabsorption. Patients with advanced histologic stage, low total cholesterol, and a low albumin are at increased risk for having fat-soluble vitamin deficiencies and should be screened appropriately. Vitamin A deficiency may manifest with symptoms such as nocturnal blindness or a history of falls. Vitamin D deficiency is common and is an independent risk factor for the development of osteoporosis. Easy bruising or bleeding may be a sign of vitamin K deficiency and may be confirmed by an increased prothrombin time. Vitamin E deficiency is rare but should be considered in the setting of ataxia, myopathies, and pigmented retinopathy.[46]

Hyperlipidemia

Increased serum lipid levels are often found in patients with PBC. Although patients may develop xanthelasma and xanthoma skin lesions, the association of hyperlipidemia with atherosclerosis in the setting of PBC remains unclear. The risk of coronary artery disease has not been extensively studied, but a study in the Netherlands showed that 12% of patients with PBC died of circulatory system diseases.[47] The increase of serum lipid levels is believed to be caused by an increase in lipoprotein-X (LP-X), which is a low-density lipoprotein particle rich in free cholesterol and phospholipids. LP-X formation is most likely caused by reduced lecithin cholesterol acyltransferase activity, leading to the accumulation of free cholesterol and phospholipids.[48] Whether this pathway leading to hyperlipidemia is a major contributor to atherogenic circulatory system disease, specifically in the PBC patient population, remains under investigation.

ASSOCIATED DISEASES

About 5% of patients with PBC may present with an AMA-negative PBC (also known as autoimmune cholangitis [AIC]).[3] These patients have the same clinical presentation and histology findings as AMA-positive patients but lack AMA by indirect immunofluorescence and immunoblotting. Such a presentation illustrates the multifactorial, and still not fully understood, nature of this illness. A liver biopsy, along with other serologic tests including PBC-specific antinuclear antibodies should be performed to confirm PBC in patients who are suspected of having the disease, but are negative for AMA.[49]

Furthermore, an overlap syndrome between PBC and autoimmune hepatitis has also been described and exists in about 5% to 19% of patients.[50] In all patients with PBC, regardless of the AMA status, a polyclonal increase of serum IgM levels can also be found.[2] Although PBC primarily involves intrahepatic bile ducts, the salivary and lacrimal glands may also be involved because of cells phenotypically similar to biliary epithelia.[51] This finding explains why PBC is associated with other autoimmune conditions such as Sjögren syndrome (70%–100% of patients), scleroderma, CREST syndrome, systemic lupus erythematosis, autoimmune hepatitis, rheumatoid arthritis, and Hashimoto thyroiditis.[3,5] Evaluation should also include anticentromere, Ro/SSA, La/SSB, Scl-70, and histone antibodies.[49]

Other diseases associated with PBC include Raynaud disease, arthropathy/ arthritis, glomerulonephritis, cutaneous disorders, celiac disease, ulcerative colitis, pulmonary fibrosis, and gallstones. There may also be an increased risk of breast cancer in women who have PBC. Although there is no consensus in this regard and this observation needs further study, it is prudent to reinforce the need for mammograms and breast cancer screening tests in accordance with standard guidelines.[52–54]

HISTOLOGY

The sentinel lesion in PBC on a liver biopsy specimen is damage to epithelial cells of the small bile ducts. The most important and only diagnostic clue in many cases is ductopenia, defined as the absence of interlobular bile ducts in greater than 50% of portal tracts. The florid duct lesion, in which the epithelium of the interlobular and segmental bile ducts degenerates segmentally, with formation of poorly defined, noncaseating epithelioid granulomas, is nearly diagnostic of PBC but is found in few cases, mainly in the early stages.[2]

The histology can be divided into 4 stages as described by Ludwig. Ludwig stage 1 disease is characterized by inflammatory destruction of the intrahepatic, septal, and interlobular bile ducts. The disease is limited to the portal triad and the tracts are usually expanded by lymphocytes. In stage 2 disease the inflammation extends from the portal tract into the hepatic parenchyma, also known as interface hepatitis or, formerly, piecemeal necrosis. Destruction of bile ducts with proliferation of bile ductules can be seen. Stage 3 disease is characterized by scarring and fibrosis. Lymphocytic involvement of the portal and periportal areas, as well as the hepatic parenchyma, can be seen, but the hallmark of this stage is the presence of fibrosis. Stage 4 disease is characterized by cirrhosis with fibrous septa and regenerative nodules.[2]

Although a liver biopsy is not necessary for the diagnosis of PBC, most patients eventually receive a liver biopsy, which may be of use in staging the disease and may also help in guiding management.[35] An instance in which a liver biopsy may be necessary is in the setting of suspected PBC in a patient lacking antimitochondrial antibodies.

NATURAL PROGRESSION OF PBC

The natural course of the classic form of PBC follows 4 phases: the preclinical, asymptomatic, symptomatic, and liver insufficiency phases. The preclinical phase consists of the identification of antimitochondrial antibodies in the absence of any other symptoms or abnormal serum liver function tests. Progression into the asymptomatic phase is defined by the development of persistently increased serum liver enzymes, with alkaline phosphatase and γ-glutamyl transpeptidase being the most commonly increased enzymes.[3,55]

The symptomatic phase of PBC is defined by the development of characteristic symptoms such as pruritus and fatigue. Disease progression can lead to advanced symptoms and complications consistent with malabsorption and cirrhosis. The final phase of liver insufficiency has symptoms related to the development of cirrhosis with subsequent portal hypertension, hepatic encephalopathy, and worsening jaundice.[55] The progression of patients through these phases, and the duration of each phase, are highly variable. Untreated, the timeline of PBC from the preclinical phase to advanced liver disease is approximately 20 years.[56] Patients with advanced disease are also at a higher risk for the development of hepatocellular carcinoma.[57]

A second form is characterized by the fluctuating or persistent presence of the features of autoimmune hepatitis. Approximately 20% of patients are affected by this variant and they have a more severe disease course, with early development of liver fibrosis and liver failure.[58] A third form, which affects 5% to 10% of patients, is referred to as the premature ductopenic variant. Its hallmark is a rapid onset of ductopenia and severe icteric cholestasis, progressing quickly toward cirrhosis in less than 5 years.[59]

TREATMENT

The only drug approved by the US Food and Drug Administration for the treatment of PBC is UDCA. UDCA is a bile acid with fewer side effects when compared with endogenous bile acids, and is used for several other cholestatic disorders. It is considered to have 3 major mechanisms of action, which include protection of cholangiocytes from cytotoxic bile acids, stimulation of hepatobiliary secretion, and protection of hepatocytes from apoptosis.[60]

Several studies have compared UDCA with placebo, showing slower disease progression and improvement in liver function tests. However, a recent meta-analysis showed that although UDCA improved liver biochemistries, jaundice, and ascites, it showed no benefit in terms of mortality or liver transplantation.[61] The inadequacy of dosage and the period of follow-up have been questioned in some of the trials used for the meta-analysis.[62] A meta-analysis of trials with appropriate dosing and follow-up showed slower disease progression, particularly in patients with stage 1 or 2 disease.[63]

The recommended dose of UDCA is 13–15 mg/kg/d.[64] Prescribing the full dose at the initiation of treatment may cause or exacerbate pruritus. Consequently, a gradual increase in the dosage over several days or weeks may be better tolerated and of more benefit to the patient. Although UDCA is most effective in patients with early stages of disease, its use is recommended for all 4 stages.[62] The most common side effect is weight gain. The average weight gain is approximately 2 kg and may be more pronounced in patients who have stopped smoking.[65] Patients may also experience gastric discomfort, reflux symptoms, and loose stool.[5]

Normalization of liver biochemistry values remains the goal of therapy. Routine evaluation of serum bilirubin, alkaline phosphatase, alanine transaminase, and aspartate transaminase are recommended. However, serum bilirubin remains the best predictor of prognosis and long-term response to UDCA treatment.[5] Normalization or a decrease of these markers to minimally increased levels leads to a normal 10-year mortality when compared with the general population. A response can be seen in a few weeks, with continued improvement over a few years.[62] UDCA treatment is highly effective in most patients but is suboptimal is approximately 40% of patients.[66] An increase in the dose was not found to be of any benefit in patients who did not respond to standard doses of treatment, and adjuvant therapy is recommended in these patients.[67]

Adjuvant Treatment

For those patients who show a suboptimal response to UDCA or have progression of their disease, additional treatment may be necessary. Several medications have been studied, particularly in combination with UDCA. However, their use and benefit remain controversial.

Immunosuppressive agents such as methotrexate alone or in combination with UDCA have been used for the treatment of PBC. Methotrexate has been shown to improve liver biochemistries, particularly in those with a suboptimal response to UDCA.[68] However, a recent Cochrane review found that methotrexate had no significant benefit in terms of mortality or need for liver transplantation.[69] Given the significant adverse effects associated with methotrexate such as fatigue and interstitial pneumonitis, its routine use cannot be recommended.

Colchicine is another medication that has been used in the treatment of PBC. Colchicine has been used as a single treatment agent because of its ability to improve liver biochemistries.[70] Like methotrexate, a recent Cochrane review found that colchicine did not show any benefit in terms of mortality or need for liver transplantation when compared with placebo, or in combination with UDCA.[71]

Several other immunosuppressive agents have also been studied. The use of glucocorticoids along with UDCA treatment may help in improving liver biochemistries and histology.[72] Budesonide in particular has been used in this setting at 6–9 mg/d.[5] However, the use of glucocorticoids is limited because of its side effects on bone mass, and consequent risk of developing or worsening osteoporosis. Budesonide should not be used and is contraindicated in patients with cirrhosis. The combination of UDCA and budesonide therapy has been shown to improve biochemical and histologic response in terms of inflammation and fibrosis in patients with PBC. Other medications that have been suggested or studied, but infrequently used because of their limited effectiveness and adverse side effects, include cyclosporine, azathioprine, penicillamine, thalidomide, and sulindac.[2,72]

Treatment of Fatigue

For extreme fatigue associated with PBC, medications such as modafinil, a stimulant used in conditions such as narcolepsy, have been shown to be effective.[73] Doses up to 400 mg/d have been well tolerated and generally effective in those with daytime somnolence and excessive fatigue.

Treatment of Pruritis

The pruritus of PBC often responds to UDCA. If pruritis continues, the next step is the use of antihistamines such as diphenhydramine or hydroxyzine. If the pruritus is refractory to these relatively innocuous medications, it warrants the use of cholestyramine, a bile-acid sequestrant. Cholestyramine is effective in alleviating symptoms in nearly 90% of patients.[2] Common side effects include bloating and constipation. When given in combination with UDCA, dosing should be spread apart by 4 hours to endure absorption and bioavailability. The antibiotic rifampin is another medication that can be used in those patients who cannot tolerate cholestyramine or do not respond to it.[74] Patients prescribed rifampin should be monitored with liver function tests to evaluate for any possible hepatotoxic side effects (increased aminotransferase and bilirubin levels).[40] In a single study, UDCA was shown to decrease pruritus when compared with placebo.[75]

It has also been suggested that the pruritus associated with PBC is mediated by endogenous opioids.[76] Opioid antagonists such as naloxone and naltrexone have subsequently been used with success in those who do not respond to cholestyramine and rifampin. Antihistamines are another option, and may help patients who are sleep deprived through their sedative effects. For those patients who do not respond to any medications, plasmapheresis may be of additional benefit.[2]

Treatment of Osteoporosis

Treatment of osteoporosis includes exercise and a healthy diet, cessation of smoking and alcohol consumption, and supplementation with calcium and vitamin D.[77] Bisphosphonates have been shown to increase bone mass. Specifically, alendronate at 70 mg/wk showed an improvement in bone mineral density of women with osteoporosis secondary to their PBC.[78] Although hormone therapy has also been suggested, the potential side effects have prevented its widespread use.[41]

Treatment of Vitamin Deficiencies

In this setting of vitamin A deficiency, patients should be supplemented with 50,000 IU/d for 1 month, followed by a maintenance dose based on serum retinol levels. Vitamin D should be supplemented regardless of a deficiency at 600 to 800 IU/d for patients older than 51 years. If vitamin D deficiency is shown, the dose may be increased to 25,000 IU to 50,000 IU 2 to 3 times per week. In cases of vitamin K deficiency, patients may be supplemented with 5 mg/d orally. Treatment of vitamin E deficiency consists of 800 to 1200 mg of α-tocopherol.[46]

Treatment of Hyperlipidemia

Treatment of hyperlipidemia in patients with PBC should be considered and continues to be an area of investigation. UDCA treatment has been shown to lower serum cholesterol.[79] In patients who continue to have increased serum cholesterol, other therapeutic measures may be considered. Statins have only recently been studied but show promising results. In 1 study, 6 patients with early-stage PBC and hyperlipidemia on UDCA treatment were placed on simvastatin 10 mg/d. Simvastatin was found to lower total cholesterol by 21% and low density lipoprotein cholesterol by 25%. Simvastatin also lowered serum levels of alkaline phosphatase and γ-glutamyl transpeptidase by 12% and 37.5%, respectively.[80]

Fibrates have had a role in lipid reduction and also been shown to reduce hepatobiliary inflammation in PBC. A study focusing on the treatment of PBC with bezafibrate monotherapy showed histologic improvement in patients taking 200 mg twice a day.[81] However, further investigation is necessary to examine the long-term effects of fibrates in PBC.

Treatment of Portal Hypertension and Cirrhosis

A few patients do not respond to medical therapy and progressively develop presinusoidal portal hypertension. Management of portal hypertension in PBC should be the same as in patients with cirrhosis from other causes. For patients with advancing disease and severe portal hypertension, decompensated cirrhosis, and liver failure, liver transplantation remains the only effective treatment. Patients should be referred to a liver transplant center for assessment once there is evidence of decompensated cirrhosis. Patients with PBC show an excellent response to liver transplantation, with 1-year and 5-year survival rates of 83% and 77%, respectively.[82] Patients continue to have antimitochondrial antibodies, and the recurrence rate of PBC is 15% at 3 years, and up to 30% at 5 years after transplantation.[83]

SUMMARY

PBC remains a widely studied, but as of yet not completely understood, disease. The female preponderance of PBC has not been fully explained by current models. However, gender plays an important role in every aspect of the disease. Environmental and chemical triggers continue to be a catalyst in the formation of disease. Diagnosis of the disease has been standardized and is highly specific. Treatment has allowed patients with PBC to have a normal life expectancy. Advanced cases of the disease can still be treated with liver transplantation, giving patients hope at every stage of the disease. Everything from the underlying genetics and cause of the disease to possible specific treatments targeted at antimitochondrial antigens remains an excellent opportunity for further research and specific intervention.

REFERENCES

1. Walker JG, Doniach D, Roitt IM, et al. Serological tests in diagnosis of primary biliary cirrhosis. Lancet 1965;285:827–31.
2. Jones DE. Pathogenesis of primary biliary cirrhosis. Postgrad Med J 2008; 84(987):23–33.
3. Angulo P, Lindor K. Primary biliary cirrhosis. In: Sleisenger MH, Feldman M, Friedman LS, et al, editors. Sleisenger & Fordtran's gastrointestinal and liver disease pathophysiology, diagnosis, management. 9th edition. St Louis (MO): MD Consult; 2009. p. 1477–87.
4. Lindor KD, Gershwin ME, Poupon R, et al. Primary biliary cirrhosis. Hepatology 2009;50:291–308.
5. Poupon R. Primary biliary cirrhosis: a 2010 update. J Hepatol 2010;52:745–58.
6. Addison T, Gull W. On a certain affection of the skin vitiligoidea-α plana, β tuberosa. Guys Hosp Rep 1851;7:265–76.
7. Dauphinee JA, Sinclair JC. Primary biliary cirrhosis. CMAJ 1949;61:1–6.
8. Ahrens EH Jr, Payne MA, Kunkel HG, et al. Primary biliary cirrhosis. Medicine 1950;29:299–364.
9. Sherlock S. Primary biliary cirrhosis (chronic intrahepatic obstructive jaundice). Gastroenterology 1959;37:574–86.
10. Feizi T, Naccarato R, Sherlock S, et al. Mitochondrial and other tissue antibodies in relatives of patients with primary biliary cirrhosis. Clin Exp Immunol 1972;10: 609–22.
11. Rubin E, Schaffner F, Popper H. Primary biliary cirrhosis: chronic non-suppurative destructive cholangitis. Am J Pathol 1965;46:387–407.
12. Douglas JG, Finlayson ND. Are increased individual susceptibility and environmental factors both necessary for the development of primary biliary cirrhosis? BMJ 1979;2:419–20.
13. Triger D. Primary biliary cirrhosis: an epidemiological study. BMJ 1980;281: 772–5.
14. Heathcote E. Primary biliary cirrhosis: historical perspective. Clin Liver Dis 2003; 7(4):735–40.
15. Kim WR, Lindor KD, Locke GR 3rd, et al. Epidemiology and natural history of primary biliary cirrhosis in a US community. Gastroenterology 2000;119: 1631–6.
16. Prince MI, James OF. The epidemiology of primary biliary cirrhosis. Clin Liver Dis 2003;7:795–819.
17. Gross R, Odin J. Recent advances in the epidemiology of primary biliary cirrhosis. Clin Liver Dis 2008;12(2):289–303.

18. Selmi C. Primary biliary cirrhosis in monozygotic and dizygotic twins: genetics, epigenetics, and environment. Gastroenterology 2004;127(2):485–92.
19. Jones D, Donaldson P. Genetic factors in the pathogenesis of primary biliary cirrhosis. Clin Liver Dis 2003;7(4):841–64.
20. Zein CO, Beatty K, Post AB, et al. Smoking and increased severity of hepatic fibrosis in primary biliary cirrhosis: a cross validated retrospective assessment. Hepatology 2006;44(6):1564–71.
21. Parikh-Patel A. Risk factors for primary biliary cirrhosis in a cohort of patients from the United States. Hepatology 2001;33(1):16–21.
22. Abdulkarim A. Primary biliary cirrhosis: an infectious disease caused by Chlamydia pneumoniae? J Hepatol 2004;40(3):380–4.
23. Selmi C. Patients with primary biliary cirrhosis react against a ubiquitous xenobiotic-metabolizing bacterium. Hepatology 2003;38(5):1250–7.
24. Leung PS, Quan C, Park O, et al. Immunization with a xenobiotic 6-bromohexane bovine serum albumin conjugate induces antimitochondrial antibodies. J Immunol 2003;170:5326–32.
25. Gershwin ME, Selmi C, Worman HJ, et al. Risk factors and comorbidities in primary biliary cirrhosis: a controlled interview-based study of 1032 patients. Hepatology 2005;42:1194–202.
26. Invernizzi P. Frequency of monosomy X in women with primary biliary cirrhosis. Lancet 2004;363(9408):533–5.
27. Parikh-Patel A, Gold E, Utts J, et al. The association between gravidity and primary biliary cirrhosis. Ann Epidemiol 2002;12(4):264–72.
28. Leuschner U. Primary biliary cirrhosis–presentation and diagnosis. Clin Liver Dis 2003;7(4):741–58.
29. Lucey MR, Neuberger JM, Williams R. Primary biliary cirrhosis in man. Gut 1986; 27:1373–6.
30. Yeaman SJ, Kirby JA, Jones DJ. Autoreactive responses to pyruvate dehydrogenase complex in the pathogenesis of primary biliary cirrhosis. Immunol Rev 2000; 174(1):238–49.
31. Kita H, Matsumura S, He XS, et al. Quantitative and functional analysis of PDC-E2-specific autoreactive cytotoxic T lymphocytes in primary biliary cirrhosis. J Clin Invest 2002;109(9):1231–40.
32. Joplin R. Membrane dihydrolipoamide acetyltransferase (E2) on human biliary epithelial cells in primary biliary cirrhosis. Lancet 1992;339(8785):93–4.
33. Invernizzi P, Mackay R. Etiopathogenesis of primary biliary cirrhosis. World J Gastroenterol 2008;14(21):3328–37.
34. Mahl T, Shockcor W, Boyer J. Primary biliary cirrhosis: survival of a large cohort of symptomatic and asymptomatic patients followed for 24 years. J Hepatol 1994; 20(6):707–13.
35. Kumagi T, Onji M. Presentation and diagnosis of primary biliary cirrhosis in the 21st century. Clin Liver Dis 2008;12(2):243–59.
36. Newton J. Fatigue in primary biliary cirrhosis. Clin Liver Dis 2008;12(2): 367–83.
37. Huet PM, Deslauriers J, Tran A, et al. Impact of fatigue on the quality of life in patients with primary biliary cirrhosis. Am J Gastroenterol 2000;95:760–7.
38. Jacoby A, Rannard A. Development, validation, and evaluation of the PBC-40, a disease specific health related quality of life measure for primary biliary cirrhosis. Gut 2005;54(11):1622–9.
39. Cauch-Dudek K, Abbey S, Stewart DE, et al. Fatigue in primary biliary cirrhosis. Gut 1998;43:705–10.

40. Bergasa N. Pruritus in primary biliary cirrhosis: pathogenesis and therapy. Clin Liver Dis 2008;12(2):385–406.
41. Pares A, Guanabens N. Osteoporosis in primary biliary cirrhosis: pathogenesis and treatment. Clin Liver Dis 2008;12(2):407–24.
42. Guanabens N, Pares A, Ros I, et al. Severity of cholestasis and advanced histological stage but not menopausal status are the major risk factors for osteoporosis in primary biliary cirrhosis. J Hepatol 2005;42(4):573–7.
43. Solaymanidodaran M, Card T, Aithal G, et al. Fracture risk in people with primary biliary cirrhosis: a population-based cohort study. Gastroenterology 2006;131(6): 1752–7.
44. Nelson H, Helfand M, Woolf S, et al. Screening for postmenopausal osteoporosis: a review of the evidence for the U.S. Preventive Services Task Force. Ann Intern Med 2002;137:529–41.
45. Pares A, Guanabens N. Treatment of bone disorders in liver disease. J Hepatol 2006;45(3):445–53.
46. Levy C, Lindor K. Management of osteoporosis, fat-soluble vitamin deficiencies, and hyperlipidemia in primary biliary cirrhosis. Clin Liver Dis 2003;7(4):901–10.
47. Van Dam GM, Gips CH. Primary biliary cirrhosis in the Netherlands: an analysis of associated diseases, cardiovascular risk, and malignancies on the basis of mortality figures. Scand J Gastroenterol 1997;32(1):77–83.
48. Sorokin A, Brown J, Thompson P. Primary biliary cirrhosis, hyperlipidemia, and atherosclerotic risk: a systematic review. Atherosclerosis 2007;194(2):293–9.
49. Hirschfield G, Heathcote E. Antimitochondrial antibody-negative primary biliary cirrhosis. Clin Liver Dis 2008;12(2):323–31.
50. Czaja AJ. Frequency and nature of the variant syndromes of autoimmune liver disease. Hepatology 1998;28(2):360–5.
51. Joplin R. Distribution of pyruvate dehydrogenase dihydrolipoamide acetyltransferase (PDC-E2) and another mitochondrial marker in salivary gland and biliary epithelium from patients with primary biliary cirrhosis. Hepatology 1994;19(6): 1375–80.
52. Wolke AM, Schaffner F, Kapelman B, et al. Malignancy in primary biliary cirrhosis. High incidence of breast cancer in affected women. Am J Med 1984;76(6): 1075–8.
53. Goudie BM, Burt AD, Macfarlane G, et al. Breast cancer in women with primary biliary cirrhosis. Br Med J 1985;291(6509):1597–8.
54. Floreani A, Baragiotta A, Baldo V, et al. Hepatic and extrahepatic malignancies in primary biliary cirrhosis. Hepatology 1999;29(5):1425–8.
55. Mayo M. Natural history of primary biliary cirrhosis. Clin Liver Dis 2008;12: 277–88.
56. Metcalf JH, Mitchison J, Palmer D, et al. Natural history of early primary biliary cirrhosis. Lancet 1996;348(9039):1399–402.
57. Nijhawan PK, Therneau TM, Dickson ER, et al. Incidence of cancer in primary biliary cirrhosis: the Mayo experience. Hepatology 1999;29(5):1396–8.
58. Poupon R. Autoimmune overlapping syndromes. Clin Liver Dis 2003;7:865–78.
59. Vleggaar FP, van Buuren HR, Zondervan PE, et al. Jaundice in non-cirrhotic primary biliary cirrhosis: the premature ductopenic variant. Gut 2001;49: 276–81.
60. Paumgartner G. Ursodeoxycholic acid in cholestatic liver disease: mechanisms of action and therapeutic use revisited. Hepatology 2002;36(3):525–31.
61. Gong Y, Huang ZB, Christensen E, et al. Ursodeoxycholic acid for primary biliary cirrhosis. Cochrane Database Syst Rev 2008;3:CD000551.

62. Lindor K. Ursodeoxycholic acid for the treatment of primary biliary cirrhosis. N Engl J Med 2007;357(15):1524–9.
63. Shi J, Wu C, Lin Y, et al. Long-term effects of mid-dose ursodeoxycholic acid in primary biliary cirrhosis: a meta-analysis of randomized controlled trials. Am J Gastroenterol 2006;101:1529–38.
64. Angulo P, Dickson ER, Therneau TM, et al. Comparison of three doses of ursodeoxycholic acid in the treatment of primary biliary cirrhosis: a randomized trial. J Hepatol 1999;30:830–5.
65. Siegel JL, Jorgensen R, Angulo P, et al. Treatment with ursodeoxycholic acid is associated with weight gain in patients with primary biliary cirrhosis. J Clin Gastroenterol 2003;37:183–5.
66. Leuschner M, Dietrich CF, You T, et al. Characterisation of patients with primary biliary cirrhosis responding to long term ursodeoxycholic acid treatment. Gut 2000;46:121–6.
67. Angulo P, Jorgensen RA, Lindor KD. Incomplete response to ursodeoxycholic acid in primary biliary cirrhosis: is a double dosage worthwhile? Am J Gastroenterol 2001;96(11):3152–7.
68. Bonis PA, Kaplan M. Methotrexate improves biochemical tests in patients with primary biliary cirrhosis who respond incompletely to ursodiol. Gastroenterology 1999;117:395–9.
69. Giljaca V, Poropat G, Stimac D, et al. Methotrexate for primary biliary cirrhosis. Cochrane Database Syst Rev 2010;5:CD004385.
70. Kaplan MM, Schmid C, Provenzale D, et al. A prospective trial of colchicine and methotrexate in the treatment of primary biliary cirrhosis. Gastroenterology 1999; 117:1173–80.
71. Gong Y, Gluud C. Colchicine for primary biliary cirrhosis. Cochrane Database Syst Rev 2004;2:CD004481.
72. Silveira M, Lindor K. Treatment of primary biliary cirrhosis: therapy with choleretic and immunosuppressive agents. Clin Liver Dis 2008;12(2):425–43.
73. Ian Gan S, de Jongh M, Kaplan MM. Modafinil in the treatment of debilitating fatigue in primary biliary cirrhosis: a clinical experience. Dig Dis Sci 2009; 54(10):2242–6.
74. Ghent CN, Carruthers SG. Treatment of pruritus in primary biliary cirrhosis with rifampin: results of a double-blind, crossover, randomized trial. Gastroenterology 1988;94:488–93.
75. Vuoristo M, Faarkkila M, Karvonen A, et al. A placebo-controlled trial of primary biliary cirrhosis treatment with colchicine and ursodeoxycholic acid. Gastroenterology 1995;108(5):1470–8.
76. Jones EA, Bergasa NV. The pruritus of cholestasis: from bile acids to opiate agonists. Hepatology 1990;11:884–7.
77. Jackson RD. Calcium plus vitamin D supplementation and the risk of fractures. N Engl J Med 2006;354(7):669–83.
78. Guanabens N, Vazquez I, Alvarez L, et al. Alendronate 70 mg once-weekly is more effective and has a better tolerability than alendronate 10 mg daily in the treatment of osteopenia associated with primary biliary cirrhosis. J Bone Miner Res 2005;20:S279.
79. Balan V, Dickson ER, Jorgensen RA, et al. Effect of ursodeoxycholic acid on serum lipids of patients with primary biliary cirrhosis. Mayo Clin Proc 1994;69:923–9.
80. Ritzel U, Leonhardt U, Nather M, et al. Simvastatin in primary biliary cirrhosis: effects on serum lipids and distinct disease markers. J Hepatol 2002;36:454–8.

81. Kurihara T, Maeda A, Shigemoto M, et al. Investigation into the efficacy of bezafi-brate against primary biliary cirrhosis, with histological references from cases receiving long term monotherapy. Am J Gastroenterol 2002;97:212–4.
82. Milkiewicz P. Liver transplantation in primary biliary cirrhosis. Clin Liver Dis 2008; 12:461–72.
83. Neuberger J. Liver transplantation for primary biliary cirrhosis: indications and risk of recurrence. J Hepatol 2003;39:142–8.

Special Considerations for Women with IBD

Stephanie M. Moleski, MD, Cuckoo Choudhary, MD

KEYWORDS

- Inflammatory bowel diseases • Crohn disease
- Ulcerative colitis • Women and IBD

Inflammatory bowel diseases (IBD), namely Crohn disease (CD) and ulcerative colitis (UC), are common in Western society, with as many as 1.4 million people in the United States and 2.2 million persons in Europe carrying these diagnoses.[1] Although there are no significant gender differences reported among patients with UC, CD does have a slight female predominance, with a male-to-female ratio of 1.0:1.8.[2] Because at least half of the patients suffering from these diseases are women, it is important that physicians are aware of their gender-specific needs. When considering matters specific to women with IBD, most discussions and articles revolve around pregnancy and IBD. There are, however, multiple other important concerns for women with UC and CD, including issues of body image and sexuality, menstruation, contraception, screening for cervical cancer, matters related to menopause and hormone replacement therapy, osteoporosis, and the overlap seen between irritable bowel syndrome (IBS) and IBD. In this article, we have addressed these important, non–pregnancy-related issues faced by women with IBD. Fertility, pregnancy, and IBD are discussed in a separate article by Dr Sunanda Kane, elsewhere in this issue.

BODY IMAGE/SEXUALITY

Many of the symptoms, morbidities, and quality-of-life issues in patients with IBD affect women's body image and sexuality.[3] Sexual dysfunction in this population was first highlighted by Moody and colleagues in 1992,[4] when they described decreased sexual activity in women with CD. They interviewed 50 women with IBD and age-matched controls. Twenty-four percent of the women with CD versus 4% of controls reported abstinence from sexual activity. The most common reason for decreased frequency of sexual activity was dyspareunia, which was reported by as many as 60% of patients with CD. Abdominal pain, diarrhea, and fear of fecal incontinence were other reasons for decreased frequency of sexual intercourse in this group of patients.

Division of Gastroenterology, Thomas Jefferson University Hospital, 132 South 10th Street, Philadelphia, PA, USA
E-mail address: Cuckoo.Choudhary@jefferson.edu

Gastroenterol Clin N Am 40 (2011) 387–398
doi:10.1016/j.gtc.2011.03.003
0889-8553/11/$ – see front matter © 2011 Published by Elsevier Inc.

gastro.theclinics.com

A year later, Moody and Mayberry[5] looked at the perceived sexual dysfunction among patients with IBD. Although differences in the frequency of sexual intercourse between the patients with IBD and controls did not reach statistical significance, patients with IBD cited numerous reasons why they limited their sexual activity, including fear of fecal incontinence, fatigue, abdominal pain, and urgency.

More recent studies have shown that women with IBD indicate that sexual function is significantly affected by their disease.[6-8] In a survey of 336 women with IBD ages 18 to 65, 63% reported low sexual activity. In this study, there was no specific feature of IBD that explained the high prevalence of sexual dysfunction. Psychosocial factors did, however, play a large role. The greatest risk factor was depressed mood, which affected all aspects of sexuality.[6]

Discussion of sexual health in the context of disease activity is essential to facilitate psychosocial adjustment to living with IBD. Unfortunately, physicians do not adequately address sexuality in women with these diseases.[7] Borum and colleagues[7] surveyed women with IBD addressing the frequency at which physicians (gastroenterologists, primary care physicians, and obstetricians/gynecologists) discuss issues related to IBD, sexuality, and sexual function. Of the 64 women surveyed, 12 (18.8%) reported that their gastroenterologist more frequently addressed issues of sexuality than their primary care physician (0%) or obstetrician/gynecologist (0%). The discussion of sexuality was reportedly initiated in all cases by the patient rather than the gastroenterologist.

It is important that physicians are aware of the impact IBD can have on women's body image and sexuality. Physicians need to do a better job at addressing issues of self-image and sexuality with their patients with IBD and provide support and disease-specific information to help with these issues. Although as gastroenterologists most of us remain focused on management of IBD disease activity, it is important to remember that issues of body image and sexuality are equally important to patients and it is our duty as physicians to make every attempt to initiate and discuss these issues with them.

MENSTRUATION

The premenstrual syndrome in women has been well described, dating back to 1973 when Timonen and Procope[9] first reported the symptoms of premenstrual irritability, depression, diarrhea, and constipation in healthy women. Fluctuations of hormonal levels during the menstrual cycle appear to influence gastrointestinal (GI) symptoms, resulting in nausea, constipation, and diarrhea. Although there are a few studies looking at the effects of the menstrual cycle on GI symptoms of patients with bowel disorders, less is available specifically with regard to IBD. One of the best studies reported in the literature to date was by Kane and colleagues,[10] in which they studied bowel symptoms and patterns in patients with IBD and IBS. In this study, patients with UC, CD, and IBS as well as healthy controls were interviewed. Reports of changes in patients' bowel habits and other symptoms during the premenstrual and menstrual phases of the cycle were compared with those of healthy women. Ninety-three percent of all patient participants reported experiencing premenstrual symptoms, the most common being emotional irritability followed by depression and weight gain. Patients with CD had more symptoms in general than controls. Premenstrual diarrhea was more common in patients with IBS and IBD than in controls, as was nausea for patients with CD or IBS versus controls. Patients with IBD and IBS were more likely to have a cyclical pattern to bowel habits, with diarrhea being the most common symptom.

Parlak and colleagues,[11] in their prospective study, investigated the difference between healthy women and those with IBD regarding GI and non-GI symptoms during the menstrual cycle. They found that GI symptoms and frequency of defecation were higher in patients with UC and CD than in controls. Patients with CD had more GI symptoms in all 3 phases of the menstrual cycle, whereas controls and patients with UC had fewer symptoms in the postmenstrual phase. The cyclic pattern present in healthy women persisted in patients with UC and CD.

These studies make it clear that the variation in GI symptoms during the menstrual cycle is prevalent. Sometimes patients with IBD may interpret the variation in bowel patterns occurring with the menstrual cycle as disease flare. Therefore, the menstrual cycle and its effect on bowel patterns should be taken into consideration when evaluating patients for disease activity.

CONTRACEPTION

Because IBD often affects women during their childbearing years, women with IBD need effective contraceptive options to avoid unintended pregnancies. Smaller family sizes and voluntary childlessness is seen more frequently in women with IBD.[12] Marri and colleagues[12] examined the considerations about pregnancy in patients with IBD. Their survey found that 18.0% of patients with CD and 14.0% with UC had a higher rate of voluntary childlessness compared with 6.2% in the general population. In addition, contraception use in the IBD population was lower than in the general population. Of all patients with IBD in this survey, 76% used contraception before the diagnosis of IBD and 82% after its diagnosis. Contraceptive options were similar to the general population with the most common choices being oral contraception (OC), barrier methods, and abstinence.

When women with IBD decide to proceed with pregnancy, it should be a planned event when the disease is well controlled. For this reason, the choice of contraception in patients with IBD is a very important issue. Ideally, it should have a very low to no failure rate and should have minimal to no effect on IBD disease activity. Although women with IBD have the same contraceptive choices as women without IBD, certain contraceptive methods may have specific cautions for patients with IBD. Barrier methods have typical user failure rates, which may make these methods inappropriate for use by women who are using teratogenic drugs. The use of intrauterine devices (IUDs) remains controversial in patients who are immunosuppressed. A literature review of immunosuppressed patients with primarily HIV or systemic lupus erythematosus found no increased risk of pelvic infection with the use of IUDs.[13] There are, however, limited case reports of patients with IBD who have exacerbation of IBD symptoms after insertion of IUDs.[14] Furthermore, Okoro and Kane[15] point out that any complication with an IUD could be misinterpreted by both the patient and the treating physician as an IBD flare up instead of possible pelvic inflammatory disease.

There are many issues specific to patients with IBD that must be considered regarding the use of OCs. Most of the absorption of OCs occurs in the small bowel. Patients with CD with inflammation or ulceration of the small bowel or those with increased transit as a result of surgery may have reduced efficacy of OCs. For patients with UC, pharmacokinetic studies have suggested that their plasma concentrations of steroid hormones are similar to that of healthy volunteers.[16,17]

There have been concerns regarding flare up of disease activity in patients with IBD who are taking OCs. Zapata and colleagues,[14] in their meta-analysis of contraceptive use among women with IBD, looked at 5 studies on this topic. None of the identified studies demonstrated a significant increased risk of disease relapse in patients with IBD who were taking OCs.

Another concern related to the use of OCs in the IBD population is that of thrombosis. There is evidence to suggest an increased risk of thrombosis in patients with

IBD, particularly in those with active or more extensive disease.[18] There are, however, no prospective studies looking at increased risk of thrombosis in patients with IBD who are taking OCs.

The risk with the use of OCs in the pathogenesis of IBD was reviewed by Cornish and colleagues.[19] Their meta-analysis found that women exposed to OCs had a pooled relative risk (RR) of 1.51 and 1.46 when adjusted for smoking and an increased RR with the length of exposure. The RR for women with UC taking OCs was 1.53 and 1.28 when adjusted for smoking. The risk for patients who stopped using OCs reverted to that of the nonexposed. The reduction in estrogen and progesterone content in OCs in the past 2 decades did not appear to reduce the RR of IBD. However, doses were not recorded in many of the studies. The investigators did not recommend that female patients stop OCs but rather that clinicians discuss possible risks with patients and consider alternative forms in patients with a strong family history of IBD.

CERVICAL SCREENING

In patients with IBD, data regarding the risk of cervical abnormality and cervical cancer has thus far been limited and inconsistent.[20–27] In a recent population-based, nested, case-control study, Huftless and colleagues[20] evaluated the risk of cervical cancer among women with IBD from 1996 to 2006. In this retrospective study, 1244 patients with IBD between the ages 15 and 68 from the Kaiser system in Northern California were assessed for a history of aminosalicylate and immunosuppressant use and the diagnosis of cervical cancer. After adjusting for age, ethnicity, and smoking history, Huftless and colleagues[20] found that women with IBD had a nonsignificant, 45% increased risk of cervical cancer over women with no IBD. They also noted a 4% increase in the number of Pap smears received by women with IBD compared with women with no IBD. Patients exposed to aminosalicylates and immune modulators and corticosteroids were found to have elevated risks of cancer but none of the associations were statistically significant. None of the patients with cervical cancer had an exposure to infliximab.

Another study looking at the positive association of cervical abnormalities and IBD is that done by Bhatia and colleagues[21] in 2006. This study demonstrated that a diagnosis of IBD in women correlates with an increased risk of abnormal Pap smear. Eighteen percent of patients with IBD had an abnormal Pap smear compared with 5% of controls. The type of IBD and exposure to immunosuppressive medications were not associated with increased risk of abnormal Pap smear. In 2008, Kane and colleagues[22] also found a significantly higher incidence of abnormal Pap smears in patients with IBD (42.5%) compared with controls (7%).

Other studies have not supported the relationship between IBD and cervical abnormalities. Lees and colleagues[23] recently published data that found no difference in rates of abnormal Pap smears between patients with IBD and controls. However, there were significantly more abnormal Pap smears in patients with IBD who were current smokers compared with ex-smokers and those who had never smoked. Similarly, Singh and colleagues[24] found no association between cervical abnormalities and UC. The increase in risk in women with CD was limited to those exposed to 10 or more prescriptions of OCs. Only the combined exposure to corticosteroids and immunosuppressants was associated with increased risk of cervical abnormalities.

Further studies are needed to assess if, in fact, women with IBD indeed have a higher incidence of cervical abnormality, and if they do, what is the underlying etiology? If women with IBD are found to have an increased incidence of cervical abnormality, there needs to be a system to ensure adequate cervical cancer screening to prevent unnecessary morbidity and mortality. Cervical testing protocols before and during immunosuppressant therapy may also be warranted.

MENOPAUSE/HORMONE REPLACEMENT THERAPY

Although IBD most commonly affects women in their reproductive years, we know that there is a bimodal peak of onset of both UC and CD and women may develop IBD for the first time after menopause. Furthermore, women whose disease onset occurred during their reproductive years will eventually go through menopause either naturally or surgically. It is important to understand the effects of IBD on menopause and vice versa. There are, however, very few data regarding menopause in patients with IBD. In 1989, Lichtarowicz and colleagues[28] surveyed women with CD regarding details of their menstrual cycles, age of menopause, history of surgery, smoking habits, and use of OCs. Of the 146 patients with CD who responded, 48 (34%) had undergone physiologic menopause at a mean age of 47.6 years compared with 49.6 years for the control group. The investigators concluded that CD was associated with premature menopause.

Conversely, Kane and colleagues,[29] in their retrospective review, sought to characterize the effects of menopause on IBD activity and identify possible modifiers of disease activity. They found a median age of menopause to be 48.2 years, similar to historical controls. In their study of 65 women, 20 with UC and 45 with CD, there was no apparent correlation between having a flare in the premenopausal state and postmenopausal state. However, when looking at hormone use, there appeared to be a protective effect in the use of hormone replacement therapy (HRT) on disease activity. Women with IBD using HRT compared with those not using HRT were 82% less likely to have a flare in the first 2 years of menopause. Those on HRT who did have a flare appeared to have less severe flares, as they did not require escalation of therapy to immunomodulator but rather required only an increased dose of mesalamine.

The use of HRT in women has recently become controversial since the Women's Health Initiative was published, showing no cardiovascular benefit with unopposed estrogen and a small increase in risk of breast cancer, coronary heart disease, stroke, and venous thromboembolism with combined therapy.[30] Until more research is available on the relationship between HRT and IBD, each individual patient's personal and family history should be considered before deciding on the use of hormones in the postmenopausal state.

OSTEOPOROSIS

Women with osteopenia or osteoporosis can potentially face severe health outcomes, including incapacitating fractures, dependency, and nursing home confinement. Over the past decade, the association between IBD and low bone mineral density (BMD) has become increasingly recognized. Patients with IBD have many risk factors for low BMD, including low body weight, frequent use of glucocorticoids, decreased intake of calcium and vitamin D owing to avoidance of dairy products, and impaired absorption of vitamin D and calcium owing to their chronic inflammatory state with elevated level of cytokines, such as interleukin (IL)-6, IL-1, and tumor necrosis factor (TNF). The prevalence of osteoporosis in IBD ranges from 15% to 42%, with osteopenia ranging from 22% to 77%. Fracture risk in patients with IBD ranges from 20% to 40%, which is greater than in the general population. Although in the general population osteoporosis is most common in postmenopausal women, in patients with IBD both men and women have a similar risk for osteoporosis and fracture.[31,32]

BMD can be measured by dual-energy X-ray absorption (DXA). The American Gastroenterological Association (AGA) and American College of Gastroenterology (ACG) guidelines published in 2003 outline recommendations on screening for osteoporosis in patients with GI diseases. The guidelines state that although DXA is a marker of low BMD and fracture risk, it is not the only consideration, and DXA should be used together with other clinical variables to predict fracture risk. They recommend screening with DXA in patients older than 50, in patients with recurrent glucocorticoid use or use for longer than 3 months, in patients with a personal history of low-trauma fracture, or in patients with hypogonadism.[32]

There has been some controversy as to whether patients who have undergone a restorative proctocolectomy (RPC) may have improved BMD. The AGA states that this procedure may be associated with an improvement in DXA score.[32] A recent study by McLaughlin and colleagues[33] that evaluated 53 patients with UC who had undergone RPC for UC found the prevalence of osteoporosis and osteopenia to be 43.4% and 13.2% respectively, similar to patients who had not undergone RPC. The investigators conclude that DXA screening should occur in line with the recommendations for the general UC population.

Although guidelines are available to help physicians in the diagnosis and treatment of osteoporosis, there is concern about the extent to which physicians implement these guidelines. A recent study by Wagnon and colleagues[34] addressed gastroenterologists' awareness and implementation of the AGA Medical Position Statement: Guidelines on Osteoporosis in Inflammatory Bowel Disease. Of the 258 gastroenterologists who responded to the survey, slightly fewer than half of the responders used the guidelines in decision making (126, 49%) or in the management (110, 42%) of their patients with IBD. Physicians whose practice was composed of more patients with IBD were more likely to follow the guidelines. The main reason physicians gave for not using the guidelines was that they felt IBD should be the focus of the visit (48, 42%); 34 (30%) reported that osteoporosis should be managed by another physician. Additional reasons included cost and lack of time and knowledge.

There are very few studies regarding treatment of low BMD and IBD. The AGA makes recommendations regarding an approach to managing bone health in patients with IBD. There should be an emphasis on patient education, prevention, and the importance of lifestyle changes such as encouraging weight-bearing exercise and avoidance of smoking, alcohol, and caffeine. Patients should be encouraged to take calcium (younger men and premenopausal women require 1000 mg/d and men and women older than 50 require 1500 mg/d). Patients generally need about 400 to 800 IU/d of vitamin D.[32]

Bisphosphonates are effective for the prevention and treatment of osteoporosis. Although most of the studies on bisphosphonates are in the general postmenopausal population, there are some that have been important in the care of patients with IBD. Alendronate, risedronate, and etidronate have been shown to be effective for the prevention and treatment of corticosteroid-induced osteoporosis.[35,36] In a prospective, double-blind placebo-controlled study by Palumba and colleagues,[37] long-term treatment with risedronate in postmenopausal osteoporotic women with IBD was shown to be effective in increasing BMD and reducing vertebral and nonvertebral fracture risk. On the other hand, studies by Bartram and colleagues looking at pamidronate and Siffledeen and colleagues using etidronate, there was no additional effect of these bisphosphonates on patients with CD and low BMD.[38,39] These studies and the side effects of bisphosphonates, including esophagitis and osteonecrosis of the jaw, make it reasonable to limit their use to that suggested by the AGA. The AGA recommends the use of bisphosphonates for the prevention and treatment of osteoporosis in patients with known osteoporosis, patients with atraumatic fractures, and patients taking corticosteroids for more than 3 consecutive months.[32]

Estrogen therapy is used to prevent osteoporosis in postmenopausal or hypogonadal women, but as mentioned previously, it is important to consider each patient's personal and family history before prescribing HRT.[40] There may be patients who require alternative therapies for low BMD, such as a selective estrogen receptor modulator or calcitonin. It may be necessary to seek the consultation of a bone disease specialist in such situations.

Finally, because inflammatory mediators in IBD, such as TNF-α, are involved in the disease process both in gut and bone, it has been proposed that anti-TNF-α could be an effective therapy for inflammation-related osteoporosis.[41] Franchimont and colleagues[42] studied 71 patients with CD who received a first dose of infliximab for refractory CD. Biochemical markers of bone formation (type-I procollagen N-terminal propeptide, bone-specific alkaline phosphatase, osteocalcin) and of bone resorption (C-telopeptide of type-I collagen) were measured in the serum before and after infliximab therapy. Eight weeks after treatment with infliximab, a normalization of bone markers was seen, as was a lower but significant decrease in resorption marker. An increase in bone formation markers was present in 30% to 61% of patients and a decrease in C-telopeptide of type-I collagen was present in 38% of patients. In a similar study, Abreu and colleagues[43] looked at the sera of 38 patients before and after infliximab therapy and evaluated the levels of markers of bone formation and markers of resorption. Infliximab therapy was associated with an increase in the marker of bone formation, bone alkaline phosphatase, but the marker of bone resorption, N-telopeptide of type I collagen, was not increased. The investigators concluded that infliximab therapy in CD may influence bone metabolism. These studies indicate that treatment with infliximab appears to be associated with increased markers of bone formation. It is unclear if this effect may be because of a beneficial effect of TNF-α blockade on bone turnover, a beneficial effect on CD activity resulting in decreased glucocorticoid dose, or both.[41–43]

It is important that clinicians identify risk factors for osteoporosis in the IBD population, that screening is properly implemented, and that prophylactic and bone density–saving measures are initiated early on.

IRRITABLE BOWEL SYNDROME AND IBD

Both IBS and IBD are common conditions in the Western world, with prevalence of IBS ranging from 9.0% to 12.0% and that of IBD from 0.1% to 0.2%.[44,45] It is therefore not surprising that both of these conditions often coexist in the same patient. Because IBD and IBS share several symptoms, such as diarrhea, abdominal pain, and bloating, it is often difficult for the physician to interpret GI symptoms in patients who carry both of these diagnoses, especially in those with IBD who, based on conventional tests, appear to be in remission but continue to frequent a physician's office with symptoms. What should physicians to do in such cases? Do physicians tell patients that their IBD is in remission and the symptoms are from IBS? And, if so, how do they support their decision with objective data, if at all? This poses a greater problem in women than in men, as IBS is more common in women. It can also be problematic in patients whose IBD is limited to the small bowel, in which case regular visualization of bowel lining to assess disease activity is not as easy. The diagnostic dilemma in previously mentioned cases has been accentuated by several recent reports of immune activation and even mild mucosal inflammation in patients with IBS leading to the age-old important question of whether IBS is nothing but a very mild form of IBD.

Shanahan and colleagues[45] addressed this issue very well in a recent prospective study in which they looked at patients with IBD (both UC and CD) who were considered to be in clinical remission on the basis of standard, well-defined criteria and looked at the prevalence of IBS-type symptoms in this group. This article also looked at the association of IBS-like symptoms in patients to levels of fecal calprotectin.[45] Calprotectin is a calcium-bound and zinc-bound protein that accounts for 60% of the soluble proteins in the granulocytes and is thought to be a very sensitive indicator of ongoing inflammation in IBD.[46] This study, which was done over 18 months, included 106 patients: 62 with CD and 44 with UC. In addition to being in clinical remission by standard criteria, 37 (60%) of the patients with CD and 17 (39%) of the patients with UC met Rome criteria for IBS **Box 1**. What was very interesting was that the fecal calprotectin levels among both patients with CD and those with UC and IBS were 8-fold to 12-fold higher than both control subjects and those with IBS. In addition, the fecal calprotectin levels were 2 to 3 times higher than those in patients with IBD without symptoms. Based on their study, the investigators concluded that the presence of IBS symptoms in patients with IBD who are otherwise considered to be in clinical remission based on standard criteria indicates ongoing mild disease activity. They go on to recommend that treating physicians should exercise caution while diagnosing IBS in patients with IBD, even when the latter appears to be in remission.[45] This study validates the utility of fecal calprotectin in differentiating IBD from IBS.

Shanahan and colleagues'[45] study is somewhat limited by the "black" or "white" interpretation of patient symptoms, ie, either the patient has IBD or IBS. Although this dichotomy is possible, it is also feasible that both the disorders coexist in the same patient, something that we have believed for years. Based on prior knowledge, we know that microscopic inflammation of the intestinal mucosa, associated cytokine activity, and the hypothalamic-pituitary-adrenal axis are all responsible for symptoms in both IBD and IBS, although the profile of cytokine activity may differ between IBD and IBS.[46,47] We are also aware that cytokine activation and release of mediators from the mast cells cause visceral hypersensitivity.[48,49] Psychological factors including stress in life can increase pain and disease activity for all medical conditions including IBD and IBS. At the peripheral level, stress can alter bacterial flora and disrupt the mucosal barrier, leading to transmigration of bacterial products, thereby increasing cytokine release and ultimately an increase in visceral hypersensitivity. This explanation of what happens at the peripheral level may be responsible for the elevated fecal calprotectin levels seen in patients with IBD who are otherwise in clinical remission. At the central level, stress can amplify pain perception and other GI symptoms. It is possible, therefore, that these patients' symptoms can actually be explained by IBS and that IBS may in fact be responsible for the mild mucosal inflammation seen in this group of patients, as in the study by Shanahan and colleagues.[45] In short, these patients have both IBS and IBD and not just one or the other. An outstanding editorial

---

Box 1
Rome II criteria for IBS

Abdominal pain or discomfort for at least 12 weeks or more in an year, which need not be consecutive, associated with any two of the following features:

1. Pain relieved by defecation
2. Onset of pain associated with change in stool frequency
3. Onset of pain associated with change in stool form

by Drossman and colleagues[50] analyzed these possible etiologies of mucosal inflammation in IBS and recommends that a larger study is needed to look at the impact of psychological stress on intestinal mucosal inflammation in IBD.

Recognition of this overlap may lead to a combined approach of treating both the IBD and the IBS components of the patient's symptoms, help physicians minimize unnecessary use of steroids and other immunomodulators in an attempt to treat the mild inflammation, and help them focus their attention on other aspects of patient treatment. Furthermore, treatment of both IBD and IBS components of the disorder in a patient will decrease both patient and physician anxiety, reduce health care costs, and ultimately lead to improvement in the quality-of-life measures in this group of patients as well.[50,51]

SUMMARY

Many characteristics of both UC and CD can have a significant impact on multiple aspects of women's lives.[3] Physicians must not only be aware of the impact IBD can have on women's health, body image, and sexuality, but they also need to address these issues with patients and provide support and disease-specific information regarding these issues. Variation in bowel patterns during the menstrual cycle is high in this population; therefore, the menstrual cycle and its effect on bowel patterns should be taken into consideration when evaluating patients for disease activity. Contraception, cervical screening, and, for perimenopausal patients, hormone replacement therapy are issues that must be paid close attention to in women patients with IBD. Osteoporosis is an additional problem that must be considered not just in postmenopausal patients but in all patients with IBD, as there are increased risk factors for low bone mineral density. Finally, there is significant overlap between symptoms in patients with IBS and IBD, such as abdominal pain and diarrhea. Distinguishing between IBD flares and IBS symptoms can be a challenge for gastroenterologists.

REFERENCES

1. Loftus EV Jr. Clinical epidemiology of inflammatory bowel disease: incidence, prevalence, and environmental influences. Gastroenterology 2004;126(6): 1504–17.
2. Andres PG, Friedman LS. Epidemiology and the natural course of inflammatory bowel disease. Gastroenterol Clin North Am 1999;28:255–81.
3. Muller KR, Prosser R, Bampton P, et al. Female gender and surgery impair relationships, body image, and sexuality in inflammatory bowel disease: patient perceptions. Inflamm Bowel Dis 2010;16(4):657–63.
4. Moody G, Probert CS, Srivastava EM, et al. Sexual dysfunction amongst women with Crohn's disease: a hidden problem. Digestion 1992;52:179–83.
5. Moody GA, Mayberry JF. Perceived sexual dysfunction amongst patients with inflammatory bowel disease. Digestion 1993;54:256–60.
6. Timmer A, Kempter D, Bauer A. Determinants of sexual function in inflammatory bowel disease: a survey-based cross-sectional analysis. BMC Gastroenterol 2008;8:45.
7. Borum ML, Igiehon E, Shafa S. Physicians may inadequately address sexuality in women with inflammatory bowel disease. Inflamm Bowel Dis 2007;13(10): 1236–43.
8. Trachter AB, Rogers AI, Leiblum SR. Inflammatory bowel disease in women: impact on relationship and sexual health. Inflamm Bowel Dis 2002;8(6):413–21.

9. Timonen S, Procope B. The premenstrual syndrome: frequency and association of symptoms. Ann Chir Gynaecol Fenn 1973;62:108–16.

10. Kane SV, Sable K, Hanauer SB. The menstrual cycle and its effect in inflammatory bowel disease and irritable bowel syndrome: a prevalence study. Am J Gastroenterol 1998;93:1867–72.

11. Parlak E, Dağli U, Alkim C, et al. Pattern of gastrointestinal and psychosomatic symptoms across the menstrual cycle in women with inflammatory bowel disease. Turk J Gastroenterol 2003;14(4):250–6.

12. Marri SR, Ahn C, Buchman AL. Voluntary childlessness is increased in women with inflammatory bowel disease. Inflamm Bowel Dis 2007;13(5):591–9.

13. Browne H, Manipalviratn S, Armstrong A. Using an intrauterine device in immunocompromised women. Obstet Gynecol 2008;112(3):667–9.

14. Zapata LB, Paulen ME, Cansino C, et al. Contraceptive use among women with inflammatory bowel disease: a systematic review. Contraception 2010;82(1): 72–85.

15. Okoro NI, Kane SV. Gender-related issues in the female inflammatory bowel disease patient. Expert Rev Gastroenterol Hepatol 2009;3(2):145–54.

16. Grimmer S, Back D, Orme M, et al. The bioavailability of ethinyloestradiol and levonorgestrel in patients with an ileostomy. Contraception 1986;33:51–9.

17. Nilsson L, Victor A, Kral J, et al. Absorption of an oral contraceptive gestagen in ulcerative colitis before and after proctocolectomy and construction of a continent ileostomy. Contraception 1985;31:195–204.

18. Miehsler W, Reinisch W, Valic E, et al. Is inflammatory bowel disease an independent and disease specific risk factor for thromboembolism? Gut 2004;53(4): 542–8.

19. Cornish JA, Tan E, Simillis C, et al. The risk of oral contraceptives in the etiology of inflammatory bowel disease: a meta-analysis. Am J Gastroenterol 2008;103(9): 2394–400.

20. Hutfless S, Fireman B, Kane S, et al. Screening differences and risk of cervical cancer in inflammatory bowel disease. Aliment Pharmacol Ther 2008;28(5): 598–605.

21. Bhatia J, Bratcher J, Korelitz B, et al. Abnormalities of uterine cervix in women with inflammatory bowel disease. World J Gastroenterol 2006;12(38):6167–71.

22. Kane S, Khatibi B, Reddy D. Higher incidence of abnormal Pap smears in women with inflammatory bowel disease. Am J Gastroenterol 2008;103(3):631–6.

23. Lees CW, Critchley J, Chee N, et al. Lack of association between cervical dysplasia and IBD: a large case-control study. Inflamm Bowel Dis 2009;15(11): 1621–9.

24. Singh H, Demers AA, Nugent Z, et al. Risk of cervical abnormalities in women with inflammatory bowel disease: a population-based nested case-control study. Gastroenterology 2009;136(2):451–8.

25. Minor MA. Is it time for increased Pap performance? Cervical cancer and Pap testing in women with inflammatory bowel disease. Inflamm Bowel Dis 2010; 16(1):175–6.

26. Moscandrew M, Mahadevan U, Kane S. General health maintenance in IBD. Inflamm Bowel Dis 2009;15(9):1399–409.

27. Kane S, Reddy D. Infliximab use does not increase the risk for abnormal Pap smears in women. Am J Gastroenterol 2005;99:S246.

28. Lichtarowicz A, Norman C, Calcraft B, et al. A study of the menopause, smoking, and contraception in women with Crohn's disease. Q J Med 1989;72(267): 623–31.

29. Kane SV, Reddy D. Hormonal replacement therapy after menopause is protective of disease activity in women with inflammatory bowel disease. Am J Gastroenterol 2008;103(5):1193–6.
30. Anderson GL, Limacher M, Assaf AR, et al, Women's Health Initiative Steering Committee. Effects of conjugated equine estrogen in postmenopausal women with hysterectomy: the Women's Health Initiative randomized controlled trial. JAMA 2004;291(14):1701–12.
31. Ezzat Y, Hamdy K. The frequency of low bone mineral density and its associated risk factors in patients with inflammatory bowel diseases. Int J Rheum Dis 2010; 13(3):259–65.
32. American Gastroenterological Association medical position statement: guidelines on osteoporosis in gastrointestinal diseases. Gastroenterology 2003;124(3): 791–4.
33. McLaughlin SD, Perry-Woodford ZL, Clark SK, et al. Osteoporosis in patients over 50 years of age following restorative proctocolectomy for ulcerative colitis: is DXA screening warranted? Inflamm Bowel Dis 2010;16(2):250–5.
34. Wagnon JH, Leiman DA, Ayers GD, et al. Survey of gastroenterologists' awareness and implementation of AGA guidelines on osteoporosis in inflammatory bowel disease patients: are the guidelines being used and what are the barriers to their use? Inflamm Bowel Dis 2009;15(7):1082–9.
35. Saag KG, Emkey R, Schnitzer TJ, et al. Alendronate for the prevention and treatment of glucocorticoid-induced osteoporosis. Glucocorticoid-Induced Osteoporosis Intervention Study Group. N Engl J Med 1998;339:292–9.
36. Bernstein CN, Leslie WD, Leboff M. AGA technical review: osteoporosis in gastrointestinal disease. Gastroenterology 2003;124:795–841.
37. Palomba S, Manguso F, Orio F Jr, et al. Effectiveness of risedronate in osteoporotic postmenopausal women with inflammatory bowel disease: a prospective, parallel, open-label, two-year extension study. Menopause 2008;15(4 Pt 1):730–6.
38. Bartram SA, Peaston RT, Rawlings DJ, et al. A randomized controlled trial of calcium with vitamin D, alone or in combination with intravenous pamidronate, for the treatment of low bone mineral density associated with Crohn's disease. Aliment Pharmacol Ther 2003;18:1121–7.
39. Siffledeen JS, Fedorak RN, Siminoski K, et al. Randomized trial of etidronate plus calcium and vitamin D for treatment of low bone mineral density in Crohn's disease. Clin Gastroenterol Hepatol 2005;3:122–32.
40. Clements D, Compston JE, Evans WD, et al. Hormone replacement therapy prevents bone loss in patients with inflammatory bowel disease. Gut 1993; 34(11):1543–6.
41. Tilg H, Moschen AR, Kaser A, et al. Gut, inflammation and osteoporosis: basic and clinical concepts. Gut 2008;57(5):684–94.
42. Franchimont N, Putzeys V, Collette J, et al. Rapid improvement of bone metabolism after infliximab treatment in Crohn's disease. Aliment Pharmacol Ther 2004; 20:607–14.
43. Abreu MT, Geller JL, Vasiliauskas EA, et al. Treatment with infliximab is associated with increased markers of bone formation in patients with Crohn's disease. J Clin Gastroenterol 2006;40:55–63.
44. Hungin AP, Whorwell PJ, Tack J, et al. The prevalence, pattern, and impact of irritable bowel syndrome: an international survey of 40,000 subjects. Aliment Pharmacol Ther 2003;17:643–50.
45. Bernstein CN, Shanahan F. Disorders of modern lifestyle: reconciling the epidemiology of IBD. Gut 2008;57:1185–91.

46. Keohane J, O'Mahoney C, O'Mahoney L, et al. IBS-type symptoms in patients with IBD: a real association or reflection of occult inflammation? Am J Gastroenterol 2010;105:1789–94.
47. Schoepfer AM, Beglinger C, Straumann A, et al. Fecal calprotectin correlates more closely with the simple endoscopic score for CD than CRP, blood leukocytes, and the CDAI. Am J Gastroenterol 2010;105:162–9.
48. Dinan TG, Quigley EMM, Ahmed SM, et al. Hypothalamic-pituitary-gut axis dysregulation in IBS: plasma cytokines as a potential biomarker? Gastroenterology 2006;130:304–11.
49. Barbara G, Stanghellini V, De Georgio, et al. Activated mast cells in proximity to colonic nerves correlate with abdominal pain in IBS. Gastroenterology 2004;126:693–702.
50. Long MD, Drossman DA. Inflammatory bowel disease, irritable bowel syndrome, or what? A challenge to the functional-organic dichotomy. Am J Gastroenterol 2010;105(8):1796–8.
51. Simrén M, Axelsson J, Gillberg R, et al. Quality of life in inflammatory bowel disease in remission: the impact of IBS-like symptoms and associated psychological factors. Am J Gastroenterol 2002;97(2):389–96.

Inflammatory Bowel Disease in Pregnancy

Dawn B. Beaulieu, MD[a], Sunanda Kane, MD, MSPH, AGAF[b],*

KEYWORDS

- Inflammatory bowel disease • IBD • Crohn's disease
- Ulcerative colitis • Pregnancy • Breastfeeding • Fertility

Crohn disease (CD) and ulcerative colitis (UC) commonly affect women in their childbearing years. Fortunately, advances in the field of inflammatory bowel disease (IBD) have made successful pregnancy outcomes a reality for many women. These advances have led to family planning as a common discussion between gastroenterologists and IBD patients. Fertility, conception, medication safety, pregnancy, delivery, and breastfeeding are common discussion topics although there are limited available data. With approximately 50% of patients less than 35 years of age at the time of diagnosis and 25% conceiving for the first time after their diagnosis of IBD,[1–3] education and patient awareness have become vital factors in successful pregnancy outcomes.

INHERITANCE

Family history is the strongest predictor for developing IBD. A Danish study looking at a population of 5.2 million found that the risk for UC and CD among offspring of patients with IBD was 2 to 13 times higher than the risk within the general population.[4] Another study looking at the lifetime risks for IBD estimated that there was a 5.2% risk for CD and 1.6% risk for UC in first-degree relatives of probands.[5] If both parents have IBD, this risk of their child having IBD has been shown as high as 36%.[6,7] Although these statistics can be intimidating to patients, it is important to emphasize that IBD is an uncommon condition and not inherited in a true mendelian fashion.

Supportive foundations: None.
Disclosures: Dawn B. Beaulieu, consultant for Abbott Laboratories; Sunanda Kane, Consultant for Abbott, Elan, Millenium, UCB, Warner Chilcott, and Shire. Research support from Elan, Shire, and Warner Chilcott.
[a] Division of Gastroenterology, Hepatology and Nutrition, Inflammatory Bowel Disease Center, Vanderbilt University, 1211 21st Avenue South, Suite 220 MAB, Nashville, TN 37232, USA
[b] Division of Gastroenterology and Hepatology, Mayo Clinic, 200 First Street South West, Rochester, MN 55905, USA
* Corresponding author.
E-mail address: kane.sunanda@mayo.edu

Gastroenterol Clin N Am 40 (2011) 399–413
doi:10.1016/j.gtc.2011.03.006
0889-8553/11/$ – see front matter © 2011 Elsevier Inc. All rights reserved.

FERTILITY

Fecundability is the ability to conceive after 1 menstrual cycle whereas infertility is the inability to conceive after 12 months of unprotected intercourse in women less than 35 years of age or after 6 months in women 35 or older. The current infertility rate for the general population has been shown to be approximately 10%, with 11.8% of women ages 15 to 44 with impaired fecundity.[8] Although older studies have estimated infertility rates as between 32% and 42% in women with CD,[9,10] more recent population-based and community-based studies indicate infertility rates as closer to 5% to 14%, which is similar to the general population.[11–13] Although one case-control study documented the increased need for infertility treatments in IBD women, this was not significant after controlling for maternal age.[14] Before surgery, age is the only independent risk factor affecting IBD fertility.[15] Voluntary childlessness in IBD women is most likely greater than in the general population, as one case-control study of 216 patients revealed that a decrease in mean number of children born to IBD women was the result of choice and not inability.[16]

Women with UC or CD seem to have fertility rates similar to the general population although this changes after surgical intervention. In 2002, Ording Olsen and colleagues[17] found that women before and after the diagnosis of UC had fecundability ratios equal to that of the general population (fecundability ratio = 1.01) but after ileal pouch–anal anastomosis (IPAA) the fecundability ratio decreased to 0.20 ($P<.001$). A meta-analysis demonstrated a 3-fold increased risk for infertility in patients who had an IPAA, with infertility increasing from 15% to 48% in women post-IPAA.[18] Among a study of 945 patients in 7 studies, the infertility rate before restorative proctocolectomy was 12% and rose to 26% after IPAA.[19] A decrease in fertility also occurs in women with familial adenomatous polyposis who undergo IPAA and those with a proctocolectomy with ileostomy.[20] In CD, surgery may decrease fertility more than medical therapy alone.[21] Fertility in CD is most likely consistent with the general population but may be impaired in those with active disease. Infertility risks should be discussed with patients along with the consideration of delaying pouch formation until after childbearing or considering an ileorectal anastomosis to possibly preserve fertility.[22]

The true rate of male IBD infertility is unknown and a difficult endpoint to measure. A survey of 106 CD men, 62 UC men, and 140 controls revealed a similar fecundability between IBD patients and controls, suggesting that the high rate of infertility in CD men was voluntary.[23] There are no definitive studies, but the general consensus is that IBD does not affect male fertility. In those men who have undergone an IPAA, there has been a small incidence of retrograde ejaculation and erectile dysfunction but overall IPAA may preserve or improve sexual function outcome.[24]

Although cervical dysplasia has been cited as a factor for reduced fertility, it is controversial whether this plays a role in women with IBD.[25,26]

Men on sulfasalazine have reversible impairment of sperm motility and sperm counts in up to 60% of patients.[27] This effect is reversible, however, within 2 full cycles of spermatogenesis or within 2 months of cessation of the drug. A small single-center study suggests that infliximab (INF) therapy decreases sperm motility and oval forms, but this has yet to be translated into a clinical decrease in male fertility rates on INF.[28]

Reproductive issues are major concerns of IBD women; recent studies reported that many IBD patients refrain from having children due to concerns of adverse reproductive outcomes.[29,30] Discussions on fertility and risk factors should be with a more positive outlook than in the past to overcome many misconceptions.

EFFECT OF IBD ON PREGNANCY

It is widely believed that the impact of IBD on pregnancy depends on disease activity at conception. Studies suggest that quiescent disease throughout pregnancy leads to risks similar to that of the general population regarding spontaneous abortion, pregnancy-related complications, and adverse perinatal outcomes.[31–33] Disease activity at conception has been associated with preterm births, low birth weight (LBW), and fetal loss.[31,34–37] In addition, active disease during pregnancy has been shown the greatest risk of adverse perinatal outcomes.[3,31,38] This risk seems higher in women with CD than with UC. Severe disease relapses during pregnancy in UC, however, are associated with shorter gestation periods and lower birth weights.[39] Reddy and colleagues[39] found a higher risk of preterm births among their study group, with the mean gestational age 35 weeks versus 38.7 weeks in the control group (without disease relapse). Despite a consistent trend of preterm delivery, most of the deliveries occurred after 35 weeks with favorable outcomes.[40]

In a cohort of 54 pregnant CD patients, patients with active disease at conception had rates of miscarriage up to 35% higher than those patients who were in remission.[13] In 2007, Norgard and colleagues[41] examined the impact of disease activity on birth outcomes in CD and reported that activity during pregnancy only increased the risk of preterm birth. It also has been shown that the presence of ileal disease in CD women was a strong predictor for LBW.[42] In a study by Dominitz and colleagues,[40] greater risk of congenital abnormalities was seen in UC women compared with controls (7.9% vs 1.7%, P<.001). This study failed to take into consideration, however, disease activity or medication use and has not been replicated by other investigators. Most studies have found no greater risk in malformations in UC or CD.[35,37,43] Lamah and Scott[44] determined that there was no increased risk of spontaneous abortions, perinatal mortality, or congenital malformations in their UC cohort.

The largest study to date on this topic is the meta-analysis by Cornish and colleagues,[45] which evaluated 12 studies in regard to the impact of IBD on pregnancy. This study comprised 3907 patients with IBD and 320,531 controls. Based on this analysis, women with IBD were more likely to experience adverse pregnancy outcomes, such as premature birth and LBW. Premature delivery was almost twice as likely compared with the general population. Women with IBD were also 1.5 times more likely to undergo cesarean section. Unfortunately, neither medication use nor disease activity was analyzed as a confounder, which makes it difficult to put the results into perspective. The meta-analysis reported a 2.37-fold greater risk of congenital abnormalities (95% CI, 1.47, 3.82; P<.001) but most of the studies included failed to differentiate between minor and major malformations.[45] In 2006, a Spanish study of 124 pregnant CD women looked at pregnancies before and after diagnosis. It concluded that the course of IBD did not adversely affect pregnancy or the postpartum time period. Furthermore, the study determined that diagnosis before pregnancy did not influence the number of cesarean sections performed or increase the presence of LBW infants.[46]

In 2007, in the largest US study to date, Mahadevan and colleagues[47] compared pregnancy outcomes between women affected with IBD and those unaffected. The study comprised 461 pregnant IBD patients and a randomly selected cohort of age-matched controls. They found that women with IBD were more likely to have an adverse pregnancy complication (stillbirth, preterm birth, or small for gestational age; odds ratio [OR] 1.54 (95% CI, 1.00, 2.38), spontaneous abortion (OR, 1.65; 95% CI, 1.09, 2.48), or complication of labor (OR 1.78; 95% CI, 1.13, 2.81) than those women without IBD. Irrespective of disease activity, there was no difference in adverse newborn outcomes or congenital abnormalities. Independent predictors of adverse outcomes included IBD diagnosis, history of IBD surgery, and nonwhite ethnicity. The use of IBD medications was not found predictive of adverse outcome in this large, nonreferral population. There also was no statistically significant difference in newborn outcomes between the IBD and control pregnancies. Furthermore, severity of disease and medical treatment were not associated with adverse outcomes.

In the general population, maternal smoking is a known risk factor for LBW infants and for disease activity in CD women.[2] Pregnant CD patients who smoke are at a substantial increased risk for LBW and preterm delivery.[2,44] Conversely, maternal smoking in UC women does not increase their risk of preterm delivery.[14] Given the known risk of maternal smoking on the mother and baby, maternal smoking cessation should be discouraged in all scenarios.

Many studies continue to associate preterm birth and IBD; however, the majority of these "preterm" deliveries occurred after 35 weeks of gestation.[14,40] It is possible that safety concerns for the mother and baby may prompt induction of early delivery, which would bias the end result of an LBW infant. These factors need to be more clearly defined. Despite many observational studies, it is difficult to determine the effect of drug and/or drug cessation versus the disease itself on pregnancy outcomes. Premature infants and LBW are consistently observed, although most studies have shown that the risk of congenital malformations shows no increase compared with the 1% to 4.8% risk seen in the general population.[32,35,40,48,49] Despite mixed data, it seems that the disease activity can be an impetus for adverse pregnancy outcomes,[50] because miscarriages are seen more frequently with active disease.[40,48,49] In the Mahadevan study, however, disease activity was not found predictive of adverse outcome.[47]

EFFECT OF PREGNANCY ON IBD

A consistent finding in recent literature has been that the rate of disease flare during pregnancy (26%–34%) is similar to nonpregnant flare rates.[34,37,51,52] An exacerbation rate of 34% per year during pregnancy in UC women and 32% per year when not pregnant was observed by Nielson and colleagues in 1983.[35] These rates of relapse were similar in the CD population.[37] In addition, the Kaiser cohort, as discussed previously, included women with inactive disease throughout their pregnancy with no sudden increase in activity postpartum.[47,51]

Ulcerative Colitis

When conception occurs during a quiescent state, 70% to 80% of UC patients remain in remission.[2,35] The rate of relapse is thus similar to nonpregnant UC patients. It was initially believed that an increase of disease flare occurred in both the first trimester and postpartum, but timing of a flare seems more related to disease activity at conception and at term. Moreover, disease flare is often related to discontinuation of medical therapy (first trimester) or resuming maternal smoking after delivery (postpartum).[2,38,53] Active disease at conception can be associated with a worse prognosis. In a cohort of UC patients, Willoughby and Truelove[16] noted that active disease during conception was more resistant to treatment.

Patients who have undergone an ileoanal anastomosis procedure present a unique situation. In 67 pregnancies in 38 UC women with IPAA, it was found that pregnancy was safe with some alteration of pouch function almost exclusively during the third trimester.[54] For most women, pouch function ultimately returns to its prepregnancy state. There was a small proportion of women who suffered long-term disturbance of pouch function. This long-term effect was not related to the method of delivery. Although the mode of delivery in a pouch patient remains disputed, the method of delivery should not be determined by the presence of a pouch but by patient and obstetric preferences and indications. There are no long-term data on pouch function after vaginal delivery but short-term data show that pouch function, continence, and quality of life are not affected by uncomplicated vaginal delivery.[2,55]

Crohn Disease

CD during pregnancy is similar to patients with UC. As with UC, the key to a good outcome is the disease state at conception and delivery. If CD is quiescent at conception, 70% of pregnant CD patients remain quiescent compared with the nonpregnant CD patient.[2,13,56] There has been some suggestion that CD symptoms may even improve during gestation, although relapse was more common in the first trimester.[2,13,14] When disease is active at the time of conception, the authors follow the rule of thirds. One-third of women get better, one-third stay the same, and one-third worsen. The biologic mechanism of this finding has yet to be fully explained, but several studies have suggested that the immune disparity between mother and fetus may play a role in immune regulation, thereby altering immune function and pathology.[57]

DELIVERY

The recommended mode of delivery in CD patients is still controversial. In comparison with the general population, CD patients undergo cesarean sections more frequently, with the rate of cesarean sections increasing after first delivery.[58,59] Using the 2005 Nationwide Inpatient Sample, Nguyen and colleagues[60] examined 2372 CD deliveries and 1368 UC deliveries. In this population-based study, the adjusted ORs of a cesarean section were higher in women with CD (adjusted OR 1.72) and UC (adjusted OR 1.29) compared with non-IBD controls. There are conflicting data concerning vaginal deliveries and perianal disease. The recommendation to avoid vaginal deliveries in the setting of active perianal disease was based on small, observational studies. In contrast, many IBD physicians feel that CD patients with uncomplicated disease should be treated like the general population when deciding on delivery, but episiotomy should be avoided. The concern with vaginal delivery is not pouch injury but potential anal sphincter damage. Although pouch function may deteriorate during pregnancy, after pregnancy it has been shown to revert back to the prepregnancy state.[61] The presence of a colostomy or ileostomy also should not designate delivery choice. Despite limited data, choice of delivery should be a collaborative decision between patient, gastroenterologist, and obstetrician.

BREASTFEEDING

Any detriment to maternal health secondary to nursing after delivery is controversial. There have been many reported associations between nursing and increased disease activity, but it is unclear whether this is related to disease course or cessation of medication. Kane and Lemieux[53] found the OR of disease flare for women who breastfeed to be 2.2 (95% CI, 1.2, 2.7) compared with those who did not breastfeed. Once medication discontinuation was factored in, however, the OR became nonsignificant. Moffatt and colleagues[62] published a population-based study of breastfeeding and found no increased risk of flare in the postpartum period and a possible protective effect once the discontinuation of medications was taken into account.

Patient concerns surrounding breastfeeding are related to secretion of medication into breast milk leading to exposure to the baby. Medications known to be safe for breastfeeding include sulfasalazine, mesalamine, and steroids with only a minimal amount secreted into the milk. There is a rare association of diarrhea in the infant with aminosalicylates.[63] Metronidazole is excreted in breast milk and suspension of breastfeeding for 12 to 24 hours after dosing is recommended. Data thus far on thiopurines suggest minimal secretion into breast milk. In the past, breastfeeding was discouraged with azathioprine (AZA)/6-mercaptopurine (6-MP) use, but current data are more positive. Four women on AZA and breastfeeding were reported by Moretti and colleagues.[64] Two of the women did not have detectable levels of AZA and all four successfully breastfed without complications. Two other studies measured metabolite levels in breastfeeding infants and found zero to low levels of drug in breast milk. They also found no signs of hematologic or clinical immunosuppression in 10 infants.[65,66] The most recent and elegant study by Christensen and colleagues[67] in 2008 revealed that the most 6-MP in breast milk was excreted in the first 4 hours after drug intake in the 8 lactating women studied. The maximum concentration was measured and it was calculated that the infant ingested less than 0.008 mg/kg bodyweight per 24 hours. Waiting 4 hours after dosing to breastfeed is warranted and one strategy is nighttime dosing with pumping and dumping of breast milk 4 hours later. Although all of this is reassuring, the risks and benefits of breastfeeding must be discussed and there does not seem to be a contraindication to breastfeeding on 6-MP/AZA. Biologics have not been detected in breast milk and are usually continued postpartum.[68]

LONG-TERM EFFECTS OF PREGNANCY ON IBD

There have not been any data to suggest a detrimental long-term effect of pregnancy on the course of IBD and there is never a role for elective termination based on a history of IBD alone. In specific cases of presence of methotrexate (MTX) or thalidomide exposure, the decision for a therapeutic abortion may need to be addressed given that these have a known association with fetal abnormalities. Pregnancy has not been shown to definitively alter disease phenotype.[59] Riis and colleagues[59] along with Castiglione and colleagues[69] demonstrated that parous IBD patients experienced a reduction in relapse rate in the 3 years after pregnancy when compared with the 3 preceding years.[2,59,70] The rate of relapse decreased in the years after pregnancy in both UC and CD. Riis and colleagues[59] looked at 580 IBD pregnancies in a European cohort. The pregnancy itself did not influence disease phenotype or surgery rates, but it was associated with a reduced number of flares in the succeeding years (UC 0.34 vs 0.18 flares/y, $P = .008$, and CD 0.76 vs 0.12 flares/y, $P = .004$). In addition, a negative correlation between increasing parity and number of resections has been demonstrated.[2,71] Nwokolo and colleagues[71] found that in parous women with CD, the need for surgical resection was inversely correlated with increasing parity. In parous IBD women, the incidence of relapses in the first 3 years after pregnancy was lower than before pregnancy.[69] Hormonal changes during and after pregnancy may account for a change in fibrosis and stricture formation.[32] Some studies suggest a down-regulation of the immune system with maternal fetal HLA disparity.[57] Maternal immune response to paternal HLA antigens may result in immunosuppression that can in turn affect the maternal immune-mediated response. Kane and colleagues[57] looked at 50 pregnancies in 38 women and found 42 disparate (84%) at the HLA-DRB1 locus, 34 (68%) at the HLA-DQ locus, and 31 (62%) at both loci. A significant difference was found in IBD activity between women mismatched at both loci versus only 1 or neither locus (OR 8.4, $P = .01$). Improvement of IBD symptoms during pregnancy was associated with disparity in HLA class II antigens between mother and fetus. When logistic regression was performed, prepartum disease activity and disparity at both HLA-DRB1 and HLA-DQ were significant predictors of overall disease activity during pregnancy. There has been no evidence to support a detrimental effect of pregnancy on IBD and, on the contrary, pregnancy has been shown to decrease disease activity and surgical need in certain patients. Given the cumulative data, pregnancy should never be discouraged or terminated on the basis of an IBD diagnosis alone but on a combination of other factors.

IBD MEDICATIONS

It is believed that the greatest risk to IBD pregnancy is active disease not active therapy. Fear of medication effect on the fetus often prompts a physician and/or patient to discontinue all medications. Pregnancy data on outcomes and disease course are complicated by the cessation of drugs, but the risk of complications during pregnancy seems primarily related to disease activity and not medication effect.[2,30] In 2010, Zelinkova and colleagues[30] addressed voluntary childlessness and found that the 2 most important reasons IBD patients chose not to have a child were fear of side effects of medication on the baby and the advice given by physicians.

Aminosalicylates

One of the earliest available drugs for the treatment of colitis, sulfasalazine, readily crosses the placenta but has not been linked to any fetal abnormalities in several large studies. Patients taking sulfasalazine, however, should be supplemented with folic acid (2 mg/d) to decrease the risk of neural tube defects. The safety of 5-ASA compounds (mesalamine, balsalazide, and sulfasalazine) during pregnancy has been demonstrated in several trials despite the fact that mesalamine and its metabolite, acetyl-5-aminosalicylic acid, have been found in cord plasma.[72,73] In two separate studies, women taking 2 to 3 g of 5-aminosalicylates per day for either UC or CD had no higher incidence of fetal abnormalities than that in normal healthy women. Recently, the Food and Drug Administration (FDA) changed the pregnancy rating on Asacol because of dibutyl phthalate, a compound found in its coating. Dibutyl phthalate has been associated with urogenital defects in male offspring of exposed mothers in rats. The dose given to rats to result in this outcome is significantly higher than that prescribed to humans, so the clinical consequences of this label change are unclear.

Steroids and Antibiotics

Corticosteroids have not been associated with teratogenicity in humans and can be used as required to control active IBD. Prednisolone crosses the placenta less efficiently than other steroid formulations and should, therefore, be the steroid preparation of choice when indicated for controlling active disease. Oral clefts in newborns were seen in a case-control study of corticosteroid use during the first trimester[74] and this was confirmed by a large case-control study and a meta-analysis,[74,75] although these studies were not IBD-specific and had few IBD patients in the study population. The overall risk of major malformations was low, however, and the reported summary for OR for case-control studies examining the risk of oral clefts was 3.35 (95% CI, 1.97, 5.69).[75] Beaulieu and colleagues[76] described a case series of 8 patients with CD treated with budesonide with no increased risk of adverse outcomes. In addition, inhaled or intranasal budesonide has not been associated with adverse outcomes.

Only limited data are available regarding the safety of antibiotics in the treatment for CD. Currently, ampicillin, cephalosporins, and erythromycin are believed low risk, as is ciprofloxacin. Although quinolones have a high affinity for bone and cartilage and may cause arthropathies in infants,[77] there have been two studies (n = 200 and n = 57) of women exposed to quinolones and there was no increased risk of congenital abnormalities.[77,78] Metronidazole has been used to treat vaginitis in women during the first trimester of pregnancy but no controlled trials have definitively shown its safety.[79] Most studies suggest that prenatal use is not associated with birth defects.

Immunomodulators

Thiopurines
The thiopurines, AZA and 6-MP, carry a pregnancy category D rating. This was in response to the original FDA submission for their use with high doses to treat leukemia. Since then, low doses have been used for autoimmune diseases and become the standard of care without a change in the FDA label, leading to misplaced fears and concerns by patients, gastroenterologists, and obstetricians. Animal studies revealing teratogenicity in mice and rats have led to recommendations of cessation during pregnancy. Although there is transplacental and transamniotic transfer of AZA and its metabolites to the fetus,[80] the oral bioavailability of AZA (47%) and 6-MP (16%) is low.[81] In addition, the early fetal liver lacks the enzyme needed to convert AZA to 6-MP, which may protect the fetus from drug exposure during the first trimester.

In a retrospective chart review, Francella and colleagues[12] (n = 79, 325 pregnancies) they compared patients on 6-MP during conception, those that stopped before conception, and those patients never exposed to 6-MP. Although they did not look at prematurity or LBW, there was no statistical difference in spontaneous abortions, major congenital abnormalities, neoplasia, or increased infection (relative risk 0.85 [0.47, 1.55], $P = .59$). Another study done by Moskovitz and colleagues[82] investigated IBD medications (including 6-MP and AZA) taken during pregnancy. In this age-controlled multivariate analysis of 113 patients with 207 conceptions, there was no evidence that medications affected pregnancy outcomes (abortions, premature birth, healthy full-term birth, ectopic pregnancy, congenital abnormalities, birth weight, or type of delivery). Norgard and colleagues[83] combined 2 large national data registries with a national prescription database to look at therapeutic drug use in women with CD and birth outcomes. Among the women who were exposed to 6-MP/AZA throughout their pregnancies, the risks of preterm birth and congenital abnormalities were 4.2 (95% CI, 1.4, 12.5) and 2.9 (95% CI, 0.9, 8.9), respectively. Preterm births were more prevalent among steroid and 6-MP/AZA–exposed women compared with the reference group. They were unable to stratify disease activity to adverse birth outcomes, however, due to the low number of hospital admissions. Because of model fitting issues, the investigators could not adjust for the disease activity when looking at the LBW infants at term.[84] Data thus far suggest that continuing AZA/6-MP during pregnancy is low risk, but given the risks of pancreatitis and leucopenia, it is advised to avoid initiation during pregnancy. One strategy when using AZA/6-MP in combination with a biologic agent is cessation of the immunomodulator during conception and pregnancy to minimize any potential risks. If this is done, the severity of the underlying IBD and the disease course of each individual patient need to be taken into consideration.

Methotrexate
MTX is potentially teratogenic and the effects can occur after exposure to a single dose, especially if the exposure had occurred during the first trimester.[85] The

pharmacokinetics of MTX is complex and it is widely distributed in body tissues, with the highest concentration in the kidneys, gall bladder, spleen, liver, and skin.[85] Its presence in the liver has been reported to last up to 116 days after an exposure[85,86] and is the reason for the theoretic risk of fetal exposure in mothers who have been treated with MTX before the current conception. In a review on the effect of MTX on pregnancy, Lloyd and colleagues[87] stated that a minimum waiting period of 6 months is needed to enable the disappearance of MTX from the tissues to avoid the potential chromosomal damage in the dividing follicle.[26,87] There is a theoretic risk of sperm mutation in men treated with MTX although there are case reports of normal children whose fathers were on low-dose MTX.[87] Oligospermia has been reported in association with MTX treatment[88] and men should avoid conception for 3 to 4 months after cessation.

MTX should be avoided in IBD women considering conception and used with caution in women of childbearing age. Recommendations of 2 forms of birth control should be conveyed to the patient and MTX should be stopped at least 6 months before attempting conception. MTX can be excreted in breast milk and is contraindicated in breastfeeding.

Cyclosporine/tacrolimus/thalidomide

Cyclosporine is used in patients with severe UC and has not been found teratogenic. It has been used extensively in transplantation and rheumatology without adverse effects noted. A meta-analysis of 15 studies involving 410 patients revealed the rate of malformations (4.1%) to be no more than the general population.[89] Cyclosporine is excreted into breast milk and is contraindicated during breastfeeding.

There is a paucity of data on tacrolimus and pregnancy. It is known to cross the placenta and is found in high concentrations in breast milk. There is one case report of a UC patient with a successful pregnancy after tacrolimus use.[90]

Thalidomide is clearly teratogenic and is contraindicated during pregnancy and breastfeeding. It has been used successfully for the treatment of CD and if needed for women during their childbearing years; 2 forms of birth control are needed before and at least 1 month after cessation of therapy.

Biologic Therapy

The first series of intentional INF use throughout pregnancy was examined by Mahadevan and colleagues,[91] who looked at the outcomes in 10 women with active CD during pregnancy. All 10 pregnancies resulted in live births, with no congenital malformations. There were 3 preterm births and 1 LBW infant, but these were not unexpected in a population of women with CD significant enough to require biologic therapy. INF is an IgG1 antibody and does not cross the placenta in the first trimester, which results in protection of exposure during crucial organogenesis. But INF is efficient at crossing during the second and third trimesters.[92] INF has been detected in the cord blood of infants born to mothers receiving INF during the third trimester of pregnancy. The long-term effect of this placental transfer is unknown[68] but there have been no reported adverse events associated with elevated INF levels in newborns thus far. Most studies suggest that INF is low risk in pregnancy, with the largest amount of data generated from the INF Safety Database and the Crohn's Therapy, Resource, Evaluation, and Assessment Tool (TREAT) registry. Despite being exposed to INF in utero, these infants have been found to have an appropriate response to standard vaccinations.[93] Given the limited data, live vaccines in infants with detectable INF levels should be avoided.

Adalimumab (ADA) is also an IgG1 antibody and is expected to cross the placenta in the second and third trimesters. At this time, there is no commercially available test to detect ADA levels. The Organization for the Teratology Information Specialists registry reports 27 women on ADA in a prospective study and 47 ADA-exposed pregnant women, and there was no increase in stillbirths or spontaneous abortion in comparison with the general population, with the rates of congenital malformations and preterm delivery within expected range.[94] A published report for the successful use of ADA in pregnancy described a patient with severely active disease at conception.[95] She was placed on ADA 1 month before conception and delivered a normal growth infant without visible congenital anomalies. A recent case series suggests its safety in fetal outcomes in women treated for CD.[96] Biologics are considered compatible with breastfeeding but there are no published human data on ADA and breastfeeding at this time.

Certolizumab pegol (CZP) is a PEGylated Fab' fragment of a humanized anti–TNF-α monoclonal antibody. The missing Fc portion results in poor transport across the placenta in the second and third trimesters, but there is a concern that CZP may be able to cross the placenta passively in low levels during the first trimester.[94] There has been a single case report of a successful pregnancy in CD[97] and in 2 CD patients reported by Mahadevan and colleagues.[98] In those 2 patients, CZP was given 2 weeks before delivery and the mothers' drug level was high (19.60) whereas the cord blood (1.65) and infant (1.02) levels were low on the day of delivery.

Natalizumab is a humanized monoclonal antibody against α4 integrin, which inhibits leukocyte adhesion and migration into inflamed tissue. Recent data presented in abstract form reported 101 patients exposed to natalizumab during pregnancy and a spontaneous abortion rate comparable with that expected in the general population.[99] The number of exposed patients, however, is too low to draw any definitive conclusions.

The general consensus is for all 3 anti-TNF agents (INF, ADA, and CZP) to be continued through conception and first and second trimesters. The cessation of third-trimester dosing is controversial and more data are needed. One strategy is to time the last dose of INF at 30 weeks, followed by re-administration immediately after delivery. For ADA, the last dose given is at 32 weeks and then re-started after delivery. CZP is considered to have minimal placental transfer and is continued throughout gestation. Although this strategy of cessation of ADA and INF in the third trimester minimizes infant exposure with the ultimate goal of low infant drug levels at birth, the risk-to-benefit ratio for each patient needs to be considered. Further observational data on the safety of biologics use during pregnancy is needed but so far the evidence is reassuring.

SUMMARY

More than 20 years ago it was recognized that IBD patients flaring at the time of conception had a higher chance of spontaneous abortion, still birth, and premature delivery. The classic article by Miller[33] from 1986 is often referenced in which patients with active disease divide into three groups—one third improve, one third stay the same and one third worsen. For patients with active disease, one-third improve, one-third stay the same, and one-third worsen. This leaves two-thirds of patients having to live with active disease during pregnancy.[84] There are potential risks involved with IBD pregnancies but also successful outcomes for both mother and baby. Remission before conception is the goal and medication choices in women of childbearing age should be discussed. IBD medications during conception and pregnancy are low risk (except MTX and thalidomide). It is crucial to understand the literature and also recognize its limitations. Conversations between a patient and her physician should occur before conception with decisions using an informed approach and a team effort between patient, obstetrician, and gastroenterologist.

REFERENCES

1. Munkholm P. Crohn's disease—occurrence, course and prognosis. An epidemiologic cohort-study. Dan Med Bull 1997;44(3):287–302.
2. Heetun ZS, Byrnes C, Neary P, et al. Review article: reproduction in the patient with inflammatory bowel disease. Aliment Pharmacol Ther 2007;26(4):513–33.
3. Baiocco PJ, Korelitz BI. The influence of inflammatory bowel disease and its treatment on pregnancy and fetal outcome. J Clin Gastroenterol 1984;6(3): 211–6.
4. Orholm M, Fonager K, Sorensen HT. Risk of ulcerative colitis and Crohn's disease among offspring of patients with chronic inflammatory bowel disease. Am J Gastroenterol 1999;94(11):3236–8.
5. Yang H, McElree C, Roth MP, et al. Familial empirical risks for inflammatory bowel disease: differences between Jews and non-Jews. Gut 1993;34(4):517–24.
6. Bennett RA, Rubin PH, Present DH. Frequency of inflammatory bowel disease in offspring of couples both presenting with inflammatory bowel disease. Gastroenterology 1991;100(6):1638–43.
7. Klement E, Reif S. Breastfeeding and risk of inflammatory bowel disease. Am J Clin Nutr 2005;82(2):486.
8. Chandra A, Martinez GM, Mosler WD, et al. Fertility, family planning and reproductive health of US women: data from the 2002 National Survey of Family Growth. Vital Health Stat 23 2005;(25):1–160.
9. Fielding JF. Pregnancy and inflammatory bowel disease. Ir J Med Sci 1982; 151(6):194–202.
10. Mayberry JF, Weterman IT. European survey of fertility and pregnancy in women with Crohn's disease: a case control study by European collaborative group. Gut 1986;27(7):821–5.
11. Andres PG, Friedman LS. Epidemiology and the natural course of inflammatory bowel disease. Gastroenterol Clin North Am 1999;28(2):255–81, vii.
12. Francella A, Dyan A, Bodian C, et al. The safety of 6-mercaptopurine for childbearing patients with inflammatory bowel disease: a retrospective cohort study. Gastroenterology 2003;124(1):9–17.
13. Khosla R, Willoughby CP, Jewell DP. Crohn's disease and pregnancy. Gut 1984; 25(1):52–6.
14. Elbaz G, Fich A, Levy A, et al. Inflammatory bowel disease and preterm delivery. Int J Gynaecol Obstet 2005;90(3):193–7.
15. Baird DD, Narendranathan M, Sandler RS. Increased risk of preterm birth for women with inflammatory bowel disease. Gastroenterology 1990;99(4):987–94.
16. Willoughby CP, Truelove SC. Ulcerative colitis and pregnancy. Gut 1980;21(6): 469–74.
17. Ording Olsen K, Juul S, Berndtsson I, et al. Ulcerative colitis: female fecundity before diagnosis, during disease, and after surgery compared with a population sample. Gastroenterology 2002;122(1):15–9.
18. Waljee A, Waljee J, Morris AM, et al. Threefold increased risk of infertility: a meta-analysis of infertility after ileal pouch anal anastomosis in ulcerative colitis. Gut 2006;55(11):1575–80.

19. Cornish JA, Tan E, Teare J, et al. The effect of restorative proctocolectomy on sexual function, urinary function, fertility, pregnancy and delivery: a systematic review. Dis Colon Rectum 2007;50(8):1128–38.

20. Olsen KO, Juul S, Bulow S, et al. Female fecundity before and after operation for familial adenomatous polyposis. Br J Surg 2003;90(2):227–31.

21. Hudson M, Flett G, Sinclair TS, et al. Fertility and pregnancy in inflammatory bowel disease. Int J Gynaecol Obstet 1997;58(2):229–37.

22. Mortier PE, Gambiez L, Karoui M, et al. Colectomy with ileorectal anastomosis preserves female fertility in ulcerative colitis. Gastroenterol Clin Biol 2006;30(4): 594–7.

23. Narendranathan M, Sandler RS, Suchindran CM, et al. Male infertility in inflammatory bowel disease. J Clin Gastroenterol 1989;11(4):403–6.

24. Gorgun E, Remzi FH, Montague DK, et al. Male sexual function improves after ileal pouch anal anastomosis. Colorectal Dis 2005;7(6):545–50.

25. Lees CW, Critchley J, Chee N, et al. Lack of association between cervical dysplasia and IBD: a large case-control study. Inflamm Bowel Dis 2009;15(11):1621–9.

26. Singh H, Demers AA, Nugent Z, et al. Risk of cervical abnormalities in women with inflammatory bowel disease: a population-based nested case-control study. Gastroenterology 2009;136(2):451–8.

27. O'Morain C, Smethurst P, Dore CJ, et al. Reversible male infertility due to sulphasalazine: studies in man and rat. Gut 1984;25(10):1078–84.

28. Mahadevan U, Terdiman JP, Aron J, et al. Infliximab and semen quality in men with inflammatory bowel disease. Inflamm Bowel Dis 2005;11(4):395–9.

29. Mountifield R, Bampton P, Prosser R, et al. Fear and fertility in inflammatory bowel disease: a mismatch of perception and reality affects family planning decisions. Inflamm Bowel Dis 2009;15(5):720–5.

30. Zelinkova Z, Mensink PB, Dees J, et al. Reproductive wish represents an important factor influencing therapeutic strategy in inflammatory bowel diseases. Scand J Gastroenterol 2010;45(1):46–50.

31. Bush MC, Patel S, Lapinski RH, et al. Perinatal outcomes in inflammatory bowel disease. J Matern Fetal Neonatal Med 2004;15(4):237–41.

32. Calderwood AH, Kane SV. IBD and pregnancy. MedGenMed 2004;6(4):14.

33. Miller JP. Inflammatory bowel disease in pregnancy: a review. J R Soc Med 1986; 79(4):221–5.

34. Morales M, Berney T, Jenny A, et al. Crohn's disease as a risk factor for the outcome of pregnancy. Hepatogastroenterology 2000;47(36):1595–8.

35. Nielsen OH, Andreasson B, Bondesen S, et al. Pregnancy in ulcerative colitis. Scand J Gastroenterol 1983;18(6):735–42.

36. Fedorkow DM, Persaud D, Nimrod CA. Inflammatory bowel disease: a controlled study of late pregnancy outcome. Am J Obstet Gynecol 1989;160(4):998–1001.

37. Nielsen OH, Andreasson B, Bondesen S, et al. Pregnancy in Crohn's disease. Scand J Gastroenterol 1984;19(6):724–32.

38. Beniada A, Benoist G, Maurel J, et al. [Inflammatory bowel disease and pregnancy: report of 76 cases and review of the literature]. J Gynecol Obstet Biol Reprod (Paris) 2005;34(6):581–8 [in French].

39. Reddy D, Murphy SJ, Kane SV, et al. Relapses of inflammatory bowel disease during pregnancy: in-hospital management and birth outcomes. Am J Gastroenterol 2008;103(5):1203–9.

40. Dominitz JA, Young JC, Boyko EJ. Outcomes of infants born to mothers with inflammatory bowel disease: a population-based cohort study. Am J Gastroenterol 2002;97(3):641–8.

41. Norgard B, Hundborg HH, Jacobsen BA, et al. Disease activity in pregnant women with Crohn's disease and birth outcomes: a regional Danish cohort study. Am J Gastroenterol 2007;102(9):1947–54.
42. Moser MA, Okun NB, Mayes DC, et al. Crohn's disease, pregnancy, and birth weight. Am J Gastroenterol 2000;95(4):1021–6.
43. Norgard B, Puho E, Pedersen L, et al. Risk of congenital abnormalities in children born to women with ulcerative colitis: a population-based, case-control study. Am J Gastroenterol 2003;98(9):2006–10.
44. Lamah M, Scott HJ. Inflammatory bowel disease and pregnancy. Int J Colorectal Dis 2002;17(4):216–22.
45. Cornish J, Tan E, Teare J, et al. A meta-analysis on the influence of inflammatory bowel disease on pregnancy. Gut 2007;56(6):830–7.
46. Ubina-Aznar E, De Sola-Earle C, Rivera-Irigoin R, et al. [Crohn's disease and pregnancy. A descriptive and retrospective study]. Gastroenterol Hepatol 2006; 29(5):277–80 [in Spanish].
47. Mahadevan U, Sandborn WJ, Li DK, et al. Pregnancy outcomes in women with inflammatory bowel disease: a large community-based study from Northern California. Gastroenterology 2007;133(4):1106–12.
48. Fonager K, Sorensen HT, Olsen J, et al. Pregnancy outcome for women with Crohn's disease: a follow-up study based on linkage between national registries. Am J Gastroenterol 1998;93(12):2426–30.
49. Kornfeld D, Cnattingius S, Ekbom A. Pregnancy outcomes in women with inflammatory bowel disease—a population-based cohort study. Am J Obstet Gynecol 1997;177(4):942–6.
50. Moscandrew M, Kane S. Inflammatory bowel diseases and management considerations: fertility and pregnancy. Curr Gastroenterol Rep 2009;11(5):395–9.
51. Dubinsky M, Abraham B, Mahadevan U. Management of the pregnant IBD patient. Inflamm Bowel Dis 2008;14(12):1736–50.
52. Mogadam M, Korelitz BI, Ahmed SW, et al. The course of inflammatory bowel disease during pregnancy and postpartum. Am J Gastroenterol 1981;75(4): 265–9.
53. Kane S, Lemieux N. The role of breastfeeding in postpartum disease activity in women with inflammatory bowel disease. Am J Gastroenterol 2005;100(1): 102–5.
54. Ravid A, Richard CS, Spencer LM, et al. Pregnancy, delivery, and pouch function after ileal pouch-anal anastomosis for ulcerative colitis. Dis Colon Rectum 2002; 45(10):1283–8.
55. Kitayama T, Funayama Y, Fukushima K, et al. Anal function during pregnancy and postpartum after ileal pouch anal anastomosis for ulcerative colitis. Surg Today 2005;35(3):211–5.
56. Caprilli R, Gassull MA, Escher JC, et al. European evidence based consensus on the diagnosis and management of Crohn's disease: special situations. Gut 2006; 55(Suppl 1):i36–58.
57. Kane S, Kisiel J, Shih L, et al. HLA disparity determines disease activity through pregnancy in women with inflammatory bowel disease. Am J Gastroenterol 2004; 99(8):1523–6.
58. Ilnyckyji A, Blanchard JF, Rawsthorne P, et al. Perianal Crohn's disease and pregnancy: role of the mode of delivery. Am J Gastroenterol 1999;94(11):3274–8.
59. Riis L, Vind I, Politi P, et al. Does pregnancy change the disease course? A study in a European cohort of patients with inflammatory bowel disease. Am J Gastroenterol 2006;101(7):1539–45.

60. Nguyen GC, Boudreau H, Harris ML, et al. Outcomes of obstetric hospitalizations among women with inflammatory bowel disease in the United States. Clin Gastroenterol Hepatol 2009;7(3):329–34.
61. Hahnloser D, Pemberton JH, Wolff BG, et al. Pregnancy and delivery before and after ileal pouch-anal anastomosis for inflammatory bowel disease: immediate and long-term consequences and outcomes. Dis Colon Rectum 2004;47(7):1127–35.
62. Moffatt DC, Ilnyckyj A, Bernstein CN. A population-based study of breastfeeding in inflammatory bowel disease: initiation, duration, and effect on disease in the postpartum period. Am J Gastroenterol 2009;104(10):2517–23.
63. Nelis GF. Diarrhoea due to 5-aminosalicylic acid in breast milk. Lancet 1989; 1(8634):383.
64. Moretti ME, Verjee Z, Ito S, et al. Breast-feeding during maternal use of azathioprine. Ann Pharmacother 2006;40(12):2269–72.
65. Gardiner SJ, Gearry RB, Roberts RL, et al. Exposure to thiopurine drugs through breast milk is low based on metabolite concentrations in mother-infant pairs. Br J Clin Pharmacol 2006;62(4):453–6.
66. Sau A, Clarke S, Bass J, et al. Azathioprine and breastfeeding: is it safe? BJOG 2007;114(4):498–501.
67. Christensen LA, Dahlerup JF, Nielsen MJ, et al. Azathioprine treatment during lactation. Aliment Pharmacol Ther 2008;28(10):1209–13.
68. Vasiliauskas EA, Church JA, Silverman N, et al. Case report: evidence for transplacental transfer of maternally administered infliximab to the newborn. Clin Gastroenterol Hepatol 2006;4(10):1255–8.
69. Castiglione F, Pignata S, Morace F, et al. Effect of pregnancy on the clinical course of a cohort of women with inflammatory bowel disease. Ital J Gastroenterol 1996;28(4):199–204.
70. Cappell MS, Colon VJ, Sidhom OA. A study at 10 medical centers of the safety and efficacy of 48 flexible sigmoidoscopies and 8 colonoscopies during pregnancy with follow-up of fetal outcome and with comparison to control groups. Dig Dis Sci 1996;41(12):2353–61.
71. Nwokolo CU, Tan WC, Andrews HA, et al. Surgical resections in parous patients with distal ileal and colonic Crohn's disease. Gut 1994;35(2):220–3.
72. Diav-Citrin O, Park YH, Veerasuntharam G, et al. The safety of mesalamine in human pregnancy: a prospective controlled cohort study. Gastroenterology 1998;114(1):23–8.
73. Marteau P, Tennenbaum R, Elefant E, et al. Foetal outcome in women with inflammatory bowel disease treated during pregnancy with oral mesalazine microgranules. Aliment Pharmacol Ther 1998;12(11):1101–8.
74. Rodriguez-Pinilla E, Martinez-Frias ML. Corticosteroids during pregnancy and oral clefts: a case-control study. Teratology 1998;58(1):2–5.
75. Park-Wyllie L, Mazzotta P, Pastuszak A, et al. Birth defects after maternal exposure to corticosteroids: prospective cohort study and meta-analysis of epidemiological studies. Teratology 2000;62(6):385–92.
76. Beaulieu DB, Ananthakrishnan AN, Issa M, et al. Budesonide induction and maintenance therapy for Crohn's disease during pregnancy. Inflamm Bowel Dis 2009; 15(1):25–8.
77. Loebstein R, Addis A, Ho E, et al. Pregnancy outcome following gestational exposure to fluoroquinolones: a multicenter prospective controlled study. Antimicrob Agents Chemother 1998;42(6):1336–9.
78. Larsen H, Nielsen GL, Schonheyder HC, et al. Birth outcome following maternal use of fluoroquinolones. Int J Antimicrob Agents 2001;18(3):259–62.

79. Rosa FW, Baum C, Shaw M. Pregnancy outcomes after first-trimester vaginitis drug therapy. Obstet Gynecol 1987;69(5):751–5.
80. de Boer NK, Jarbandhan SV, de Graaf P, et al. Azathioprine use during pregnancy: unexpected intrauterine exposure to metabolites. Am J Gastroenterol 2006;101(6):1390–2.
81. Polifka JE, Friedman JM. Teratogen update: azathioprine and 6-mercaptopurine. Teratology 2002;65(5):240–61.
82. Moskovitz DN, Bodian C, Chapman ML, et al. The effect on the fetus of medications used to treat pregnant inflammatory bowel-disease patients. Am J Gastroenterol 2004;99(4):656–61.
83. Norgard B, Pedersen L, Christensen LA, et al. Therapeutic drug use in women with Crohn's disease and birth outcomes: a Danish nationwide cohort study. Am J Gastroenterol 2007;102(7):1406–13.
84. Friedman S. Medical therapy and birth outcomes in women with Crohn's disease: what should we tell our patients? Am J Gastroenterol 2007;102(7):1414–6.
85. Yedlinsky NT, Morgan FC, Whitecar PW. Anomalies associated with failed methotrexate and misoprostol termination. Obstet Gynecol 2005;105(5 Pt 2):1203–5.
86. Svirsky R, Rozovski U, Vaknin Z, et al. The safety of conception occurring shortly after methotrexate treatment of an ectopic pregnancy. Reprod Toxicol 2009;27(1):85–7.
87. Lloyd ME, Carr M, McElhatton P, et al. The effects of methotrexate on pregnancy, fertility and lactation. QJM 1999;92(10):551–63.
88. Sussman A, Leonard JM. Psoriasis, methotrexate, and oligospermia. Arch Dermatol 1980;116(2):215–7.
89. Bar Oz B, Hackman R, Einarson T, et al. Pregnancy outcome after cyclosporine therapy during pregnancy: a meta-analysis. Transplantation 2001;71(8):1051–5.
90. Baumgart DC, Sturm A, Wiedenmann B, et al. Uneventful pregnancy and neonatal outcome with tacrolimus in refractory ulcerative colitis. Gut 2005;54(12):1822–3.
91. Mahadevan U, Kane S, Sandborn WJ, et al. Intentional infliximab use during pregnancy for induction or maintenance of remission in Crohn's disease. Aliment Pharmacol Ther 2005;21(6):733–8.
92. Simister NE. Placental transport of immunoglobulin G. Vaccine 2003;21(24):3365–9.
93. Mahadevan U, Kane S, Church J, et al. The effect of maternal peripartum infliximab use on neonatal immune response [abstract]. Gatroenterology 2008;134(4 Suppl 1):A69.
94. Mahadevan U. Pregnancy and inflammatory bowel disease. Med Clin North Am 2010;94(1):53–73.
95. Vesga L, Terdiman JP, Mahadevan U. Adalimumab use in pregnancy. Gut 2005;54(6):890.
96. Mishkin DS, Van Deinse W, Becker JM, et al. Successful use of adalimumab (Humira) for Crohn's disease in pregnancy. Inflamm Bowel Dis 2006;12(8):827–8.
97. Oussalah A, Bigard MA, Peyrin-Biroulet L. Certolizumab use in pregnancy. Gut 2009;58(4):608.
98. Mahadevan U, Siegel C, Abreu M. Certolizumab use in pregnancy: low levels detected in cold blood [abstract]. Gastroenterology 2009;136(5):960.
99. Mahadevan U, Nazareth M, Cristiano L, et al. Natalizumab use during pregnancy. Am J Gastroenterol 2008;103(4 Suppl 1):A1150.

Issues Related to Colorectal Cancer and Colorectal Cancer Screening Practices in Women

Brenda Jimenez, MD*, Nicole Palekar, MD, Alison Schneider, MD

KEYWORDS

- Colorectal cancer • Colorectal cancer screening
- Colon polyps • Colonoscopy

Colorectal cancer (CRC) has the second highest cancer-related mortality rate in the United States and is the third most common cause of cancer in women.[1] It is believed that there is an adenoma-cancer paradigm, and target interventions for CRC focus on adenoma detection and removal, primarily with optical colonoscopy. In fact, colonoscopy is considered to be the most effective method for screening and diagnosis of CRC. Studies have shown that CRC incidence is equal between men and women. However, several studies have demonstrated lower adenoma detection rates in women than in men. Many questions arise about differences in adenomas, CRC, and screening practices between men and women: should screening be the same for both sexes, are there differences in risk factors in the formation of colon cancer, should special groups of women be screened differently from the general population, are colonoscopies tolerated differently in women and why, and what determines if a woman will undergo colonoscopy? This article reviews these issues.

COLORECTAL CANCER IN WOMEN

The lifetime risk of developing CRC is 5.12% in men and women. It is estimated that 142,570 men and women (72,090 men and 70,480 women) will be diagnosed with CRC in 2010, accounting for 10% of all new cancer cases in women. This figure translates to a 41.7 per 100,000 incidence rate in women per year. The cancer burden is sizeable; for example, on January 1, 2007, in the United States there were

Department of Gastroenterology and Hepatology, Cleveland Clinic Florida, 2950 Cleveland Clinic Boulevard, Weston, FL 33331, USA
* Corresponding author.
E-mail address: jimeneb2@ccf.org

Gastroenterol Clin N Am 40 (2011) 415–426
doi:10.1016/j.gtc.2011.03.001
0889-8553/11/$ – see front matter © 2011 Elsevier Inc. All rights reserved.

gastro.theclinics.com

approximately 1,112,493 men and women alive who had a history of cancer of the colon and rectum, more than half of these being women.[2]

The incidence rates of CRC have decreased from 1998 through 2004 in both men and women, likely from the increased use of colonoscopy driving the increase in CRC screening.[3] Despite the decreased incidence rates, it is still the third most common cancer in the United States and the second leading cause of cancer death among men and women. An estimated 50,000 men and women die each year from CRC; 25,000 of these deaths occur in women, accounting for 9% of all cancer deaths in women.[4] Data on cancer cases collected by the Surveillance Epidemiology and End Results (SEER) database and data on United States population collected by the US Census Bureau suggest that the incidence and mortality are slightly lower in women than in men, with a decline in mortality of 1.1% per year over 10 years in both men and women.[5]

Since 1990, there has been a dramatic decline in mortality, by 32% in men and 28% in women. At the same time, there has been an increase in CRC screening among individuals 50 years of age and older. It is estimated that currently 50% of the population in the United States undergo screening.[3] Other factors that may have contributed to a decrease in CRC mortality include hormone replacement therapy given to many women at the onset of menopause during the 1970s and 1980s (which might protect against CRC),[6] and the increased use of aspirin for cardiovascular disease and nonsteroidal anti-inflammatory drugs for musculoskeletal disorders, which reduce the risk of colon polyps and CRC.[7] The role of estrogen in the development of CRC is discussed later in the article.

COLON POLYPS IN WOMEN

There are gender differences in the prevalence and location of colorectal polyps and tumors. There are reports noting a lower rate of colorectal adenomas in women as compared with men, with similar rates of colon cancer.[8]

Several large studies have indicated that there is a significantly lower adenoma detection rate in women than men. A recent meta-analysis by Nguyen and colleagues[9] that included 924,932 asymptomatic, average-risk adults undergoing screening colonoscopy reports that men had greater age-specific risk for advanced colorectal neoplasia than women, with a relative risk of advanced neoplasia in men versus women of 1.83 (95% confidence interval [CI] 1.69–1.97). Advanced neoplasia was defined as any adenoma equal to or greater than 10 mm, with any villous histology or high-grade dysplasia, or invasive adenocarcinoma. Given these findings, the aforementioned study also showed that the number needed to endoscope to detect one patient with advanced neoplasia in women is larger than in men. This finding has also been shown before in a study by Lieberman and colleagues,[10] which showed that among patients younger than 50 years undergoing asymptomatic screening colonoscopy, 42 women and 28 men would need to be screened to identify 1 patient with a mass or polyp greater than 9 mm. After age 50, the risk of masses or polyps greater than 9 mm increases progressively with age in both men and women, with a decline in the number needed to endoscope in men from 18 (50–59 years) to 10 (>80 years); in women, the number needed to endoscope declines from 28 (50–59 years) to 14 (>80 years). Review of these data suggests that there is a lag time of about 7 to 8 years between risk in asymptomatic men and women, such that a 50-year-old man has roughly the same risk for CRC as a 58-year-old woman.

Gender differences in colorectal polyps and tumors are also seen in regard of location within the colon. Several retrospective studies have suggested that women have more right-sided tumors as compared with men.[11] A recent retrospective analysis of a national endoscopic database showed that women had a greater risk of developing pure right-sided polyps and tumors (defined as located in the cecum, ascending, and hepatic flexure). However, this gender difference was lost with increasing age, with significant differences seen between the group aged 60 to 69 years and not those older than 69 years.[12]

Does this location difference have clinical significance? A study by Elsaleh and colleagues[13] published in 2000 compared response to chemotherapy in CRC; findings suggested that there were survival benefits for patients who had right-sided tumors and who received adjuvant chemotherapy (48% vs 27%), whereas those with left-sided tumors had only a minimal benefit.

RISK FACTORS RELATED TO COLORECTAL CANCER IN WOMEN

Several mechanisms have been suggested to account for the lag time in the development of polyps and tumors in women. One theory is that estrogen may have a protective role in prevention of polyp formation by mechanisms of estrogen receptor genes, decreased secondary bile acid production, and decreased serum levels of insulin-like growth factors.[6] There is evidence that women have a relatively low risk of CRC until menopause, and might receive continued protection from hormone replacement therapy after menopause. When women age, reduced estrogen production may alter the bile acid composition, resulting in more toxic secondary bile acids, exposing the proximal colon to these neoplastic promoters.[14]

In observational studies, postmenopausal hormone replacement therapy has been associated with a decreased incidence of CRC. A meta-analysis of 18 studies involving postmenopausal women showed a 20% reduction in the incidence of CRCs among women who had ever taken hormones and a 34% reduction among women who were taking them at the time of the study, as compared with women who had never taken hormones.[15] In the Women's Health Initiative, a randomized controlled trial of estrogen plus progestin in nearly 17,000 postmenopausal women, the results reported in observational studies were confirmed.[6] After an average follow-up of 5.6 years, women in the hormone group had fewer large colorectal adenomas and CRCs than women in the placebo group; an overall 37% reduction in CRC risk was also seen. However, more women in the hormone group had lymph node involvement, advanced cancer stage, and metastasis at diagnosis. The benefit was not shown in estrogen-alone hormone replacement.

Other risk factors for the development of CRC such as diets high in fat and low in fiber have been extensively studied. Several large United States cohort studies (the Nurses' Health Study [NHS] and the Health Professionals Follow-Up Study [HPFS]) found no benefit between fiber consumption and colon cancer risk.[16,17] Data from the Women's Health Initiative also failed to show a reduction in CRC in postmenopausal women on a low-fat diet.[18] However, a diet high in red meat has been shown to increase the risk of CRC. Chao and colleagues[19] studied a large cohort of patients enrolled in the Cancer Prevention Study II Nutrition Cohort, and found that prolonged consumption of red and processed meat increased the risk of CRC (relative risk [RR] = 1.41 and 1.33, respectively), with the highest association in distal cancers (RR = 1.75). The risk increased significantly with the amount of red meat consumed, with a 17-fold difference in women observed between the lowest and highest quintiles of red meat consumption. Subsequently, in one study of asymptomatic women undergoing colonoscopy, red meat consumption was associated with a higher rate of colorectal adenomas (odds ratio [OR] = 2.02).[20]

Over the last decade with the increased incidence of obesity in the United States, there have been many studies showing an increased risk for gastrointestinal diseases such as nonalcoholic fatty liver disease. Multiple studies have now shown obesity as a risk factor for the development of both CRCs and adenomas. The Framingham Study showed that a body mass index (BMI; calculated as weight in kilograms divided by height in meters squared, ie, kg/m^2) of 30 or more led to a 50% increase in CRC in middle age (30–54 years) and a 2.4-fold increase in older (55–79 years) adults; however, the effect was stronger for men than for women.[21] This was confirmed by the European Prospective Investigation into Cancer and Nutrition (EPIC) study, which showed BMI as a risk factor (RR = 1.55) for men but not for women.[22] However, both the Framingham and EPIC studies demonstrated that waist circumference, an indicator of central obesity, was strongly associated with colon cancer risk in both men and women. The risk increased linearly with increasing waist size and was evident for both proximal and distal cancers. More recently, Anderson and colleagues[23] reported a significant correlation between BMI and colonic adenomas in women. This cross-sectional study of 2493 asymptomatic patients undergoing screening colonoscopy found the highest risk patients were women with a BMI greater than 40 (OR = 4.26). In this group of women, almost one-quarter had significant colorectal neoplasia (polyp $\geq$1 cm, villous tissue, high-grade dysplasia).

It has been postulated that insulin resistance and hyperinsulinemia is the common pathway for environmental risk factors such as obesity, increased waist-to-hip ratio, sedentary lifestyle, and a diet high in meat and saturated fats to promote the development of CRC. Insulin is a growth factor that has been shown to promote proliferation of colon cancer cells in vitro and to promote colonic tumors in experimental animals.[24–26] A cross-sectional analysis by Elwing and colleagues[27] focused on the impact that type 2 diabetes mellitus may have on the risk of colorectal adenoma in women. A total of 600 estrogen-negative women were included in the analysis (100 diabetic, 500 nondiabetic). The study showed an increased prevalence of adenomas (37% vs 24%; OR = 1.82, 95% CI 1.16–2.87, P = .009) and advanced adenomas (defined as villous or tubulovillous features, size >1 cm, or high-grade dysplasia) in women with diabetes (14% vs 6%; OR = 2.38, 95% CI 1.22–4.65, P = .009). Several observational studies in large cohorts of women have also supported that there is an increased risk of CRC with type 2 diabetes and hyperinsulinemia.[28–30]

Lifestyle factors such as tobacco, alcohol, and exercise have all been studied with varying results. Initial studies of tobacco did not find an increased risk for CRC. However, several meta-analyses have found statistically significant results with an approximate 20% risk increase, although the association appears stronger for rectal cancers.[31] Analysis of 8 prospective cohort studies showed a multivariate risk of CRC of 1.24 with alcohol consumption of 30 g or more per day.[32] In the HPFS, men who drank more than 2 drinks per day had twice the risk of developing CRC than men who drank less than 0.25 drinks per day, and there was an increased risk of colorectal adenomas with heavy alcohol use.[33] Lastly, physical activity has been shown in both the HPFS and NHS to be inversely associated with the risk of CRC, decreasing the risk approximately twofold between those in the lowest quintile and those in the highest quintile of activity.[34,35]

Studies have shown that women diagnosed previously with gynecologic cancers may have an increased risk for the development of CRC. Hereditary nonpolyposis CRC (HNPCC), a familial CRC syndrome with the early development of CRC, is associated with the development of both endometrial and ovarian cancer. Forty percent of women with HNPCC are affected with endometrial cancer and 10% develop ovarian cancer, which is 4 times that of women without HNPCC. Weinberg and colleagues[36] evaluated the risk for CRC after gynecologic cancer in women enrolled in the SEER registry. In total 21,222 patients with cervical cancer, 51,680 patients with endometrial cancer, and 28,832 patients with ovarian cancer were evaluated for subsequent incidence of colon or rectal cancer from 1974 to 1995 and then compared with the general female population. Women who were diagnosed with endometrial or ovarian cancer before age 50 years were more than 3 times more likely to have subsequent CRC (RR = 3.39 and 3.67, respectively). Women aged 50 to 64 years with ovarian cancer also had an increased risk of CRC (RR = 1.52). Cervical cancer did not increase the risk of CRC.

Whether the occurrence of colon tumors is increased in women with a history of breast cancer is controversial. The SEER registry failed to show an increase in CRC risk in those women with a previous history of breast cancer.[37] Similarly, no increase in CRC was found in relatives of Ashkenazi Jews with BRCA1 and BRCA2.[38]

Should we screen women with gynecologic cancers earlier or more often for CRC? Official guidelines exist to begin screening earlier and perform surveillance every 1 to 2 years for individuals with a diagnosis of or who are at increased risk for HNPCC. However, there are no guidelines or recommendations for women with gynecologic cancers. Given the data presented here, it would be reasonable to screen more often. Some experts advocate colonoscopy every 3 to 5 years for women with a history of ovarian or endometrial cancer diagnosed before age 50 years, even without a history of HNPCC. If the cancer is diagnosed after age 50 or if there is history of breast cancer alone, these women should be screened according to recommendations for the average risk population.

COLONOSCOPY ISSUES IN WOMEN

Colonoscopy is considered the gold standard screening test for CRC, yet colonoscopy may be technically more difficult in women than in men. One of the main differences documented in several studies is longer colonic length in women as compared with men. A longer colonic length likely leads to more looping of the colonoscope and more difficult examinations. Saunders and colleagues[39] looked at a barium enema series from 183 female and 162 male patients. Mean colonic length was 155 cm for women and 145 cm for men ($P \leq .005$). The transverse colon was the primary area found to have a longer length, and extended into the true pelvis more often in women than in men (62% vs 26%, $P<.001$). In a study cohort of 505 computed tomographic colonography examinations, women had significantly longer colons than men ($P<.002$) and the transverse colon was again shown to be the section that was primarily longer.[40,41] Older age ($P<.001$) and female gender ($P<.01$) were also more likely to have incomplete conventional colonoscopy. General factors associated with incomplete colonoscopy included greater colonic length, tortuosity, and advanced diverticular disease.[42] Rowland and colleagues[43] used a technique with magnetic drive coils to visualize the path of a colonoscope, and found longer colon length and significantly more looping in the sigmoid colon in women than in men ($P<.05$).

Other anatomic features can make colonoscopy more difficult, including previous abdominal surgeries (particularly hysterectomy), pelvic irradiation, diverticulosis, and BMI. Postsurgical pelvic adhesions can lead to a more fixed sigmoid colon, which may be hard to traverse. A study evaluating flexible sigmoidoscopy in women cited hysterectomy and women younger than 70 years as more likely to have incomplete procedures.[44] In a prospective study comparing women with and without hysterectomy, sigmoidoscopy in those with hysterectomy was more difficult ($P<.001$), painful ($P<.001$), and less complete ($P<.0001$).[45] Church[42] found adjusted completion rates of colonoscopy to be lower in women after hysterectomy (92.8% vs 98.3%). Takashi and colleagues[46] found that the two factors predictive of pain and difficult cecal intubation in a series of consecutive unsedated colonoscopies were female gender and previous hysterectomy. There was, however, an overall high completion rate in this study (99.6%). Of interest, one study has shown that women who have had hysterectomy had significantly longer procedures, lower completion rates (89.2% vs 98.1%), and higher sedation requirements with benzodiazepine (88.7% vs 43%) than women who had a hysterectomy and sigmoid resection in the past ($P<.05$).[47] Anderson and colleagues[48] found lower adjusted completion rates for colonoscopy in women (94.8%) than in men (98.2%) ($P<.005$). Lower BMI and diverticular disease were predictive of more difficult examinations with longer times to cecal intubation ($P<.001$) in this study.

All the aforementioned features make colonoscopy more challenging to do, leading not only to lower completion rates but also reduced patient comfort. Procedures can require more time, leading to the use of more air insufflation, more external abdominal pressure, and thus a greater risk for procedural pain and complications. More medications may be used for sedation and analgesia for these reasons, and can also be associated with complications, particularly cardiopulmonary adverse events. Several studies have found that women experience more pain with colonoscopy than men.[49–51] One study prospectively looked at the incidence of minor complications and time lost from normal activities after screening or surveillance colonoscopy. Of 504 patients, 34% reported complications before day 7 and 6% between days 7 and 30. The most common complications were bloating (25%) and abdominal pain (11%), and were reported significantly more often in women than men ($P = .0020$).[52]

Various ways to improve colonoscopy in women have been studied. The use of thinner-diameter scopes with more flexibility, such as pediatric colonoscopes, can traverse fixed angulations in the colon more easily. In a study of 100 randomized colonoscopies in women, cecal intubation was shown to be higher with pediatric colonoscopes than with standard colonoscopes (96.1% vs 71.4%; $P<.001$), although procedure time and use of meperidine and midazolam were no different.[53] Other methods used to obtain higher completion rates for those with a previous incomplete colonoscopy include use of push enteroscopes, upper endoscopes, overtube placements, external stiffeners, and the use of propofol sedation.[54,55] Most recently, double-balloon colonoscopy and double-balloon enteroscopy have been shown to achieve full colonoscopy in previously incomplete procedures. In a series of 29 patients with previous incomplete colonoscopies, 28 of 29 were able to have repeat procedures reaching cecum with a double-balloon retrograde technique.[56] Reasons cited for higher completion rates with a double balloon included smaller scope diameter and improved flexibility, better loop fixation and control by overtubes, and greater tip deflection through angles.[57,58]

BARRIERS TO COLON CANCER SCREENING PRACTICES IN WOMEN

In 1996 the US Preventive Services Task Force published guidelines recommending CRC screening.[59] Two years later, colorectal screening became a covered Medicare benefit.[60] There is now some data to state that CRC screening rates are increasing,[3,61] but the overall number of patients who undergo screening remains low among both men and women. In general, men are more likely than women to undergo CRC screening.[62] A reason for lower screening rates among women may be attributable to barriers that exist in their participation and acceptance of colonoscopy for CRC screening. Such barriers likely stem from the fact that these procedures are considered to be invasive and embarrassing. In the United States, gender preferences for a female endoscopist have been well documented. Women may delay or avoid colorectal screening until they have the endoscopist of their choice. Fidler and colleagues[63] found that 48% of female patients preferred a female endoscopist to perform their sigmoidoscopy. Similarly, Varadarajulu and colleagues[64] found a gender preference of 45% among women awaiting colonoscopy versus 4.3% of men. Menees and colleagues[65] surveyed women in a primary care setting and showed that 43% had a preference for a female endoscopist; 87% of these were willing to wait longer than 30 days to have the preference of their choice. Schneider and colleagues[66] found that women surveyed at an outpatient endoscopy center in an urban inner city were more likely to have a gender preference than men (42.3% vs 21%; $P<.001$). Of these women who had a preference, 92% preferred a female endoscopist. Multivariate analysis showed that female gender, lower income level, and history of physical/emotional abuse were significant factors related to gender preference. Gender preference is also seen among specific ethnic groups. Lee and colleagues[67] found 32.7% of Korean women recruited from a digestive disease center had a gender preference for upper endoscopy and that 45.5% of women had a preference for colonoscopy. Zapatier and colleagues[68] found that among a Hispanic population in the southeastern United States, Hispanic women (35%) were more likely to have a gender preference than men (20.4%; $P<.05$). There was also a greater ethnic preference among these Hispanic women for Hispanic endoscopists compared with Hispanic men as well as Caucasian men and women.

These studies all highlight that a major obstacle to CRC screening practices among women may be the preference for health care providers of their own gender and even perhaps of similar ethnic backgrounds. Reasons cited as to why women prefer female endoscopists include less embarrassment when the same sex is performing the examination, better communication with women, and that women are more empathetic.[69] Of interest, studies that have included men have rarely noted a gender preference among them. However, even though women are more likely to report pre-colonoscopy embarrassment, in a 2005 National Health Interview Survey (NHIS) on CRC test use, less than 5% of patients cited fear of pain or embarrassment as a reason for not being up to date with CRC screening. The most common reported reason for not having CRC screening was "never thought about it," suggesting that other barriers exist to CRC screening among women.[70] Thus, physician recommendation is likely to have a major impact on CRC screening practices. It should be noted that certain groups of women appear more likely to undergo screening for colon cancer. Women who undergo other screening practices such as mammography and Papanicolaou tests are more likely to sign up. Again, recommendations from primary care providers were found to be a strong predictor that women will undergo colonoscopy.[71]

The findings of this survey are further supported by a recent prospective cohort study in which screening colonoscopies were offered to women aged 50 to 69 years who were eligible for colonoscopy through an outreach program. The study used a nonrandomized trial comparison group, in which women in the study group were verbally offered a female endoscopist to perform their colonoscopy. The aim of the study was to determine whether the availability of a female endoscopist would increase the likelihood of completing screening colonoscopy. The study found that women who were offered a female endoscopist were more likely to request one than those who were not (44.2% vs 4.8%, $P<.001$), but women who requested a female endoscopist were not more or less likely to undergo screening colonoscopy than those who did not ($P = .9$).[72]

Another important issue that should not be overlooked is access to health care and patient education. In another NHIS that included data from 1987 to 2003, female minority groups had the lowest screening rates of all groups studied, with 31.4% of Hispanic women and 37.5% of black women undergoing any screening test for colon cancer. Reasons may be related to lower socioeconomic status and access to care. Those patients with higher educational levels were former smokers and had health insurance, and access to medical care providers was significantly associated with use of CRC tests.[73] Much of the emphasis on CRC screening is through the use of colonoscopy. Colonoscopy is the preferred test for CRC screening by many gastrointestinal organizations, but it is costly and can only be performed by a physician. Patients of lower socioeconomic standing may not be able to obtain this modality.

These data suggest that there are several obstacles to CRC screening practices in women. These barriers could be overcome by ensuring adequate numbers of female endoscopists, and incorporating a team approach to CRC screening, in which primary care physicians and nonphysician members of a practice participate in educating eligible patients when screening is due. This approach could lead to an increase in CRC screening among women.

SUMMARY

Colorectal cancer is the third most common cause of cancer in women, and a significant number of deaths in women are attributed to it. There are many factors related to CRC that are intrinsic to women, as described in this article. The risk for CRC in women, although thought to be lower in women than in men, is in fact similar, but there is a lag time of about 7 to 8 years, which is likely secondary to protection from estrogens. Although it seems reasonable to recommend hormone replacement therapy to prolong this protective effect after menopause, the cardiovascular risk carried by hormone replacement therapy precludes this recommendation. Obese women and women with previous gynecologic cancers are at increased risk for CRC. However, national screening guidelines do not include these as risk factors for CRC. The data presented here provide support for incorporating obesity and previous gynecologic cancers into future recommendations for CRC screening guidelines. There are issues unique to performing colonoscopy in women, such as longer colonic lengths and previous abdominal surgeries, making the procedure more challenging to perform. Different techniques should be considered when attempting to perform colonoscopy in women, including the use of upper endoscopes, pediatric colonoscopes, or push enteroscopes. Lastly, women tend to prefer female endoscopists and while female gastroenterologists are becoming more prevalent, it still remains a male-dominated field, and this may lead to limited choices for women. Being able to offer women more choices such as the ability to choose the gender of their endoscopist will likely improve colorectal screening acceptance. Overall, not enough women screen for CRC. More education is needed to increase this practice.

REFERENCES

1. National Cancer Institute. SEER cancer statistics review 1950–2007. Available at: http://seer.cancer.gov/. Accessed October 11, 2010.
2. Altekruse SF, Kosary CL, Krapcho M, et al (eds). SEER cancer statistics review, 1975–2007, National Cancer Institute. Bethesda (MD). Available at: http://seer.cancer.gov/csr/1975_2007/. Accessed October 11, 2010.
3. US Preventive Services Task Force. Screening for colorectal cancer: US Preventive Services Task Force recommendation statement. Ann Intern Med 2008;149: 627–37.

4. Jemal A, Siegel R, Ward E, et al. Cancer statistics 2008. CA Cancer J Clin 2008; 58:71–96.
5. Available at: www.cancer.org. Accessed November 10, 2010.
6. Chlebowski RT, Wactawski-Wende J, Ritenbaugh C, et al, Women's Health Initiative Investigators. Estrogen plus progestin and colorectal cancer in postmenopausal women. N Engl J Med 2004;350:991–1004.
7. Rostom A, Dube C, Lewin G, et al, U.S. Preventive Services Task Force. Nonsteroidal anti-inflammatory drugs and cyclooxygenase-2 inhibitors for primary prevention of colorectal cancer: a systemic review prepared for the U.S. Preventive Services Task Force. Ann Intern Med 2007;146:376–89.
8. Brenner H, Hoffmeister M, Arndt V, et al. Gender differences in colorectal cancer: implications for age at initiation of screening. Br J Cancer 2007;96:828–31.
9. Nguyen SP, Bent S, Chen YH, et al. Gender as a risk factor for advanced neoplasia and colorectal cancer: a systematic review and meta-analysis. Clin Gastroenterol Hepatol 2009;7(6):676–81.
10. Lieberman DA, Holub J, Eisen G, et al. Prevalence of polyps greater than 9 mm in a consortium of diverse clinical practice settings in the United States. Clin Gastroenterol Hepatol 2005;3:798–805.
11. Nelson RL, Dollear T, Freels S, et al. The relation of age, race, AJG—March, 2001 and gender to the subsite location of colorectal carcinoma. Cancer 1997;80:193–7.
12. McCashland T, Brand R, Lyden E, et al. Gender differences in colorectal polyps and tumors. Am J Gastroenterol 2001;96:882–6.
13. Elsaleh H, Joseph D, Grieu F, et al. Association of tumour site and sex with survival benefit from adjuvant chemotherapy in colorectal cancer. Lancet 2000; 355:1745–50.
14. Everson GT, McKinley C, Kern F. Mechanisms of gallstone formation in women. Effects of exogenous estrogen and dietary cholesterol on hepatic lipid metabolism. J Clin Invest 1991;87:237–46.
15. Grodstein F, Newcomb PA, Stampfer MJ. Postmenopausal hormone therapy and the risk of colorectal cancer: a review and metaanalysis. Am J Med 1999;106: 574–82.
16. Fuchs CS, Giovannucci EL, Colditz GA, et al. Dietary fiber and the risk of colorectal cancer and adenoma in women. N Engl J Med 1999;340:169–76.
17. Michels KB, Fuchs CS, Giovannucci E, et al. Fiber intake and incidence of colorectal cancer among 76,947 women and 47, 279 men. Cancer Epidemiol Biomarkers Prev 2005;14(4):842–9.
18. Beresford SA, Johnson KC, Ritenbaugh C, et al. Low-fat dietary pattern and risk of colorectal cancer. JAMA 2006;295:643–54.
19. Chao A, Thun MJ, Connell CJ, et al. Meat consumption and risk of colorectal cancer. JAMA 2005;293:172–82.
20. Ferrucci LM, Sinha R, Graubard BI, et al. Dietary meat intake in relation to colorectal adenoma in asymptomatic women. Am J Gastroenterol 2009;104:1231–40.
21. Moore LL, Bradlee ML, Singer MR, et al. BMI and waist circumference as predictors of lifetime colon cancer risk in Framingham Study adults. Int J Obes 2004;28: 559–67.
22. Pischon T, Lahmann PH, Boeing H, et al. Body size and risk of colon and rectal cancer in the European Prospective Investigation into Cancer and Nutrition (EPIC). J Natl Cancer Inst 2006;98:920–31.
23. Anderson JC, Messina CR, Dakhllalah F, et al. Body mass index: a marker for significant colorectal neoplasia in a screening population. J Clin Gastroenterol 2007;41:285–90.

24. Tran TT, Medline A, Bruce WR. Insulin promotion of colon tumors in rats. Cancer Epidemiol Biomarkers Prev 1996;5:1013–5.

25. Koenuma M, Yamori T, Tsuruo T. Insulin and insulin-like growth factor 1 stimulate proliferation of metastatic variants of colon carcinoma 26. Jpn J Cancer Res 1989;80:51–8.

26. Koohestani N, Tran TT, Lee W, et al. Insulin resistance and promotion of aberrant crypt foci in the colons of rats on a high-fat diet. Nutr Cancer 1997;29: 69–76.

27. Elwing JE, Gao F, Davidson NO, et al. Type 2 diabetes mellitus: the impact on colorectal adenoma risk in women. Am J Gastroenterol 2006;101(8):1866–71.

28. Kaaks R, Toniolo P, Akhmedkhanov A, et al. Serum C peptide, insulin-like growth factor (IGF)-I, IGF-binding proteins, and colorectal cancer risk in women. J Natl Cancer Inst 2000;92:1592–600.

29. Limburg PJ, Anderson KE, Johnson TW, et al. Diabetes mellitus and subsite-specific colorectal cancer risks in the Iowa Women's Health Study. Cancer Epidemiol Biomarkers Prev 2005;14:133–7.

30. Hu FB, Manson JE, Liu S, et al. Prospective study of adult onset diabetes mellitus (type 2) and risk of colorectal cancer in women. J Natl Cancer Inst 1999;91: 542–7.

31. Liang PS, Chen TY, Giovannucci E. Cigarette smoking and colorectal cancer incidence and mortality: systematic review and meta-analysis. Int J Cancer 2009; 124:2406–15.

32. Cho E, Smith-Warner S, Ritz J, et al. Alcohol intake and colorectal cancer: a pooled analysis of 8 cohort studies. Ann Intern Med 2004;140(8):603–14.

33. Giovannucci E, Rimm EB, Ascherio A, et al. Alcohol, low-methionine, low-folate diets, and risk of colon cancer in men. J Natl Cancer Inst 1995;87:265–73.

34. Giovannucci E, Ascherio A, Rimm EB, et al. Physical activity, obesity, and risk for colon cancer and adenoma in men. Ann Intern Med 1995;122:327–34.

35. Giovannucci E, Colditz GA, Stampfer MJ, et al. Physical activity, obesity, and risk of colorectal adenoma in women. Cancer Causes Control 1996;7:253–63.

36. Weinberg DS, Newschaffer CJ, Topham A. Risk for colorectal cancer after gynecologic cancer. Ann Intern Med 1999;131:189–93.

37. Newschaffer CJ, Topham A, Herzberg T, et al. Risk of colorectal cancer after breast cancer. Lancet 2001;357:837–40.

38. Niell BL, Rennert G, Bonner JD, et al. BRCA1 and BRCA2 founder mutations and the risk of colorectal cancer. J Natl Cancer Inst 2004;96(1):15–21.

39. Saunders BP, Fukumoto M, Halligan S, et al. Why is colonoscopy more difficult in women? Gastrointest Endosc 1996;43:124–6.

40. Hanson ME, Pickhardt PJ, Kim DH, et al. Anatomic factors predictive of incomplete colonoscopy based on findings at CT colonoscopy. Am J Roentgenol 2007;189:774–9.

41. Kashab MA, Pickhardt PJ, Rex DK. Colorectal anatomy in adults at computed tomography colonography: normal distribution and the effect of age, sex, and body mass index. Endoscopy 2009;41:674–8.

42. Church JM. Complete colonoscopy: how often? And if not, why not? Am J Gastroenterol 1994;89(4):556–60.

43. Rowland RS, Bel GD, Dogramadzi S, et al. Colonoscopy aided by magnetic 3D imaging: is the technique sufficiently sensitive to detect differences between men and women? Med Biol Eng Comput 1999;37:673–9.

44. Ramakrishan K, Scheid DC. Predictors of incomplete flexible sigmoidoscopy. J Am Board Fam Pract 2003;16:478–84.

45. Adams C, Cardwell C, Cook C, et al. Effect of hysterectomy status on polyp detection rates at screening flexible sigmoidoscopy. Gastrointest Endosc 2003; 57:848–53.
46. Takashi Y, Yanaka H, Kinjo M, et al. Prospective evaluation of factors predicting difficulty and pain during sedation-free colonoscopy. Dis Colon Rectum 2005; 48:1295–300.
47. Garrett KA, Church J. History of hysterectomy: a significant problem for colonoscopists that is not present in patients who have had sigmoid colectomy. Dis Colon Rectum 2010;53:1055–60.
48. Anderson JC, Gonzalez JD, Messina CR, et al. Factors that predict incomplete colonoscopy: thinner is not always better. Am J Gastroenterol 2000;95:2784–7.
49. Anderson JC, Messina CR, Cohn W, et al. Factors predictive of difficult colonoscopy. Gastrointest Endosc 2001;54:558–62.
50. Schutz SM, Lee JG, Schmitt CM, et al. Clues to patient dissatisfaction with conscious sedation for colonoscopy. Am J Gastroenterol 1994;89:1476–9.
51. Hull T, Church JM. Colonoscopy: how difficult, how painful? Surg Endosc 1994;8: 784–7.
52. Ko CW, Riffle S, Shapiro JA, et al. Incidence of minor complications and time lost from normal activities after screening or surveillance colonoscopy. Gastrointest Endosc 2007;65:648–56.
53. Marshall JB, Perez RA, Madsen RW. Usefulness of pediatric colonoscopy for routine colonoscopy in women who have undergone hysterectomy. Gastrointest Endosc 2002;55:838–41.
54. Rex DK. Achieving cecal intubation in the very difficult colon. Gastrointest Endosc 2008;67:938–44.
55. Rex DK, Chen SC, Overhiser AJ. Colonoscopy technique in consecutive patients referred for prior incomplete colonoscopy. Clin Gastroenterol Hepatol 2007;5:879–83.
56. Gay G, Delvaux M. Double-balloon colonoscopy after failed conventional colonoscopy: a pilot series with a new instrument. Endoscopy 2007;39:788–92.
57. Yamato H, Kita H, Sugano K. Other applications of double balloon technique. In: Sugano K, Yamamoto H, Kita H, editors. Double balloon endoscopy. Heidelberg (Germany): Springer; 2006. p. 101–13.
58. May A, Nachbar L, Ell C. Push-and-pull enteroscopy using a single balloon technique for difficult colonoscopy. Endoscopy 2006;38:395–8.
59. U.S. Preventive Services Task Force. Guide to clinical preventive services. Alexandria (VA): International Medical Publishing; 1996.
60. Available at: http://healthservices.cancer.gov/seermedicare/considerations/testing.html. Accessed November 17, 2010.
61. Lieberman DA. Screening for colorectal cancer. N Engl J Med 2009;361:1179–87.
62. Brawarsky P, Brooks DR, Mucci LA. Correlates of colorectal cancer testing in Massachusetts men and women. Prev Med 2003;36:659–68.
63. Fidler H, Hartnett A, Cheng Man K, et al. Sex and familiarity of colonoscopist. Gastrointest Endosc 2000;32:481–2.
64. Varadarajulu S, Petruff C, Ramsey WH. Patient preference for gender of endoscopists. Gastrointest Endosc 2002;56:170–3.
65. Menees SB, Inadomi JM, Korsens S, et al. Women patients/preference for women physicians is a barrier to colon cancer screening. Gastrointest Endosc 2005;62: 219–23.
66. Schneider A, Kanagarajan N, Anjelly D, et al. Importance of gender, socioeconomic status, and history of abuse on patient preference for endoscopist. Am J Gastroenterol 2009;104:340–8.

67. Lee SY, Yu SK, Kim JH, et al. Link between preference for women colonoscopists and social status in Korean women. Gastrointest Endosc 2008;67:273–7.
68. Zapatier JA, Kumar AR, Perez A, et al. Preferences for ethnicity and gender of endoscopists within a Hispanic population in the United States. Gastrointest Endosc 2011;73:89–97.
69. Elta GH. Women are different from men. Gastrointest Endosc 2002;56:308–9.
70. Shapiro JA, Seeff LC, Thompson TD, et al. Colorectal cancer test use from the 2005 National Health Interview Survey. Cancer Epidemiol Biomarkers Prev 2008;17:1623–30.
71. Stockwell DH, Woo P, Jacobson BC, et al. Determinants of colorectal cancer screening in women undergoing mammography. Am J Gastroenterol 2003;98: 1875–80.
72. Denberg TD, Kraus H, Soenken A, et al. Rates of screening colonoscopy are not increased when women are offered a female endoscopist in a health promotion outreach program. Gastrointest Endosc 2010;72:1014–9.
73. Meissner HI, Breen N, Klabunde CN, et al. Patterns of colorectal cancer screening uptake among men and women in the United States. Cancer Epidemiol Biomarkers Prev 2006;15:389–94.

A Global Perspective on Gastrointestinal Diseases

Radha Menon, MD[a], Andres Riera, MD[b], Asyia Ahmad, MD, MPH[c],*

KEYWORDS

• Global • Gender • International

Common gastrointestinal diseases often exhibit interesting geographic, cultural, and gender variations. Diseases that were previously less prevalent in certain areas of the world have shown a recent increase in prevalence. Industrialization has traditionally been noted as a major cause for this epidemiologic evolution. However, environmental factors such as diet, hygiene, and exposure to infections may also play a major role. Moreover, the way one disease presents in a certain location may vary significantly from the way it manifests in another culture or location. In this article the authors discuss the global variations of inflammatory bowel disease, *Helicobacter pylori*, irritable bowel disease, fecal incontinence, hepatitis B, and hepatocellular cancer.

INFLAMMATORY BOWEL DISEASE

Over the past few decades, inflammatory bowel disease (IBD) has become increasingly recognized in diverse populations around the world. The prevalence and incidence rates of IBD have historically been higher in developed countries, with a decreasing prevalence from north to south latitudes. These demographics have started to change recently as a significant portion of underdeveloped countries have begun to modernize. The increase in incidence and prevalence of IBD has paralleled the social and economic development and adoption of the Western lifestyle.[1,2]

The incidence of ulcerative colitis (UC) has been increasing in developed countries since World War II; however, over the past few decades studies have suggested that it may be starting to plateau or even decrease. The highest prevalence rates of IBD

The authors have nothing to disclose.

[a] Division of Gastroenterology, Department of Medicine, Drexel University College of Medicine, 245 North 15th Street, MS 487, 6104 New College Building, Philadelphia, PA 19102, USA
[b] Division of Internal Medicine, Department of Medicine, Drexel University College of Medicine, 245 North 15th Street, MS 427, 6218 New College Building, Philadelphia, PA 19102, USA
[c] Division of Internal Medicine, Department of Medicine, Drexel University College of Medicine, 219 North Broad Street, 5th Floor, Philadelphia, PA 19107, USA
* Corresponding author.
E-mail address: asyia.ahmad@drexelmed.edu

Gastroenterol Clin N Am 40 (2011) 427–439
doi:10.1016/j.gtc.2011.03.002
0889-8553/11/$ – see front matter © 2011 Elsevier Inc. All rights reserved.

gastro.theclinics.com

worldwide have been documented in the Israeli Jewish population. In a recent study that surveyed physicians in Israel, the prevalence of Crohn disease (CD) was found to be 113 per 100,000, and the prevalence of UC in the same population was noted to be 216.6 per 100,000.[3,4] The United States and the northern and western countries of Europe have also traditionally documented high prevalence rates of IBD, especially when compared with southern European countries. A study conducted in Northern California found the point prevalence per 100,000 of CD and UC to be 96.3 and 155.8, respectively.[5] Similar rates have been documented in western Europe. A study that prospectively identified patients who were newly diagnosed with IBD in 20 European centers between 1991 and 1993 showed that the incidence rates for UC and CD were 40% and 80% higher in the northern centers than in the southern centers.[6] This previously described north to south gradient of IBD seems to be changing over the past few decades, as shown in more recent studies performed in European populations. Recent studies suggest that Europe has seen a stabilization of IBD incidence rates in northern and western countries with a corresponding increase in incidence rates of southern and eastern countries. A prospective study published in 2005 reported the incidence of UC in central Greece to be 11.2 per 100,000.[7] This finding suggests an increase in the incidence of IBD in this previously low-incidence area of the world. A similar increase was documented in the Croatian population in a recent prospective study. The incidence rates for UC and CD were found to be 4.3 and 7 per 100,000, respectively, in this study performed from 2000 to 2004, suggesting a threefold increase in the incidence of UC and a tenfold increase in the incidence of CD in Croatia over the past 24 years.[8]

Similarly, studies indicate that previous low-incidence areas of eastern Europe, Asia, and Central and South America have demonstrated a recent increase in the incidence and prevalence of IBD. One of the first studies on the prevalence and incidence of IBD in the Indian population was conducted in Punjab, India by Sood and colleagues.[9] Almost 52,000 people were screened for signs or symptoms of UC using a questionnaire. Anyone who was suspected to have UC received further workup with a sigmoidoscopy/colonoscopy and biopsies. The incidence rate of UC in this population was determined to be 6.0 per 100,000 inhabitants with a prevalence rate of 44.3 per 100,000 inhabitants.[9] This study was the first published to document prevalence rates of UC in this population, and it noted a surprisingly high rate in this previously "low-prevalence" country. The incidence of IBD has also been noted to increase in South Korea and Japan over the past few decades. A large population-based study was performed in South Korea over a period of 20 years between 1986 and 2005. The mean annual incidence rates of CD and UC increased significantly from 0.05 and 0.34 per 100,000 in 1986 to 1990, to 1.34 and 3.08 per 100,000 in 2001 to 2005.[10] Studies also show that the presenting features may vary based on geography. In India, colonic involvement in CD is more common and fistulization is less common. In Pakistan, few patients with CD have perianal or fistulizing disease, and there is much less extraintestinal disease compared with what is reported in the West.[11]

During the past few decades, there have been large migrations from the Indian subcontinent into western Europe and the United States. This unique population of immigrants and their children, or first-generation immigrants, provides an opportunity to ponder possible environmental etiologic factors that may play a role in the pathogenesis of IBD. These environmental factors may also help to explain why the incidence of IBD seems to be higher among these immigrant populations when compared with data from studies conducted in their native countries. Of interest, it seems that individuals who migrate to developed countries before adolescence, who initially belong to traditionally low-incidence populations, have a higher incidence of IBD, this being comparable with that of the developed country to which they migrated. Multiple studies report that those who move from an area of low prevalence to one of high prevalence after childhood retain a similar rate of IBD as before, but their children (first-generation immigrants) have an increased risk of IBD.[12] Changes in diet and the changing prevalence of previously common infections are 2 proposed mechanisms that may explain the increasing incidence of IBD in not only migrant populations but also in native populations in what were previously considered "low-incidence" countries.

It has long been accepted that immune dysregulation is a large contributory factor to the onset and pathogenesis of many allergic disorders. IBD likely results from dysregulated immune responses to intestinal contents. Some common pathogens have been proposed to stimulate the normal development of regulatory immune mechanisms. Examples of such organisms include saprophytic mycobacteria, bifidobacteria, lactobacilli, and helminths. These organisms are recognized by the immune system as innocuous, and they therefore gear immune responses toward regulatory modulation. Helminths are multicellular worm parasites that infect more than 1 billion people around the world, but helminth carriage is much less frequent in westernized societies.[13,14] Most helminths stimulate the production of Th2 cytokines. IBD, along with a few other immunodysregulatory disorders, is predominantly a Th1-driven disease. In addition, helminthiasis also prevents Th2-driven allergic reactions. Therefore, the ability of some helminths to induce regulatory cytokines, including interleukin-10 and transforming growth factor β, via stimulation of both regulatory T cells and regulatory type non-T cells suppresses both Th1 and Th2 arms of immunity.[14] A combination of these factors probably accounts for the seemingly protective and possibly therapeutic role played by helminths in patients with IBD. Genetically susceptible people who are never exposed to helminths may lack a counteractive Th2 response, and this may be vital in preventing the onset of IBD.

The possibility that intestinal helminths might protect against development of IBD led to the consideration by one group in Iowa to use helminths in the treatment of IBD. These investigators chose *Trichuris suis*, as it is not a human parasite but the ova are capable of colonizing a human host for several weeks and then are eliminated from the body on their own without any specific therapy. A single dose of 2500 live *T suis* eggs was administered to a small number of patients with active CD and UC, following which a majority of subjects entered remission.[15] The worldwide distribution of *Trichuris trichiura* (a human parasite) is chiefly tropical, with infection being more common in Asia, Africa, and South America than in Western nations. Within the United States, infection is rare overall, with the highest infection rate affecting the southeastern area of the country. Infection with *T trichiura* is associated with poor hygiene and consumption of soil or food that may have been fecally contaminated. There have been mass public health initiatives worldwide to decrease the incidence of *T trichiura* infections in underdeveloped countries, and this may correspond to the increase in IBD in these countries.

Changing diet in developing countries has been proposed as a risk factor for the development of IBD in certain populations, and this has been most extensively documented in South Asian populations. Almost 2 decades ago, Chuah and colleagues[16] reported that westernization of the Indian diet may be linked to IBD. In a questionnaire study conducted in the United Kingdom, investigators found that Hindu patients with IBD were less likely to use spices and eat flour than age-matched and ethnicity-matched controls.[17] One spice that may play an integral role is turmeric, a spice used in cooking by most South Asians. Turmeric is derived from the herb *Curcuma longa*, a member of the ginger family. Curcuminoids are polyphenolic compounds that give turmeric its yellow color, and curcumin is the principal curcuminoid in turmeric. Several studies have shown that curcumin has both anti-inflammatory and antioxidant properties. It has also been shown to reduce colonic inflammatory responses.[18] A few studies to date have also studied curcumin's therapeutic potential in patients with IBD. Investigators in a pilot study published in 2005 administered curcumin to 10 patients with either UC or CD, and reported a marked improvement of symptoms and disease activity in 9 of the 10 patients.[19] In addition, a slightly larger randomized placebo-controlled trial from Japan reported significantly lower recurrence rates among patients with quiescent UC who were administered curcumin when compared with placebo controls.[20] These studies suggest that curcumin, the active ingredient in the commonly known spice termed turmeric, may have significant therapeutic benefits in the treatment of IBD. However, large randomized controlled studies should be performed to better determine whether curcumin can actually play a significant role in the management of IBD.

IRRITABLE BOWEL SYNDROME

Irritable bowel syndrome (IBS) is classified as a functional bowel disorder, and is one of the most frequent reasons for consultation with a gastroenterologist. However, it remains an underdiagnosed entity, especially in developing societies. Assessment of the prevalence of IBS based on studies conducted over the past 20 years is difficult given the varying populations and assessment criteria used by researchers.[21] The Manning criteria were introduced in the 1970s, which identified 4 symptoms thought to differentiate patients with IBS from those with other disorders: visible abdominal distention, pain relieved by bowel movement, more frequent stools with the onset of abdominal pain, and looser stools with the onset of pain. Investigators also found that IBS sufferers were more likely to suffer from rectal passage of mucus and sensation of incomplete evacuation. An international committee met to specify time dimensions to this symptom classification system, and this became known as the Rome criteria.[22] Over time, this classification has been revised and currently the Rome III questionnaire is used.

The prevalence of IBS ranges from 3% to 20%, and is quoted as being between 10% and 15% in most studies conducted in the Western population. It is commonly recognized to have a high female to male ratio (2:1 in most studies), with a typical onset of symptoms before age 45 years and an increase in prevalence again in the elderly.[21] Some studies use both the Manning and Rome criteria and report a markedly different prevalence (20.4% with Manning vs 8.5% with Rome criteria). Saito and colleagues[23] concluded that the prevalence of IBS varied substantially depending on the specific definition of IBS used.

The global picture of IBS is far from complete, with limited data, if any, available from certain regions of the world.[24] It is clear, however, that significant global differences in demographics and clinical presentation of IBS do exist. Based on the literature, the prevalence of IBS seems to be higher than previously thought in Asian countries. By Rome II criteria, the prevalence of IBS in places like Singapore and Japan are 8.6% and 9.8%, respectively, which is comparable to Europe (9.6%), though not as high as in the Unites States, Canada, and England (12%).[25] Interpretation of some of these data is problematic, due to the use of varying diagnostic criteria already mentioned, with many studies reporting varying prevalence rates based on different diagnostic criteria. The largest and most recent study in Japan, which surveyed 10,000 subjects, estimated the prevalence of IBS to be 13% by Rome III criteria.[26] This figure represents a notable increase compared with the prevalence of IBS based on Rome II criteria of 6.1%, which was reported 4 years earlier.[27] South Asian prevalence rates are slightly lower when compared with data available on other Asian countries. A prospective national study conducted in India recently estimated the prevalence of IBS in India to be 4.2%.[28] However, this study did not use the standard Rome II or III criteria in its assessment. In a population-based survey from Pakistan, 13% of subjects met Rome II criteria for IBS.[29] It is unclear whether these seemingly rising prevalence rates in recent studies from Asia reflect a true increase in prevalence, or whether IBS is now becoming more easily recognized and diagnosed in these countries.

Although IBS is more prevalent among women in Western societies, this trend has not proved to be true in other countries. For example, a recent large population-based study from Mumbai, India reported a significant male predominance.[30] Another study conducted in Hong Kong, a telephone survey that used the Rome II diagnostic criteria, revealed there was no significant difference between men and women regarding prevalence of IBS.[31] In one of the most recent and largest studies from India, investigators again reported a higher prevalence of IBS in men (4.3% vs 4.0%). However, the diagnostic criteria used to classify patients as having IBS were less well defined.[28] These statistics do not hold true for a majority of studies published in Asian countries, however. Several studies from other Asian countries did not report a male predominance, but rather no significant difference in prevalence between genders.[32] Similar to much of the Western data, a Japanese study published in 2008 documented a predominant female to male ratio (16% vs 10%) that was statistically significant.[26] Although apparent differences in gender distribution may arise from the use of varying diagnostic criteria, one must ponder why there seems to be such a lack of female predominance in most Asian IBS studies while data from the West suggest that IBS has consistently been more common among women. Are these true gender differences, or are these data a manifestation of cultural factors that make it easier for men to seek medical care? And if cultural factors in these male-dominated societies are not influencing the apparent gender disparity, are there other factors that may make men in these cultures more prone to developing IBS?

There also appear to be differences in socioeconomic status and clinical presentation between Asians and westerners with IBS. Asian patients with IBS tend to come from more affluent classes of their society and are better educated when compared with patients without IBS. By contrast, data from the Unites States reveal that patients with functional bowel disorders are more likely to belong to a lower household income group.[32] Studies reveal that location of abdominal pain is also a factor that seems to vary between Asian and non-Asian IBS patients. Lower abdominal pain is more frequently reported in Western studies, whereas Asian patients are much more likely to present with upper abdominal pain.[32] Clinical overlap between functional dyspepsia and IBS is more common in certain Asian countries. This overlap may result in an underestimation of IBS prevalence in some studies, especially if patients are being classified as having dyspepsia rather than a combination of dyspepsia and IBS. Overall, pain seems to play a bigger role than bowel function in disease perception in Asian societies. What may be perceived as normal in certain Asian populations may really be "abnormal" based on standard Western criteria. For example, a national Indian study found there was a wide mismatch between patient perception of constipation and diarrhea and physicians' rating based on standard Western diagnostic criteria. A majority of their control population admitted to having bowel movements once or twice a day. On average, this is significantly higher than what is deemed as normal according to Western criteria whereby 3 or more movements per week is considered normal.[28] Similarly, in a study conducted in Singapore, when subjects were asked to describe their bowel habits over the preceding 3 months, a majority of those who met diagnostic criteria for IBS believed they had normal bowel habits.[33] Even if the defecatory disturbances were relatively mild in subjects who participated in these two studies, their data suggest that IBS may be missed in certain populations where the threshold for perception of altered bowel habits is higher.

Helicobacter pylori

Helicobacter pylori is linked to a variety of gastric pathologies including gastritis, peptic ulcer disease, and gastric cancer. Affecting more than half of the world's population, it is one of the most common chronic bacterial infections in humans. Studies involving genetic sequence analysis suggest that our species has been infected with *H pylori* since we first migrated from Africa around 58,000 years ago.[34] Most individuals infected with *H pylori* are asymptomatic. It is estimated that 15% to 20% of infected individuals will develop peptic ulcer disease, and fewer than 1% will develop gastric cancer.

There are definite distinct geographic, racial, and social differences in the prevalence of *H pylori* infection. The rate of *H pylori* infection traditionally has differed geographically, specifically divided into low prevalence in developed countries and high prevalence in developing countries. However, this division is changing rapidly with the increase of socioeconomic level in many developing nations and the increasing movement toward treatment of *H pylori* globally. At present, the overall global prevalence of *H pylori* is thought to be around 50%, although the prevalence of *H pylori* has been shown to be decreasing in many countries over the past couple of decades.

Age, ethnicity, geography, and socioeconomic status are all factors that influence prevalence of *H pylori* infection. A recent study performed in Canada revealed that prevalence of infection increased significantly with age and number of siblings. It is interesting that non-Caucasians and immigrants who moved to Canada after age 20 years were also more likely to have *H pylori* infection.[35] A smaller retrospective study in the United States[36] also reported that *H pylori* prevalence varies based on race, finding that a higher percentage of Hispanics (40%) were infected with *H pylori* when compared with Caucasians and African Americans (24% and 28%, respectively). Racial differences in prevalence of *H pylori* within the same country were also proved soon after its discovered link to gastric pathology. In an epidemiologic study performed almost 20 years ago, researchers found that frequency of *H pylori* infection was significantly higher in African Americans when compared with Caucasians (70% vs 34%).[37] However, these trends may be more reflective of socioeconomic status rather than a true racial disparity.

Sanitation, water quality, hygiene, and living conditions have been linked to prevalence of *H pylori* infection. In general the populations in developing countries live in conditions that are highly conducive to the acquisition of microorganisms. Poor hygiene, substandard sanitation, and crowded household conditions are a reality for many in these countries. These factors may help to explain the geographic and population-based differences in the prevalence of *H pylori* infection. In a study conducted in South India,[38] investigators studied the roles of household hygiene and water source in the prevalence and transmission of *H pylori* infection. It was concluded that prevalence of *H pylori* infection was significantly higher among people who drank from wells compared with those who drank tap water. Water from wells is thought to be more susceptible to contamination from nearby excretory/toilet facilities and from animal contamination. The investigators also found a higher prevalence of infection among people with a lower clean water index (a numerical categorization based on a combination of 3 factors: regularity of boiling drinking water, frequency of restoring and reusing water, and frequency of bathing and showering), lower socioeconomic status, and higher crowding index. Similarly, Nurgaleiva and colleagues[39] from Kazakhstan reported a higher prevalence of *H pylori* infection among those with a lower clean water index, river water users, those with outdoor toilet facilities, and those of lower socioeconomic status. Lower socioeconomic status and crowded living conditions are likely etiologically linked risk factors for *H pylori* infection because of their association with less hygienic environments. Interfamilial transmission of *H pylori* has also been documented, with higher rates of *H pylori* prevalence among children with infected mothers.[40] All of the aforementioned findings suggest that the most likely sources of transmission are person to person and exposure to a common source of infection.

Epidemiologic studies around the world have suggested that *H pylori* infection in developing nations is characterized by a rapid acquisition of the infection, such that approximately 80% of the population is infected by age 20 years.[41] On the other hand, prevalence of infection in developed countries tends to peak in the third decade of life. Despite high pockets of *H pylori* infection in certain countries around the world, the frequency of *H pylori* infection is declining worldwide. Most importantly, studies conducted in countries with high prevalence of *H pylori* infection have documented this decline. Seroprevalence in South Korea fell from 66.9% in 1998 to 59.6% in 2005.[42] Another study from Southern China reported a decrease in prevalence from 62.5% to 49% between 1993 and 2003, and a study from the Czech Republic revealed a dramatic decline in *H pylori* prevalence from 70% to 35% over a 13-year period.[43,44] Chinese researchers were also able to demonstrate an improvement in prevalence of peptic ulcer disease along with the decline in *H pylori* prevalence.[45] However, these results were not reproduced in the United States, likely because of persistent use of nonsteroidal anti-inflammatory medications.[46]

To briefly comment on gender, studies performed until now have not demonstrated a significant gender difference in the prevalence of *H pylori*. However, in their population-based study Naja and colleagues[35] did report that men had a higher prevalence of *H pylori* infection when compared with women (29.4% vs 14.9%). Also, a Chinese study found that men and *H pylori*–positive patients were much more likely to develop peptic ulcer disease than women and *H pylori*–negative patients. However, these data represent a minority of results from epidemiologic studies on the prevalence of *H pylori* infection. Overall, it is safe to say that gender differences have not been documented among those with *H pylori*.

FECAL INCONTINENCE

Fecal incontinence is defined as the involuntary passage of solid or liquid stool or mucus. In the United States, the prevalence of fecal incontinence is believed to be 2% to 7%.[47,48] In high-risk populations, such as nursing home residents, the prevalence approaches 50%.[48] Despite these impressive numbers, the true prevalence of fecal incontinence is likely underreported and underestimated. Patients are often embarrassed about their symptoms and are thus less likely to seek help from medical professionals. Lastly, many physicians tend to shy away from asking their patients about symptoms of fecal incontinence.

Female gender is believed to be a risk factor for fecal incontinence, perhaps because underlying conditions such as multiple sclerosis, scleroderma, and IBS that predispose a person to fecal incontinence are also more prevalent among women. Gynecologic surgery, pregnancy, and obstetric trauma are also well-documented and significant causes of fecal incontinence in women.[49] Gender differences in anorectal anatomy, physiology, and hormones also predispose the female gender to this condition. Conversely, men are less willing to report fecal incontinence to a medical professional and are therefore underrepresented in this overall group.[47]

Despite these compelling facts, studies have failed to consistently show that fecal incontinence is more common in women. Whitehead and colleagues[50] conducted a national survey in the United States on approximately 2300 participants. Besides reporting that the prevalence of fecal incontinence increases significantly with age, they also found no significant difference in prevalence between men (7.7%) and women (8.9%). Nelson and colleagues[48] conducted a survey of Wisconsin nursing home residents, and found that urinary incontinence was most strongly associated with the presence of fecal incontinence. This group did not, however, find gender to be a strong risk factor. Moreover, a meta-analysis, which aimed to determine prevalence of anal incontinence according to age and gender, showed that age, but not gender, had a significant influence on rates of solid and liquid fecal incontinence.[51] Lastly, a population-based study conducted in Australia found that men were significantly more likely to have fecal incontinence than women. In their discussion of the findings in their study, the investigators noted that there were a few other population-based studies that also reported a higher male prevalence, but a majority of these studies were postal questionnaires and not interview based. Limited data exists on the prevalence of fecal incontinence in the developing world. A majority of the studies conducted on fecal incontinence are from North America and Europe, with a few from Japan as well.

One region that has been uniquely studied is the Middle Eastern Islamic nations. These cultures are described as being pro-natal, with a high average total fertility rate and female life expectancy. Thus, a high prevalence of pelvic floor disorders would be expected in women from this region of the world due to multiparity and long postmenopausal life span.[52] Despite a higher prevalence of pelvic floor disorders, a study from the United Arab Emirates showed that only 41% of women with fecal incontinence actually sought medical advice. Reasons for not seeking medical advice included embarrassment, male gender of physician, preference to discuss the matter with close friends or relatives and, surprisingly, the belief that fecal incontinence is normal with aging or perceived by some to be the consequence of a neurologic or senile disorder.[53] The intimate and sensitive nature of incontinence may also hinder a woman from seeking medical advice from a physician who is likely to be of the opposite gender, especially in a culture where the gender roles are so clearly delineated.

HEPATITIS B

Hepatitis B is a viral infection considered endemic around the world. Two billion people have serologic evidence of current or previous hepatitis B infection, and approximately 350 million have chronic infection. Between 15% and 40% of patients with chronic infection will develop cirrhosis as part of the course of the disease, and it is estimated that 500,000 to 1,200,000 deaths per year are attributable to hepatitis B virus (HBV) infection.[54] It is well recognized that the prevalence of HBV infection varies significantly between different regions around the world. To facilitate the understanding of this distribution, most of the literature divides the different areas of the world into high, medium, and low endemicity. The prevalence of chronic infection ranges from less than 1% in western Europe and North America to 10% in South-East Asia, China, sub-Saharan Africa, and the Amazon area. It is estimated that around 45% of the total population of the world live in areas of high endemicity. It is noteworthy that because of the globalization process, individuals from areas of high endemicity may migrate to areas of low endemicity and be largely unnoticed.

The wide range of prevalence of chronic HBV infection around the world is closely related to the age of infection. When the infection occurs perinatally (vertical infection), the chance of becoming chronically infected is 70% to 90%. If the infection occurs during early childhood (younger than 5 years), the chance of the infection becoming chronic is 20% to 50%. In immunocompetent adults, the chance of developing chronic hepatitis B after the initial infection ranges between 1% and 3%. It is very likely that in areas with a high prevalence of chronic HBV infection, people are most often infected via vertical transmission. For this reason, worldwide initiatives for vaccination against hepatitis B are of the utmost importance. Routine vaccination of infants was first recommended in China in 1992.[55] To date, 88% of World Health Organization Member States have introduced the vaccine for at least some of their population. It is estimated that approximately 93% of Africa and close to 100% of Southeast Asia have implemented a vaccination policy. In 2007, 92% of the 1-year-old children in the United States were immunized.[56] Continued movement toward population-based vaccination against hepatitis B should help to decrease the vertical transmission of this virus.

HEPATOCELLULAR CARCINOMA

One of the most dangerous complications of liver disease is the development of hepatocellular carcinoma (HCC). HCC currently is the sixth most common malignancy worldwide and the third leading cause of cancer deaths. HCC is the fifth most common type of cancer in men, and eighth among women. In some regions of Africa and Asia, HCC has been found to be the most common type of malignancy. It is estimated that around 50% of the deaths due to HCC occur in China alone. A majority of the remainder of cancer deaths from HCC occur in sub-Saharan Africa, another region with limited resources.[57] These findings are likely secondary to failure to recognize the population at risk, low awareness of ways to prevent liver disease, lack of surveillance programs, and high prevalence of risk factors in these populations, all of which lead to lack of early diagnosis and treatment.

In the United States, Japan, western Europe, and Latin America, cirrhosis secondary to hepatitis C infection is the most common underlying risk factor for HCC. On the other hand, in Asia, Africa, and some eastern European countries, chronic hepatitis B is the most common underlying risk factor for HCC. In China and Africa alone, close to 75% of patients with HCC have chronic hepatitis B infection.[57] One unique environmental factor for HCC is the ingestion of food contaminated with aflatoxins. Aflatoxins were first described in the 1960s, and they have been proven to be carcinogenic. Hyperendemic areas like sub-Saharan Africa, Southeast Asia, and southern China have dietary staples highly contaminated with aflatoxin. During the 1960s and 1970s, many epidemiologic studies in Africa and Asia focused on the correlation between high aflatoxin exposure and increased incidence of HCC.[58] These studies found an increase in the incidence of HCC when there is a high intake of food that is contaminated with aflatoxin. One of the limitations of initial studies was the inability to account for confounding factors such as HBV or hepatitis C virus infection. Within the past 20 years, many studies have been published on the correlation of aflatoxin exposure and HCC. Bulatao-Jayme and colleagues[59] found that patients with confirmed HCC were exposed to a 4.5 times higher aflatoxin load per day when compared with matched controls. These investigators also compared alcohol, and found a synergistic and statistically significant effect on the relative risk of HCC with aflatoxin exposure and alcohol intake. A study conducted in Swaziland[60] showed that the prevalence of HBV infection was high across the different geographic regions analyzed. Of note, there was a more than a fivefold variation in aflatoxin exposure between the different regions, and this was strongly associated with a fivefold increase in the incidence of HCC. Yeh and colleagues[61] examined the interaction between HBV infection and aflatoxin exposure in Guangxi province, China. Their results showed that people with positive hepatitis B surface antigen (HBsAg) and heavy aflatoxin exposure had a tenfold higher incidence of HCC than people from areas with low aflatoxin contamination. Also, HBsAg-negative people who were exposed to heavy aflatoxin load had a rate of HCC comparable to that of the HBsAg-positive people with low aflatoxin load. These findings suggest that an increased effort in both HBV immunization programs and programs to lower aflatoxin exposure will lower the incidence of HCC.

SUMMARY

There are distinct global differences in the prevalence of many gastrointestinal disorders. These variations are a result of diet, sanitation, genetics, and environmental exposures. As Third World countries become more industrialized, these disparities will begin to diminish. This article highlights IBD, H pylori, IBS, fecal incontinence, hepatitis B, and HCC. However, global variations exist for most medical diseases, which should be recognized by all physicians.

REFERENCES

1. Logan I, Bowlus C. The geoepidemiology of autoimmune intestinal diseases. Autoimmun Rev 2010;9:A372–8.
2. Yamamoto T, Nakahigashi M, Saniabadi AR. Review article: diet and inflammatory bowel disease—epidemiology and treatment. Aliment Pharmacol Ther 2009;30:99–112.
3. Zvidi I, Hazazi R, Birkenfeld S, et al. The prevalence of Crohn's disease in Israel: a 20-year survey. Dig Dis Sci 2009;54:848–52.
4. Birkenfeld S, Zvidi I, Hazazi I, et al. The prevalence of ulcerative colitis in Israel: a twenty-year survey. J Clin Gastroenterol 2009;43(8):743–6.
5. Herrinton LJ, Liu L, Lewis J, et al. Incidence and prevalence of inflammatory bowel disease in a northern California managed care organization 1996–2002. Am J Gastroenterol 2008;103:1998–2006.
6. Shivnanda S, Lennard-Jones J, Logan R, et al. Incidence of inflammatory bowel disease across Europe: is there a difference between north and south? Results of the European Collaborative Study on Inflammatory Bowel Disease. Gut 1996;39(5):690–7.
7. Ladas SD, Mala E, Giorgiotis K, et al. Incidence of ulcerative colitis in Central Greece: a prospective study. World J Gastroenterol 2005;11:1785–7.
8. Sincic BM, Vucelic B, Persic M, et al. Incidence of inflammatory bowel disease in Primorsko-Goranska County, Croatia, 2000–2004: a prospective population-based study. Scand J Gastroenterol 2006;41(4):437–44.
9. Sood A, Midha V, Sood N, et al. Incidence and prevalence of ulcerative colitis in Punjab, North India. Gut 2003;53(11):1587–90.
10. Yang SK, Yun S, Kim JH, et al. Epidemiology of inflammatory bowel disease in Songpa-Kangdong district, Seoul, Korea. Inflamm Bowel Dis 2008;14(4):542–9.
11. Bernstein CN, Fried M, Krabshuis JH, et al. Inflammatory bowel disease: a global perspective. Global Guidelines. World Gastroenterology Organization; 2009.

Available at: http://www.worldgastroenterology.org/assets/downloads/en/pdf/guidelines/21_inflammatory_bowel_disease.pdf. Accessed March 21, 2011.

12. Pinsk F, Lemberg D, Grewal K, et al. Inflammatory bowel disease in South Asian pediatric population of British Columbia. Am J Gastroenterol 2007;102: 1077–83.

13. Maizels RM, Yazdanbakhsh M. Immune regulation by helminth parasites: cellular and molecular mechanisms. Nat Rev Immunol 2003;3:733–44.

14. Guarner F, Bourdet-Sicard R, Brandtzaeg P, et al. Mechanisms of disease: the hygiene hypothesis is revisited. Nat Clin Pract Gastroenterol Hepatol 2006;3(5): 275–84.

15. Summers R, Elliott D, Khurram Q, et al. *Trichuris suis* seems to be safe and possibly effective in the treatment of inflammatory bowel disease. Am J Gastroenterol 2003;98(9):2034–41.

16. Chuah SY, Jayanthi V, Lee CN, et al. Dietary fats and inflammatory bowel disease in Asians. Ital J Gastroenterol 1992;24:336–88.

17. Probert C, Bhakta P, Bhamra B, et al. Diet of South Asians with inflammatory bowel disease. Arq Gastroenterol 1996;33(3):132–5.

18. Plummer SM, Holloway KA, Manson MM, et al. Inhibition of cyclo-oxygenase 2 expression in colon cells by the chemopreventive agent curcumin involves inhibition of NF-KB activation via the NIK/IKK signaling complex. Oncogene 1999;18: 6013–20.

19. Holt PR, Katz S, Kirshoff R. Curcumin therapy in inflammatory bowel disease: a pilot study. Dig Dis Sci 2005;50(11):2191–3.

20. Hanai H, Iida T, Takeuchi K, et al. Curcumin maintenance therapy for ulcerative colitis: randomized, multicenter, double-blind, placebo-controlled trial. Clin Gastroenterol Hepatol 2006;4:1502–6.

21. Grundmann O, Yoon SL. Irritable bowel syndrome: epidemiology, diagnosis, and treatment: an update for health-care practitioners. J Gastroenterol Hepatol 2010; 25:691–9.

22. Hahn BA, Saunders WB, Maier WC. Differences between individuals with self-reported irritable bowel syndrome (IBS) and IBS-like symptoms. Dig Dis Sci 1997;42(12):2585–90.

23. Saito YA, Locke R, Talley N, et al. A comparison of the Rome and Manning Criteria for case identification in epidemiological investigations of irritable bowel syndrome. Am J Gastroenterol 2000;95(10):2816–24.

24. Quigley E, Fried M, Gwee KA, et al. Irritable bowel syndrome: a global perspective. Global Guideline. World Gastroenterology Organization; 2009. Available at: http://www.worldgastroenterology.org/assets/downloads/en/pdf/guidelines/20_irritable_bowel_syndrome.pdf. Accessed March 21, 2011.

25. Gwee KA, Lu CL, Ghoshal UC. Epidemiology of irritable bowel syndrome in Asia: something old, something new, something borrowed. J Gastroenterol Hepatol 2009;24:1601–7.

26. Miwa H. Prevalence of irritable bowel syndrome in Japan: internet survey using Rome III criteria. Patient Prefer Adherence 2008;2:143–7.

27. Kumano H, Kaiya H, Yoshiuchi K, et al. Comorbidity of irritable bowel syndrome, panic disorder, and agoraphobia in Japanese representative sample. Am J Gastroenterol 2004;99:70–6.

28. Ghoshal UC, Abraham P, Bhatt C, et al. Epidemiological and clinical profile of irritable bowel syndrome in India: report of the Indian Society of Gastroenterology Task Force. Indian J Gastroenterol 2008;27:22–8.

29. Husain N, Chaudhry IB, Jafri F, et al. A population-based study of irritable bowel syndrome in a non-Western population. Neurogastroenterol Motil 2008;20(9): 1022–9.
30. Shah SS, Bhatia SJ, Mistry FP. Epidemiology of dyspepsia in the general population in Mumbai. Indian J Gastroenterol 2001;20(3):103–6.
31. Kwan ACP, Hu WH, Chan YK, et al. Prevalence of irritable bowel syndrome in Hong Kong. J Gastroenterol Hepatol 2002;17(11):1180–6.
32. Gwee KA. Irritable bowel syndrome in developing countries—a disorder of civilization of colonization? Neurogastroenterol Motil 2005;17:317–24.
33. Gwee KA, Wee S, Wong ML, et al. The prevalence, symptom characteristics, and impact of irritable bowel syndrome in an Asian urban community. Am J Gastroenterol 2004;99(5):924–31.
34. Linz B, Balloux F, Moodley Y, et al. An African origin for the intimate association between humans and Helicobacter pylori. Nature 2007;445:915.
35. Naja F, Kreiger N, Sullivan T. Helicobacter pylori infection in Ontario: prevalence and risk factors. Can J Gastroenterol 2007;21(8):501–6.
36. Smith JG, Li W, Rosson RS. Prevalence, clinical and endoscopic predictors of Helicobacter pylori infection in an urban population. Conn Med 2009;73(3): 133–7.
37. Graham DY, Malaty HM, Evans DG, et al. Epidemiology of Helicobacter pylori in an asymptomatic population in the United States. Effect of age, race, and socioeconomic status. Gastroenterology 1991;100(6):1495–501.
38. Ahmed KS, Khan AA, Ahmed I, et al. Impact of household hygiene and water source on the prevalence and transmission of Helicobacter pylori: a South Indian perspective. Singapore Med J 2007;48(6):543–9.
39. Nurgalieva ZZ, Malaty HM, Graham DY, et al. Helicobacter pylori infection in Kazakhstan: effect of water source and household hygiene. Am J Trop Med Hyg 2002;67(2):201–6.
40. Fujimoto Y, Furusyo N, Toyoda K, et al. Intrafamilial transmission of Helicobacter pylori among the population of endemic areas of Japan. Helicobacter 2007;12: 170–6.
41. Malaty HM. Epidemiology of Helicobacter pylori infection. Best Pract Res Clin Gastroenterol 2007;21(2):205–14.
42. Yim JY, Kim N, Choi SH, et al. Seroprevalence of Helicobacter pylori in South Korea. Helicobacter 2007;12(4):333–40.
43. Chen J, Bu XL, Wang QY, et al. Decreasing seroprevalence of Helicobacter pylori infection during 1993–2003 in Guangzhou, Southern China. Helicobacter 2007; 12(2):164–9.
44. Bures J, Kapacova M, Rejchrt S. Decrease of prevalence of Helicobacter pylori infection in the Czech Republic. Cas Lek Cesk 2008;147(5):255–7 [in Czech].
45. Wu HC, Tuo BG, Wu WM, et al. Prevalence of peptic ulcer in dyspeptic patients and the influence of age, sex, and Helicobacter pylori infection. Dig Dis Sci 2008; 53:2650–6.
46. Manuel D, Cutler A, Goldstein J, et al. Decreasing prevalence combined with increasing eradication of Helicobacter pylori infection in the United States has not resulted in fewer hospital admissions for peptic ulcer disease-related complications. Aliment Pharmacol Ther 2007;25(12):1423–7.
47. Drossman DA, Li Z, Andruzzi E, et al. U.S. householder survey of functional gastrointestinal disorders. Prevalence, sociodemography, and health impact. Dig Dis Sci 1993;38(9):1569–80.

48. Nelson R, Norton N, Cautley E, et al. Community-based prevalence of anal incontinence. JAMA 1995;274(7):559–61.
49. Hawes SK, Ahmad A. Fecal incontinence: a woman's view. Am J Gastroenterol 2006;101:S610–7.
50. Whitehead WE, Borrud L, Goode PS, et al. Fecal incontinence in US adults: epidemiology and risk factors. Gastroenterology 2009;137:512–7.
51. Pretlove SJ, Radley S, Toozs-Hobson PM, et al. Prevalence of anal incontinence according to age and gender: a systematic review and meta-regression analysis. Int Urogynecol J Pelvic Floor Dysfunct 2006;17:401–17.
52. Rizk DE, El-Safty MM. Female pelvic floor dysfunction in the Middle East: a tale of three factors—culture, religion and socialization of health role stereotypes. Int Urogynecol J Pelvic Floor Dysfunct 2006;17:436–8.
53. Rizk DE, Hassan MY, Shaheen H, et al. The prevalence and determinants of health care-seeking behavior for fecal incontinence in multiparous United Arab Emirates females. Dis Colon Rectum 2001;44(12):1850–6.
54. Heathcote J, Abbas Z, Alberti A, et al. Hepatitis B. Global Guidelines. World Gastroenterology Organization; 2008. Available at: http://www.worldgastroenterology.org/assets/downloads/en/pdf/guidelines/12_hepatitis_b_en.pdf. Accessed March 21, 2011.
55. Centers for Disease Control and Prevention (CDC). Progress in hepatitis B prevention through universal infant vaccination—China, 1997-2006. MMWR Morb Mortal Wkly Rep 2007;56(18):441–5.
56. Viral hepatitis: global policy: World Hepatitis Alliance; 2010.
57. Ferenci P, Fried M, Labrecque D, et al. Hepatocellular Carcinoma (HCC): a global perspective. Global Guidelines. World Gastroenterology Organization; 2009. Available at: http://www.worldgastroenterology.org/assets/downloads/en/pdf/guidelines/24_hepatocellular_carcinoma_en.pdf. Accessed March 21, 2011.
58. Groopman JD, Scholl P, Wang JS. Epidemiology of human aflatoxin exposures and their relationship to liver cancer. Prog Clin Biol Res 1996;395:211–22.
59. Bulatao-Jayme J, Almero EM, Castro MC, et al. A case-control dietary study of primary liver cancer risk from aflatoxin exposure. Int J Epidemiol 1982;11(2):112–9.
60. Peers F, Bosch X, Kaldor J, et al. Aflatoxin exposure, hepatitis B virus infection and liver cancer in Swaziland. Int J Cancer 1987;39(5):545–53.
61. Yeh FS, Yu Mc, Mo CC, et al. Hepatitis B virus, aflatoxins, and hepatocellular carcinoma in southern Guangxi, China. Cancer Res 1989;49(9):2506–9.

The Challenges of Being a Female Gastroenterologist

Grace H. Elta, MD

- Gastroenterologist • Women • Gastroenterology • Challenges

Gastroenterology (GI) has been one of the slowest fields in medicine to be embraced by women (**Fig. 1**). It has been nearly 20 years since medical schools in the United States were populated almost 50% by women (**Fig. 2**). Despite that fact, GI has only started attracting significant numbers of female physicians in the past 5 years. Of graduating medical students, a large percentage of women have chosen internal medicine as a career. More female than male internists choose to stay in primary care rather than subspecialize. Of the women who do decide to pursue a fellowship, few have historically chosen gastroenterology or cardiology. The percentage of female first-year gastroenterology fellows is still hovering around 25% to 30% (**Fig. 3**). The reasons for this lack of interest in GI have not been well studied, although the assumption is that many women seek careers that are lifestyle friendly. Both GI and cardiology are perceived as subspecialties that have significant on-call responsibilities. This explanation is not completely satisfying because obstetrics and gynecology have long attracted many female medical students and yet clearly have an on-call requirement that is greater than GI. Another explanation is that the culture of GI has not been inviting to women, similar to what has occurred in surgery.[1] A study performed many years ago found that 39% of female GI fellows perceived gender discrimination and 19% perceived sexual harassment during their training.[2] Sexual stereotypes and biases against women can have a profound influence on a woman's professional experience. Female medical students and residents are less likely to choose a profession if they do not receive the verbal encouragement and opportunities for advancement afforded to their male colleagues.

HURTLES UNIQUE TO FEMALE GASTROENTEROLOGISTS
Combining Child Rearing and Career

Perhaps the biggest hurtle to all female physicians is trying to combine career advancement and child rearing. Because of the length of medical training, many

Division of Gastroenterology, University of Michigan, 3912 Taubman Center, Ann Arbor, MI 48109-5362, USA
E-mail address: gelta@umich.edu

Gastroenterol Clin N Am 40 (2011) 441–447
doi:10.1016/j.gtc.2011.03.004
0889-8553/11/$ – see front matter © 2011 Elsevier Inc. All rights reserved.

gastro.theclinics.com

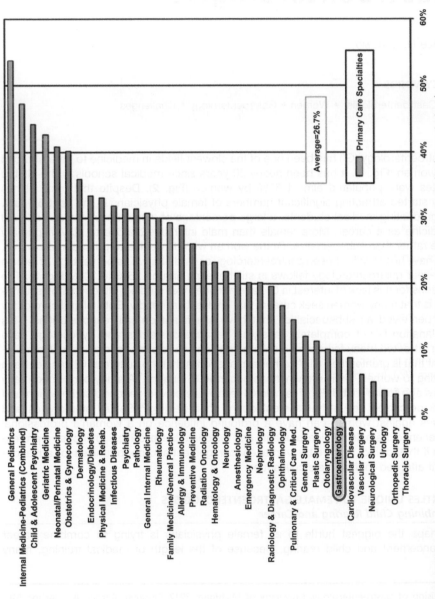

Fig. 1. Percentage of active physicians who are female by specialty. (*Data from* the American Medical Association.)

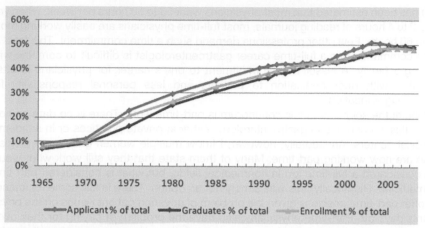

Fig. 2. Percentage of medical students who are female. (*Data from* the Association of American Medical Colleges.)

female physicians put off starting a family until they have finished their training, which takes them into their early 30s. At that age there is already a decreasing fertility rate giving a sense of urgency to starting a family. Although it is never easy to combine career and family for either gender, the burden of organizing childcare and family activities still tends to fall to the mother more than the father. This traditional female role is actually a full-time job in itself as exemplified by many full-time stay-at-home mothers. To combine this complex but rewarding job with a demanding medical career is daunting at best, and overwhelming at other times. In a survey of GI fellows, female fellows were more likely to choose programs according to parental leave policies and family reasons than the male fellows.[2] Female fellows were also more likely than men to alter their family planning because of training program restrictions (20% vs 7%). In addition, they were more likely to remain childless or have fewer children at the end of training despite marital status, not unlike their male colleagues.

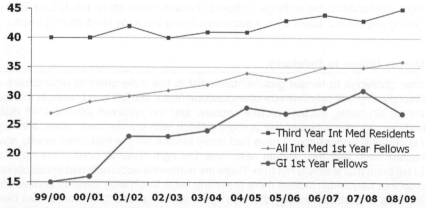

Fig. 3. Percentage of trainees who are female. (*Data from* the American Board of Internal Medicine.)

It has been estimated that most physicians work 55 to 60 hours per week; when you add 2 to 4 hours of reading journals, most full-time physicians are easily working more than 60 hours. Few other professions demand such a time commitment. This level of time commitment as a full-time career gastroenterologist is difficult to combine with raising a family. A lesser time commitment to one's career for physicians is often equated with poor dedication to patients and less personal responsibility for continuing education.

One of the solutions to this conundrum is part-time work. There is no data on how often this is occurring in gastroenterology, either in private practices or in academic medical centers. Anecdotally, however, I know multiple women gastroenterologists who are now working part time. Many of them state that they still work what would be considered a full-time job in nonmedical fields, but what is considered part time in medicine. Historically, this was simply not an option. There is still some reluctance to offer part-time positions given the problem of covering patient issues on the physician's days off. Part-time physicians also have the problem of paying for their overhead. Generally, the malpractice and support personnel needs are not easily scaled back for part-time physicians. There is no data looking at the competence of physicians who choose to work part time. However, given the large number of physicians who work part time clinically and spend the rest of the time in research or administration, it would appear that part-time clinical work does not adversely affect quality of care.

In a study that addressed the work satisfaction of part-time female physicians compared with their full-time counterparts, the part-time workers had lower career satisfaction if their marital and parental satisfaction was low; whereas, this correlation did not exist for the full-time physicians. The part-time female physicians were also more likely to consider leaving their employment entirely depending on interference of career with family. Both career satisfaction and intention to leave their employment were correlated with the quality of home life for reduced-hours physicians.[3]

What are the solutions to this problem? First, it is important that female gastroenterologists support the reasonable work-hour demands of each other. For example, conferences should not be scheduled in early morning or evening hours. Family time and family responsibilities need to be respected. Second, it is important that female physicians be allowed to choose the number of hours that they want to work and to be paid appropriately, which is really quite simple in an relative value unit-based system. Lastly, there are 25 years of productive work after children enter school and 10 years after children are no longer at home. It would be unreasonable to lose 50% of our young physicians' talent by not accommodating the early child-rearing years.

Challenges Unique to Endoscopy

Another challenge to female gastroenterologist is the male-oriented ergonomics of endoscopy. There is only one size of endoscope head. The left hand controls multiple functions: air, water, suction, picture capture, and the up/down and right/left dials. Nobody has studied whether this is more difficult with smaller hand sizes, although that is certainly conceivable. I have had many fellows tell me that other faculty have instructed them that they should *never* use the right hand to control the right/left dial; I tell them that is simply not true. There are numerous accomplished endoscopists who do that frequently. Indeed there are many ways to expertly perform endoscopy.

One area of gastroenterology that has had a particular dearth of women has been interventional endoscopy. Because there is clearly no evidence that men have greater dexterity or stamina than women, this dearth is most likely explained by the lack of encouragement of female GI fellows or frank discrimination. There have also been few role models available.

For female interventionalists, there is always the question of radiation exposure in the endoscopic retrograde cholangiopancreatography suite during pregnancy. Only recently the public and the press have come to realize that radiation exposure received by patients with medical imaging, such as computed tomography scanning, affects future cancer risk. There is even less data on the issue of radiation exposure of health care workers, particularly during pregnancy. Although the data suggests that the risk is either nonexistent or small, there are still several women in health care fields who avoid all radiation exposure during pregnancy. At many medical centers, the radiation safety departments recommend wearing a second radiation badge at abdominal level under the lead apron. Careful radiation control should of course be part of all of our work experience, although concerns about fetal exposure are greater. The National Council on Radiation Protection recommends limiting exposure to 100 mrem during the first trimester and 500 mrem during the entire pregnancy. Doses significantly lower than this should be obtained in the fluoroscopy room if the equipment is up to date and appropriate radiation control measures are taken. All interventional endoscopists should understand the basics of radiation safety in procedure rooms.

Is there a Glass Ceiling?

Although few women have chosen gastroenterology as a career, a disproportionally small percentage of them have been promoted to leadership positions in academic medical centers and in professional societies. Has this poor advancement been caused by discrimination or the old boys' network, or is it caused by a lack of personal promotion and drive in many women, qualities that are simply not a part of the traditional female gender role? The author's suspicion is that this lack of leadership positions is caused by both of the previously mentioned reasons, although one of the reasons that women do not promote themselves is that they have not been rewarded equally with men. When academic women have been surveyed, a high percentage of them feel that they have been discriminated against.[4] Discrimination encountered by female physicians are often nonactionable micro-inequities, such as conscious and unconscious slights, including ignoring women at rounds or in discussions of patients and not crediting women's ideas.[5]

Discrimination has clearly happened in salary structures. Female medical school faculty neither advance as rapidly nor are compensated as well as professionally similar male colleagues. Deficits for female physicians are greater than those for nonphysician female faculty, and for both physicians and nonphysicians, women's deficits are greater for faculty with more seniority.[6] Female gastroenterologists are paid less even when number of hours worked are accounted for.[7] A survey of gastroenterologists who were 3 and 5 years out of their training showed that academic female gastroenterologists made an average of 77% of their male colleagues salaries at 3 years and 76% at 5 years. A similar wage disparity occurs in nonacademic practices at 3 years post-training, although the differences improved at 5 years out of fellowship; whereas, it did not for academic women. However, it is also true that women do not tend to ask for much, whether it be salary raises or office and research space. Because the squeaky wheel tends to get greased, it is not surprising that women have not thrived; they do not tend to be self-promoters. Despite this difference in gender personalities, it is hard to deny that basic fairness should have equalized these wage gaps but failed to do so because of serious ongoing discrimination issues.

The flip side of the glass-ceiling problem is that women have also been highly sought after for positions of prominence. The low number of women in gastroenterology has historically helped promote some aspects of their careers. Many boards and committees have sought diversity in their ranks for more than 20 years and there have been few women to choose from. It is difficult to ascertain if this reverse discrimination has been sufficient to balance out the true discrimination that has occurred.

Sexual Harassment

Sexual harassment is characterized by unwelcome sexual advances, requests for sexual favors, and other verbal or physical conduct of a sexual nature where submission is made either explicitly or implicitly a condition of an individual's success. In a study of residents in internal medicine, 73% of women and 11% of men who responded reported that they had been sexually harassed at least once during their training.[8] Many of the men who report harassment are gay men. About half of the reported incidents occurred during medical school and half during residency. Despite the frequency of sexual harassment, appropriate responses are rare because of either underreporting or noncorrective action.

ADVANTAGES TO BEING A FEMALE GASTROENTEROLOGIST

There are several advantages to being a woman in a male-dominated field. First, male professions have traditionally garnered higher incomes than female-predominant professions. This finding is clearly true of medicine in general and especially true of gastroenterology. One of the fears in American medicine is that the salaries will start to drop significantly as they have in some European countries where women now outnumber men in medicine.

Another advantage in being a female gastroenterologist and endoscopist is that many female patients prefer to see a female physician. This phenomenon has been described in multiple medical fields. In Gastroenterology, this female physician preference has been best studied for the performance of colonoscopy. In several studies, almost half of female patients prefer having a women endoscopist.[8–10] In contrast, few men state that they have a preference and the few that do often also prefer a female physician. Recognition of this fact has led many large GI private practices to actively recruit women to their group so they can remain competitive in the market place. The reasons for this female physician preference have included less embarrassment and the common societal thought that women are more compassionate and better communicators.

SUMMARY

Women have started to enter gastroenterology in significant numbers over the past 5 years, although they are still underrepresented compared with the proportion of female graduating medical students. This underrepresentation is most likely caused by the culture of GI where female students and residents have felt undervalued and unwelcome. This type of discrimination is difficult to fight because it is behind the scenes. However, with increasing female role models in GI, this underrepresentation will likely change in the coming years. Change in medicine comes slowly but does occur.

Career options are bright for women who do decide to enter gastroenterology. Many patients have a preference for female physicians, which has made them sought-after hires in private practices. A greater emphasis on embracing diversity has promoted the careers of women in academic and salaried positions.

REFERENCES

1. Sonnad SS, Colletti LM. Issues in the recruitment and success of women in academic surgery. Surgery 2002;132:415–9.
2. Arlow FL, Raymond PL, Karlstadt RG, et al. Gastroenterology training and career choices: a prospective longitudinal study of the impact of gender and of managed care. Am J Gastroenterol 2002;97:459–69.
3. Barnett RC, Gareis KC, Carr PL. Career satisfaction and retention of a sample of women physicians who work reduced hours. J Womens Health 2005;14:146–53.
4. Carr PL, Ash AS, Friedman RH, et al. Faculty perceptions of gender discrimination and sexual harassment in academic medicine. Ann Intern Med 2000;132: 889–96.
5. Lenhart SA, Evans CH. Sexual harassment and gender discrimination: a primer for women physicians. JAMA 1991;46:77–82.
6. Ash AS, Carr PL, Goldstein R, et al. Compensation and advancement of women in academic medicine: is there equity? Ann Intern Med 2004;141:205–12.
7. Burke CA, Sastri SV, Jacobsen G, et al. Gender disparity in the practice of gastroenterology: the first 5 years of a career. Am J Gastroenterol 2005;100:259–64.
8. Komaromy M, Bindm AB, Haber JH, et al. Sexual harassment in medical training. N Engl J Med 1993;328:322–6.
9. Varadarajulu S, Petruff C, Ramsey WH. Patient preferences for gender of endoscopists. Gastrointest Endosc 2002;56:170–3.
10. Menees SB, Inadomi JM, Korsnes S, et al. Women patients' preference for women physicians is a barrier to colon cancer screening. Gastrointest Endosc 2005;62:219–23.

Gastrointestinal Issues in the Older Female Patient

Tobias Zuchelli, MD[a],*, Scott E. Myers, MD[b,c]

KEYWORDS

- Anorexia of aging • Fecal incontinence • Constipation
- Female • Motility

As the body ages, it undergoes a multitude of changes. Some of these changes are visible, whereas others are not and may be elicited during the patient encounter. Some gastrointestinal issues may be more common in the elderly population and possibly in older women. These issues range from motility disorders, such as fecal incontinence (FI) and constipation, to changes in neuropeptide function and its effect on the anorexia of aging. This article comprehensively reviews gastrointestinal issues that commonly afflict the elderly female population.

ANOREXIA

Enjoying food depends on a combination of factors including taste, olfaction, pain, temperature, sensation, learned responses, cultural beliefs, and prior experiences. This information is gathered, integrated, and processed at the cortical level to yield what we recognize as taste. Alterations of these processes may occur with aging, thereby affecting taste, smell, and ultimately appetite. With aging, many physiologic and pathologic factors may contribute to these alterations and influence both the ability to sense and process information. These factors are examined in this article. It is not clear if gender contributes to anorexia with aging. However, gender may exert an independent influence.

Olfaction has been recognized as the major component involved in tasting food. Over time, olfactory receptors are lost at a rate of approximately 10% per decade.[1]

The authors have nothing to disclose.

[a] Drexel University College of Medicine, 245 North 15th Street, 5th Floor New College Building, Philadelphia, PA 19107, USA

[b] Division of Gastroenterology and Hepatology, Drexel University College of Medicine, 219 North Broad Street, 5th Floor, Philadelphia, PA 19107, USA

[c] Internal Medicine Residency Program, Drexel University College of Medicine, Philadelphia, PA, USA

* Corresponding author.

E-mail address: tobias.zuchelli@drexelmed.edu

Gastroenterol Clin N Am 40 (2011) 449–466

doi:10.1016/j.gtc.2011.03.007

Studies have also shown that olfactory potentials decrease with age.[2] These anatomic and physiologic changes lead to a diminished sense of smell that, in combination with processing and interpretive changes, lead to an altered taste perception, especially in cognitively impaired older patients. No clear gender differences have been observed.

Studies have shown that the threshold for taste declines with age and the male gender, especially with respect to saltiness and unami.[3] Besides salty, sweet, bitter, and sour, unami is the fifth taste sensation and is sensitive to amino acids. The effects of mixtures of food products, solubility properties in water, and olfactory preservation must be considered when interpreting data and reviewing studies. Although some studies suggest that changes in both the sensitivity and the actual number of taste buds are factors in determining taste, it is generally accepted that function, rather than number, is of prime importance. Other factors that contribute to the perception include dental or periodontal disease, medications, tobacco use, and alterations in saliva.

The concept of anorexia of aging can be traced back to Morley and Silver[4] whose 1988 article pointed toward the decline in caloric intake with aging. More recent studies confirm that elderly patients typically experience earlier satiety and have difficulty upregulating caloric intake after a period of abstinence from food when compared with their younger counterparts.[5,6] Sturm and colleagues[7] found that early satiety in the elderly is secondary to decreased nitric oxide synthase activity in the stomach, causing decreased fundal compliance and a heightened antral stretch response. Therefore, less food triggers antral stretch and thus satiation signals that lead to early satiety.[8] The 2 commonly studied satiety hormones seen with aging are leptin and cholecystokinin (CCK). This section reviews the basic mechanisms of various neuropeptides and their relation to appetite, satiety, and the anorexia of aging in elderly women.

Leptin is a peptide hormone that is produced by white adipose tissue and monitors energy stores. Leptin inhibits the expression of orexigenic neuropeptides, leading to the upregulation of anorexigenic neuropeptides and satiety. This effect is referred to as leptin-induced inhibition of food intake.[9] Studies have reported high fasting concentrations of leptin in the elderly.[10–12]

Some studies suggest that men experience greater anorexia of aging than women. This trend may be related to a decrease in testosterone levels associated with age, which triggers an increase in levels of circulating leptin.[13,14] Postmenopausal women experience a decrease in adrenal androgens and testosterone as well, although to a lesser degree than men. This decrease may also lead to an increase in levels of leptin because the 2 hormones are inversely related. Di Francesco and colleagues[15] reported that there were higher serum concentrations of leptin in the elderly (aged 74–82 years) than in the younger patients (aged 25–38 years), that body mass indexes (BMIs, calculated as the weight in kilograms divided by the height in meters squared) were not significantly different in elderly and younger patients, and that satiety was more prolonged in the elderly cohort. This study also suggested that the elderly had less postprandial hunger and higher fasting and postprandial insulin concentrations but these values did not quite attain statistical significance.[15] Elevated plasma insulin levels are thought to amplify the anorexigenic effect of leptin through stimulating central leptin action and sensitivity.[16] This study was limited, however, by the small number (n = 8) of elderly adults studied, all of who were healthy.

The release of CCK from I cells occurs when nutrients such as fatty acids and aromatic amino acids enter the duodenum.[17] CCK is also present in the hypothalamus, cortex, and midbrain. This neuropeptide acts as a satiety hormone[4] by triggering the contraction of gallbladder, relaxing the sphincter of Oddi, and slowing the rate of gastric emptying.[17] With age, there is an increased basal release of CCK and a heightened release in response to fatty acids in the duodenum. The satiating effects of CCK therefore increase with age.[18,19] Martinez and colleagues[20] examined elderly patients with idiopathic anorexia and found that they had significantly higher plasma levels of CCK than healthy age-matched controls. Other studies have also shown that the intravenous administration of CCK-8 suppressed food intake twice as much in the elderly as in the young.[21] Understanding the biochemistry of CCK and its role in anorexia of aging have led many to study the effects of CCK antagonists in countering anorexia of aging.

Opioids comprise another class of neuropeptides that are frequently considered in the anorexia of aging. Animal studies have shown that the exogenous administration of opioid agonists causes increased food intake, whereas opioid antagonists inhibit food intake in animals and humans.[22] The role of opioids in the elderly, however, remains unclear. Martinez and colleagues[20] found a correlation between anorexia in the elderly, decreased cerebrospinal fluid (CSF) levels of β endorphin, and increased plasma concentrations of CCK-8. Silver and Morley[23] studied the effect of intraperitoneal injections of morphine and naloxone in mice and found that morphine increased food intake in younger but not older mice, whereas naloxone led to decreased food intake in the same respective groups of mice. MacIntosh and colleagues[19] evaluated energy intake after naloxone infusions in adults and found that 16% of older adults had suppressed energy intake, whereas only 8% of younger adults were affected, suggesting that aging is not associated with a significant reduction of the endogenous feeding drive. Although this study was double-blinded and randomized, it was limited by a small sample size (N = 24) and did not attain full statistical significance. Multiple studies have revealed conflicting evidence regarding the opioid response to food in aging. However, it remains a critical neuropeptide in understanding the anorexia of aging.[22]

Neuropeptide Y (NPY) is abundant in the central and peripheral nervous systems. NPY is a potent orexigenic molecule that promotes feeding and weight gain.[24] It is released during states of low energy or starvation from the hypothalamus and peripheral nervous system. It was previously thought that NPY activity was reduced in patients with anorexia. Martinez and colleagues[20] reported that elderly patients with senile anorexia actually had increased levels of NPY in both plasma and CSF when compared with age-matched controls. The results from this study challenge the postulated role and mechanism of action of this neuropeptide, and further studies elucidating the definitive role of NPY in the anorexia of aging are needed.

Galanin is yet another neuropeptide that stimulates food intake.[25] A study by Baranowska and colleagues[26] suggests that the mechanism behind galanin's relationship to anorexia is not from a decrease in secretion but rather from a decrease in sensitivity over time. Previous studies have also shown that growth hormone (GH) secretion is diminished in response to galanin in older women compared with younger women. This effect is thought to be secondary to higher circulating estrogen levels in young women, which has been shown to enhance galanin-induced GH secretion. As estrogen levels drop in postmenopausal women, the ability of galanin to enhance GH secretion is diminished, leading to decreased food intake in elderly women.[27] Further research into the mechanism of action of galanin is warranted to better understand and elucidate its role in the anorexia of aging and its mechanism of action.

Orexins or hypocretins are synthesized in the hypothalamus as either orexin A or orexin B and constitute another group of neuropeptides studied in relation to the anorexia of aging. Orexin A and B secretion help regulate feeding and sleep patterns.[28] Deficiency of these neuropeptides causes narcolepsy and contributes to decreased appetite and subsequent weight loss in animal models.[29] Interestingly, studies have found that orexin levels actually increase rather than decrease with aging. This finding confounds the role of orexins in the anorexia of aging,[29] although their effect on receptor sensitivity over time has yet to be determined.

Peptide YY (PYY) is released from the brain when fats and carbohydrates reach the small intestine. Batterham and colleagues[30] found a 30% reduction in food intake in obese and nonobese patients younger than 50 years on injecting intravenous PYY. The exact role of PYY in anorexia of aging and gender preferences has yet to be defined.

Glucagon-like peptide-1 (GLP-1) is an incretin that is released from the intestinal epithelium in response to nutrient and carbohydrate ingestion. In turn, GLP-1 stimulates insulin secretion, reduces glucagon secretion, slows gastric emptying, and decreases appetite.[18] Flint and colleagues[31] discovered that when GLP-1 was injected into 20 young healthy men, it reduced energy intake and improved satiety. The effects on the elderly, however, have yet to be studied, and there are no clear gender-based observations.

Ghrelin is an endocrine peptide hormone produced primarily by the enteroendocrine cells of the stomach as well as the placenta, pituitary, and hypothalamus. It seems to be an orexigenic regulator of appetite. Levels of ghrelin are highest in fasting states and at nadir during meals.[9,32] Ghrelin also stimulates the release of GH, and is inhibited by leptin, insulin, GH, a high-fat diet, and insulinlike growth factor-1.[33] Ghrelin is upregulated by fasting, a low protein diet, and a malnourished state.[34-36] The stomach produces ghrelin in 2 forms: active acylated ghrelin that stimulates food intake and desacyly ghrelin that is thought to have no hormonal action. Research has shown that in animal models, the des-acyl ghrelin released by the stomach actually decreases food intake.[37,38] This observation begs the question whether ghrelin in the elderly is the primary des-acyl ghrelin with appetite inhibitory properties. Rigamonti and colleagues[33] suggest that there is an age-related decline in plasma ghrelin concentrations. Another theory is that elevated fasting and postprandial insulin levels in elderly patients suppress ghrelin activity and sensitivity.[24] Some studies purport that fasting ghrelin levels are lower in the elderly.[39] However, Di Francesco and colleagues[15] revealed that neither basal nor postprandial ghrelin levels differed significantly between the young and elderly groups. This study also showed that in the elderly patients there was no postprandial increase in the ghrelin concentration. Further studies must be done to better elucidate this relationship.

Interleukin (IL)-1, IL-6, and tumor necrosis factor α are inflammatory cytokines that are present in higher levels in cachectic patients and lead to decreased food intake and body weight. In older cachectic patients, IL-1 and IL-6 levels have been shown to be elevated.[25] Roubenoff and colleagues[40] revealed that plasma IL-6 levels increase with aging and are inversely correlated with functionality in the elderly. Levels of these cytokines also increase with stress, malignancy, and infection and lead to a decrease in appetite, body weight, and functional capacity in the elderly.[25]

The interplay of receptor dysfunction, olfactory and taste decline, gastric motility and compliance, hormonal influence, and centrally mediated mechanisms involving neurotransmitters may contribute to anorexia and weight loss in the older patient. Investigating the individual effects of these mechanisms is difficult because of the multitude of other confounding factors, such as the ability to purchase and prepare food, loss of functional status, and other psychological and socioeconomic issues that may hinder oral intake. Studies at the neuronal and cellular level attempt to more clearly define the approach and management of such issues but are not yet clearly conclusive. Although anorexia of aging may manifest differently in men and women, the aforementioned factors likely play a more substantial role.

GASTROESOPHAGEAL REFLUX DISEASE

The prevalence of gastroesophageal reflux disease (GERD) does not seem to demonstrate an age-related gender preference. Although overt symptoms may be less common or less frequently reported in the older population,[41] complications related to GERD such as peptic stricture, esophagitis, and Barrett esophagus do seem to worsen with age.[41–45] A true understanding of the prevalence is difficult because of conflicts in the definition of GERD (esophagitis vs no esophagitis), as well as the relatively sparse number of international studies when compared with the magnitude of the problem. Differences in race, BMI, diet, central adiposity, acid production, and presence of *Helicobacter pylori* may be confounding factors in determining the presence of GERD.[46,47] Current literature, however, cites an overall prevalence of about 20% for weekly symptoms and 40% to 45% for monthly symptoms.[48] It is to be noted that there is significant worldwide variation.

Factors that contribute to the development and expression of GERD, such as anti-reflux barriers, lower esophageal sphincter (LES) pressure, esophageal clearance, acid production, gastric emptying, duodenogastric reflux, and esophageal resistance, may be influenced by age. Medications commonly used in the elderly may alter these factors and exacerbate reflux. There is a paucity of long-term studies that examine the effects of medications and other contributing factors within the elderly population. The pathogenesis of GERD is multifactorial and, as noted earlier, involves both anatomic and physiologic factors, which may be influenced by both age and gender.

Salivary secretion and bicarbonate concentration are decreased in the older population when compared with their younger counterparts.[49] Saliva and bicarbonate production is also affected by medications, tobacco usage, and the presence of GERD itself but has not been shown to be gender specific. Some medications, such as anticholinergics, may affect esophageal clearance of saliva in the older patient. This is especially true with regard to nocturnal acid exposure, a time when basal salivary output is at its lowest point, which may partly help to explain the higher rates of esophagitis in the elderly as well as the higher rate of GERD-related complications.

The role of hiatal hernia in GERD has evolved. Although the presence of a hernia is often associated with more severe GERD, erosive esophagitis, and esophageal injury, as well as reflux-associated complications, its presence alone is not always a cause.[50] Despite a higher incidence of hiatal hernia with aging and the female gender, the clinical correlation with respect to GERD and its complications is not clearly evident.[51–56]

Acid clearance is paramount in preventing reflux damage through both volume clearance and restoration of a normal esophageal pH. These actions do not prevent reflux but rather attempt to prevent damage and restore basal homeostasis; they depend on both effective peristalsis and action of saliva. The amplitude and effectiveness of peristalsis may also be decreased in some older individuals, leading to more prolonged acid exposure and, potentially, to more subsequent esophagitis.

LES plays the most important role in the generation of reflux in many individuals. Transient lower esophageal sphincter relaxation (tLESR) accounts for reflux in most patients. Gastric distention is the major stimulus for this event, although medications such as cholinergic drugs, stress, and certain foods such as fats may contribute to tLESRs.[57,58] Hypotensive LES pressures are less common causes of GERD. There are no studies to date that document alterations in tLESRs or basal LES pressures with either aging or gender. Such studies are needed to help clarify the importance of these factors in GERD in the older individual.

Acid and pepsin are 2 components of gastric refluxate that cause esophagitis. Although gastric emptying may be altered in the older individual, it is not clear whether this delay is clinically relevant. Acid production in the older individual may also be decreased but seems to be a consequence of atrophic gastritis and H pylori infections rather than a function of aging per se.[59–62] These mitigating factors may contribute to symptoms in some patients, but the effects on any particular individual may be too variable to predict a defined and reproducible clinical response and effect.

Clinical Presentation

Older patients are often less symptomatic with GERD. This may be associated with less acid production, decreased pain perception or esophageal sensitivity, or failure to report symptoms altogether.[41] It is, in part, a consequence of this lack of recognition or underreporting of symptoms that complications such as Barrett esophagitis and peptic strictures occur more commonly in the elderly.[42,60,63] There are no clear gender-based differences in the clinical presentation of GERD. Extraintestinal symptoms such as atypical chest pain and pulmonary issues are seen equally in the older population with GERD without any gender preference or difference.

Management

Treatment strategies and management do not significantly differ in the older patient when compared with the younger patient with GERD. Acid suppression remains the cornerstone of therapy. When placing an older female patient on acid-suppressing medications, concerns for malabsorption of calcium and vitamins, as well as bacterial overgrowth, arise. Clinicians must be cognizant of the potential risk of osteopenia, osteoporosis, and resultant fractures associated with decreased calcium absorption. Also, when the gastric pH is increased via acid suppressants, patients are more susceptible to bacterial overgrowth, which can be complicated by vitamin B_{12} deficiency and subsequent anemia and neuropathy. Although endoscopic treatment modalities have been largely abandoned because of safety and efficacy concerns, surgical approaches remain plausible for managing GERD in the older patient. Functional status and comorbidities are more important risk stratifiers than age in determining appropriateness for antireflux surgery. There do not seem to be gender differences with regard to efficacy of treatment modalities, outcomes, mortality, and morbidity.

MOTILITY

Aging has been associated with alteration in motility of the gastrointestinal tract. Changes in esophageal peristalsis, gastric emptying, colonic transit, and sphincter pressure and function may contribute to symptoms in the older patient. However, there is no clear evidence of alteration in small intestinal motility with either age or gender. Colonic transit time and FI in the elderly are discussed in the subsequent sections.

Esophageal motility is clearly affected by aging. Many individuals older than 80 years have a decline in the amplitude of peristaltic waves, as well as an increased frequency of nonpropulsive contractions.[64,65] There may also be less secondary peristalsis. Many studies cite these findings in patients older than 80 years, although a clear correlation with gastrointestinal symptoms is lacking. This findings may be secondary to diminished pain perception and an overall failure to report symptoms in this cohort, as previously mentioned.[66] Ren and colleagues[67] recognized an inverse relationship between age and both upper and lower esophageal sphincter pressures, lengths, and peristaltic wave amplitudes and velocities. This relationship may contribute to lengthier reflux episodes in older patients.[68] No gender difference was noted.

Gastric emptying times may be delayed in older individuals. Although initial studies did not clearly demonstrate age- or gender-related differences,[69,70] later studies demonstrated a delay in gastric emptying of solid food in older patients.[71-73] Electromyographic studies have shown a decrease in contractile force and peristalsis in the stomach. In addition, the lipid component of the meal may independently exert a profound effect on gastric emptying in the older individual.[74] Methodology and clinical relevance are 2 factors that are important and germane to the interpretation of these studies. At present, it does not seem that aging or gender plays a significant role in gastric emptying and its relationship with GERD.

Changes in esophageal and gastric motility may certainly contribute to symptoms such as GERD, dyspepsia, and anorexia in the elderly. Motility abnormalities, if present, in the small intestine and colon may also contribute to these symptoms. Definitive studies that account for underreporting and confounding factors are needed to ascertain whether these changes can predict clinical symptoms.

CONSTIPATION
Background

Constipation is one of the most common gastroenterological complaints. The prevalence of constipation in elderly patients is 50% in the general community and up to 74% in nursing home residents, which may be due, in part, to insufficient caloric intake or several other comorbidities in this population.[75] The Rome III criteria for functional constipation were developed to more clearly define this disorder. Older patients, however, may commonly present with symptoms of constipation that may not fit the Rome III criteria. Despite this presentation, clinicians must be able to recognize and treat such symptoms.

Self-reported constipation in the United States is more common among women, non-Caucasians, and those older than 65 years.[76,77] Studies have also shown a positive correlation with minimal physical activity, poor diet, low income, limited education, polypharmacy, history of sexual abuse, and depression.[78-81] Furthermore, severe constipation, defined as bowel movements occurring twice per month, is almost exclusively seen in women.[78]

Constipation can be primary or secondary. Symptoms of constipation can be secondary to underlying disorders such as primary diseases of the colon (strictures, cancer, anal fissure, proctitis), metabolic disturbances (hypercalcemia, hypothyroidism, diabetes mellitus), and neurologic disorders (parkinsonism, spinal cord lesions/injury, multiple sclerosis).[82,83] Some of these issues may be more common in the aging individual without clear gender difference, and treatment should be targeted at the primary disorder. There are 3 known subtypes of constipation: normal transit, dyssynergic defecation (DD), and slow transit. The first subtype, normal transit constipation, is the most common form of constipation treated by physicians.[82] These patients have normal stool transit times and pelvic floor function; however, they often feel constipated.[84,85] This feeling may be because of the perceived presence of hard stools and difficulty with subsequent evacuation. These patients may complain of bloating and abdominal pain[80] and many may also have irritable bowel syndrome.[84,86] The second subtype of constipation, DD, is described as difficulty expelling stool from the anorectum.[87] DD results from the failure to relax the puborectalis muscle or inappropriate contraction of the puborectalis and external anal sphincter muscles. This behavior is acquired in two-thirds of patients.[88] The final subtype, slow transit constipation, is defined as the delay of stool transit from the proximal to distal colon.[89] This delay may be caused by colonic myopathy or neuropathy.[87] Within this category, patients can either have (1) colonic inertia, associated with decreased frequency of high-amplitude colonic contractions, accounting for impaired propulsion of colonic contents especially after meals or (2) increased, uncoordinated motor activity of the distal colon, causing retropulsion of colonic contents. Frequently, patients may also have a combination of both.[90] The relationship between colonic transit and aging is somewhat controversial because some studies have found a slowing in the elderly,[69,91] whereas others have found no difference.[92–95]

Studies that delineate which type of constipation is more common in the elderly are lacking. However, it is known that constipation in the elderly is multifactorial, including polypharmacy, endocrine and metabolic disorders, neurologic disorders, myopathic disorders, depression, disability, and limited mobility. In elderly patients with multiple illnesses, cancer, and chronic pain, opioid-induced constipation is the most common.[83] A study by Towers and colleagues[96] revealed that elderly patients who consume fewer meals and calories are more inclined to have constipation. These patients can also develop fecal impaction with overflow incontinence.[97] Slow transit constipation can result from a myopathy, neuropathy, or DD in the elderly population.[87] With aging, the enteric nervous system undergoes age-related neurodegenerative changes.[75] In patients older than 65 years, there is a 37% loss of enteric neurons when compared with people aged 20 to 35 years. This loss is associated with an increase in the elastic and collagen fibers in the myenteric ganglia of older subjects.[75] Although enteric neuron loss has been documented in the elderly,[75] cases of Hirschsprung disease in this population are rarely reported.[98]

Diagnostic Approach

Regardless of the cause, a thorough history and physical examination is of paramount importance in the diagnosis of constipation. Discussion should focus on the nature and duration of constipation, medication history, surgical history, systemic and neurologic disorders, and history of malignancy. A psychosocial history should also be assessed. This multifaceted approach is especially important in the elderly because of the multiple factors that predispose to constipation, such as decreased mobility, poor nutrition, lack of independence, and social isolation.[75] Elderly patients may ignore the urge to defecate, for example, because they are unable to mobilize for toileting. This process may lead to the suppression of fecal rectal sensation and a decreased desire to defecate. In turn, this can exacerbate constipation because fecal retention can lead to large volume hard stools, which are difficult to evacuate.[99]

Colonic transit time is commonly assessed with the Hinton (sitz marker) test, which delineates colonic inertia from outlet delay and normal transit. Gastroenterologists may also use a wireless motility capsule, a viable and safe option for the elderly population that does not use radiation or require radiographs.[100] Anorectal manometry is another diagnostic test used in the setting of DD. It provides a method to determine pressures in both the rectum and the anal sphincters, allows assessment of rectal sensation and rectoanal reflexes, and evaluates rectal compliance as well. The balloon expulsion test is another useful study to assess rectal sensation and the ability to relax the pelvic floor in defecation.[87] Care must be taken in choosing the least embarrassing and least uncomfortable diagnostic tool for the older female patient. These studies are not mutually exclusive and a combination may be most helpful in the delineation of the cause for constipation in a specific individual.

Treatment

Patients with constipation can face 3 inextricable problems: significant financial burden, diminished quality of life,[88] and negative self-perception. For an older woman, these factors may lead to unnecessary stress, psychological burden, and awkward social encounters. These factors have also been associated with significant psychological distress. Multiple studies show a higher prevalence of depression, anxiety, obsessive compulsiveness, paranoia, and somatization in the constipated population.[85] Studies in adults with constipation have also elucidated sexual abuse in 22% to 48% of subjects and physical abuse in 31% to 74%.[88,101] Multiple studies also demonstrate a positive correlation between bowel function and quality of life.[85] Constipation can also be a social handicap, causing some patients to never leave their homes for fear of unpredictable bowel movements or urges.

One of the first steps in treating constipation in the elderly is to increase fiber intake. Daily fiber intake should optimally range between 20 and 35 g, ideally in the form of fruits, vegetables, and whole grains.[82] If increased ingestion of dietary fiber is unsuccessful, fiber supplements may be added. Side effects may limit usage, and supplements are better tolerated when starting with smaller amounts with subsequent gradual increments. It is important to educate older patients about dose adjustments to help enhance compliance. Excessive intake may exacerbate constipation.[102] A written outline or plan for management of the older individual with constipation may also be helpful.

Laxatives can also be used in the elderly population. Bulk-forming laxatives are natural or synthetic polysaccharides or cellulose derivatives that lead to water absorption, increased fecal mass, and increased stool frequency. Although the efficacy of bulk laxatives has not been well studied, there is considerable clinical experience with these agents.[103] Osmotic laxatives, such as polyethylene glycol, lactulose, and magnesium citrate, are available for patients who do not respond to increased fiber intake. These laxatives are poorly absorbed agents that act as hyperosmolar solutions and increase secretion of water into the gut lumen.[75,90] In the elderly patient with underlying renal or cardiac dysfunction, these agents must be used with caution because of disturbances in the absorption of magnesium.[82] Osmotic laxatives can also cause dehydration, making them a less-attractive option for the elderly. Stimulant laxatives, such as bisacodyl and senna, produce an increase in intestinal motility and secretions via alteration of electrolyte transport by the intestinal mucosa. Stimulant laxatives are commonly used in patients who are unresponsive or intolerant of osmotic laxatives or those with specific issues or needs requiring an increase in motility and secretions.[104,105]

Other agents are available and may be efficacious in the older individual with constipation. Lubiprostone is an oral bicyclic fatty acid that activates type 2 chloride channels on intestinal epithelial cells, leading to secretion of chloride and water into the gut lumen.[106] Several randomized controlled trials have shown that lubiprostone when compared with placebo leads to increased spontaneous bowel movements per week, improved consistency and patient-perceived treatment efficacy, and decreased straining and severity.[107–109] In the study by Johanson and Ueno[109] 10% of the participants were elderly. Alvimopan and methylnaltrexone are newer medications used for the treatment of opioid-induced constipation. These agents work peripherally as μ-opioid receptor antagonists, inhibiting opioid-induced gastrointestinal hypomotility without crossing the blood-brain barrier.[83] This class of medication allows elderly patients with chronic pain the benefit of pain control without the debilitating effects of constipation.[83]

The treatment of choice for pelvic floor dysfunction is biofeedback, a conditioning treatment that helps patients learn how to control pelvic floor movements. There are different therapeutic approaches to biofeedback, including anorectal electromyography, manometry, and balloon expulsion. These modalities are commonly used to highlight normal coordination for successful defecation.[75,82,83] This therapy does require compliance and active participation in the therapeutic process, which may be challenging for some older individuals. The efficacy of biofeedback in the elderly is thus contingent on an initial assessment of both the physical and mental aptitudes of the patient and must be individualized.

Surgery is an option in patients with refractory constipation. In patients with slow transit constipation refractory to medical management, a subtotal colectomy with ileorectal anastomosis may be considered.[110,111] As with any surgical procedure, there are side effects, including diarrhea, incontinence, bowel obstruction, and prolonged ileus.[75,112,113]

Summary

Constipation is a widespread disorder, affecting nearly one-fifth of people worldwide. If left untreated, it can have a deleterious effect on functionality and quality of life, especially in the elderly female population. Obtaining a thorough patient history is paramount in distinguishing between slow and normal transit constipation, and can be confirmed using the Hinton test and anal manometry for DD. Therapy is individualized and may start with dietary fiber intake and can be supplemented with physical activity, adequate fluid intake, laxatives, opioid antagonists, biofeedback, and, for refractory cases, surgery (depending on the cause of the constipation). Through recognition of symptoms, goal-directed therapy can be initiated and implemented early and efficaciously.

FI

The true prevalence of FI is difficult to state with certainty but seems to range between 1% and 18% in the general population.[114–116] Methodology and study design, definitions of FI, and social stigma attached to this disorder are among the factors that account for this variable range. The prevalence is higher in certain populations such as older adults, hospitalized patients, those residing in long-term care facilities, and, possibly, in middle-aged women.[117–119] Although female gender was previously associated with a perceived higher prevalence rate, many studies do not support this suggestion, and there may well be an overall equal distribution among men and women.[116,120] The prevalence does seem to increase with age and is more common in hospitalized patients.[99,121,122]

Mechanisms for FI include abnormal sphincter muscle function; puborectalis dysfunction; pudendal nerve damage or dysfunction; spinal cord dysfunction, damage, or injury; alteration of stool consistency or characteristics; loss of rectal accommodation and sensation; immobility; alteration in cognitive function; presence of fecal impaction; pelvic floor dyssynergy; and use of medication, which may all play a role in the pathophysiology of FI. Individuals may often have more than 1 factor or abnormality contributing to incontinence,[123,124] and aging may affect some of these factors.

There are particular issues germane to the development and expression of FI in older individuals. The thickness of the internal anal sphincter (IAS) increases with age and is related to an increase in collagen deposition. This anatomic change, however, does not seem to have major influence on the development or presence of FI. Anal sphincter function exhibits little change with aging.[125] However, there is a decrease in anal sphincter pressure in older individuals, with a rapid decrease in women at or after menopause.[126] The sphincter pressure decreases by 30% to 40% in both men and women older than 70 years.[125] There is also a decrease in anal squeeze pressure with age.[126] These changes along with a lesser degree of rectal pressure required to produce sphincter relaxation in the older individual may produce or contribute to FI.

Anal sphincter tear during childbirth is also associated with FI and can manifest itself later in life.[127–130] Labor and delivery may also damage or disrupt the pudendal nerve. Estrogen seems to play a role in the manifestation of FI.[131,132] Whether the pelvic floor muscles can compensate for sphincter tears or damage until menopause when hormonal levels decline or, alternatively, the sphincters are under some protective effect from estrogen or other hormones is not clear. Age-related drops in the pelvic floor musculature may also be a factor that may not manifest until later in life. Pudendal nerve dysfunction and terminal motor latency time may be abnormal in older individuals, and pelvic floor descent may be excessively contributing to FI.[133]

Changes in stool consistency or frequency may also contribute to FI in the older individual. Fecal impaction in this population may lead to FI.[134] This impaction may impair rectal sensation and lead to dysfunction of the IAS causing a prolonged relaxation allowing liquid stool to flow around an impaction.[135] Chronic constipation may be a predisposing factor. Chronic diarrhea may also lead to FI. If the stool is especially loose and voluminous, it may overcome the ability of the rectum to sense and distend in accommodation and of the external anal sphincter to more forcefully contract.[123] There is no clear gender difference for these causes of FI in the older individual.

Medications may also contribute to or cause incontinence. Many of these medications, such as anticholinergics to control urinary incontinence, muscle relaxants, narcotics, antidepressants, and laxatives, are used by the authors' older patients. These medications may interfere or negatively influence sphincter tone or function, pelvic floor function, and rectal sensation; may alter stool consistency; and predispose to or produce FI. Their use should always be considered when managing and treating the older individual who may already have some continence issues and also in approaching patients with unexplained FI. There does not seem to be any gender difference with respect to the effect of these medications producing FI in the older patient.

A significant number of older individuals with FI have no clearly demonstrable physiologic or pathologic abnormality that could account for FI. Other factors such as immobility, depression, dementia, and lack of easy access to toileting facilities may play an important role in the development and expression of FI in the older patient.[136–138] There is no gender difference with respect to these factors causing or contributing to FI in the older patient.

Although many of these factors may be present in the older population, it is not clear that they are clinically relevant for each individual. It is to be viewed as a spectrum of effects, both physiologic and pathologic, that may express themselves differently in individuals. Current studies are not sensitive enough to determine or predict which factors are of paramount importance for each individual.

SUMMARY

The geriatric population is predisposed to multiple gastrointestinal issues because of anatomic and physiologic changes associated with aging. As clinicians, it is imperative to identify and treat these disorders to preserve quality of life in this population. Research is lacking in elderly women, especially in regard to the anorexia of aging, GERD, and FI. More clearly defining the causative and treatable factors within these disorders will be paramount in successfully caring for the elderly population.

REFERENCES

1. Loo AT, Youngetob SL, Kent PF, et al. The aging olfactory epithelium: neurogenesis, response to damage, and odorant-induced activity. Int J Dev Neurosci 1996;14:881–900.
2. Stuckk BA, Frey S, Freiburg C, et al. Chemosensory event-related potentials in relation to side of stimulation, age, sex, and stimulus concentration. Clin Neurophysiol 2006;117:1367–75.
3. Mojet J, Christ-Hazelhof E, Heidema J. Taste perception with age: generic or specific losses in threshold sensitivity to the five basic tastes? Chem Senses 2001;26:845–60.
4. Morley JE, Silver AJ. Anorexia in the elderly. Neurobiol Aging 1988;9:9–16.
5. Cook CG, Andrews JM, Jones KL, et al. Effects of small intestinal nutrient infusion on appetite and pyloric motility are modified by age. Am J Physiol 1997; 273(2 Pt 2):R755–61.
6. Roberts SB, Fuss P, Heyman MB, et al. Control of food intake in older men. JAMA 1994;272:1601–6.
7. Sturm K, Parker B, Wishart J, et al. Energy intake and appetite are related to antral area in healthy young and older subjects. Am J Clin Nutr 2004;80:656–67.
8. Jones KL, Doran SM, Hveem K, et al. Relation between postprandial satiation and antral area in normal subjects. Am J Clin Nutr 1997;66:127–32.
9. Molina PE, Molina PE. Endocrine physiology, 3e. "Chapter 10. Endocrine integration of energy & electrolyte balance" (Chapter). Available at: http://www.accessmedicine.com/content.aspx?aID=6169115. Accessed November, 2010.
10. Gomez JM, Maravall FJ, Gomez N, et al. Interactions between serum leptin, the insulin-like growth factor-1 system, and age, anthropometric and body composition variables in a healthy population randomly selected. Clin Endocrinol 2003; 58:213–9.
11. Ruhl CE, Everhart JE. Leptin concentrations in the United States: relations with demographic and anthropometric measures. Am J Clin Nutr 2001;74:295–301.
12. Zamboni M, Zoico E, Fantin F, et al. Relation between leptin and the metabolic syndrome in elderly women. J Gerontol A Biol Sci Med Sci 2004;59:396–400.
13. Boggiano MM, Chandler PC, Oswald KD, et al. PYY3-36 as an anti-obesity drug target. Obes Rev 2005;6(4):307–22.
14. Morley JE. Androgens and aging. Maturitas 2001;38:61–71.
15. Di Francesco V, Zamboni M, Zoico E, et al. Unbalanced serum leptin and ghrelin dynamics prolong postprandial satiety and inhibit hunger in healthy elderly: another reason for the "anorexia of aging." Am J Clin Nutr 2006;83(5):1149–52.
16. Doucet E, St-Pierre S, Alméras N, et al. Fasting insulin levels influence plasma leptin levels independently from the contribution of adiposity: evidence from both a cross-sectional and an intervention study. J Clin Endocrinol Metab 2000;85:4231–7.
17. Barrett KE, Barrett KE. Gastrointestinal physiology. "Chapter 4. Pancreatic and Salivary Secretion" (Chapter). Available at: http://www.accessmedicine.com/content.aspx?aID=2306914. Accessed November, 2010.

18. Davis Stephen N, Brunton LL, Lazo JS, et al. Goodman & Gilman's The pharmacological basis of therapeutics, 11e. "Chapter 60. Insulin, Oral Hypoglycemic Agents, and the Pharmacology of the Endocrine Pancreas" (Chapter). Available at: http://www.accessmedicine.com/content.aspx?aID=958974. Accessed November, 2010.

19. MacIntosh CG, Andrews JM, Jones KL, et al. Effects of age on concentrations of plasma cholecystokinin, glucagon-like peptide 1, and peptide YY and their relation to appetite and pyloric motility. Am J Clin Nutr 1999;69(5):999–1006.

20. Martinez M, Hernanz A, Gomez-Cerezo J, et al. Alterations in plasma and cerebrospinal fluid levels of neuropeptides in idiopathic senile anorexia. Regul Pept 1993;49(2):109–17.

21. MacIntosh CG, Morley JE, Wishart J, et al. Effect of exogenous cholecystokinin (CCK)-8 on food intake and plasma CCK, leptin, and insulin concentrations in older and young adults: evidence for increased CCK activity as a cause of the anorexia of aging. J Clin Endocrinol Metab 2001;86(12):5830–7.

22. MacIntosh CG, Sheehan J, Davani N, et al. Effects of aging on the opioid modulation of feeding in humans. J Am Geriatr Soc 2001;49(11):1518–24.

23. Silver AJ, Morley JE. Role of the opioid system in the hypodipsia associated with aging. J Am Geriatr Soc 1992;40:556–60.

24. Reid Ian A, Katzung BG. Basic & clinical pharmacology, 11e. "Chapter 17. Vasoactive Peptides" (Chapter). Available at: http://www.accessmedicine.com/content.aspx?aID=4511993. Accessed November, 2010.

25. Chapman IM. The anorexia of aging. Clin Geriatr Med 2007;23(4):735–56, v. Review.

26. Baranowska B, Radzikowska M, Wasilewska-Dziubinska E, et al. Relationship among leptin, neuropeptide Y, and galanin in young women and in postmenopausal women. Menopause 2000;7(30):149–55.

27. Giustina A, Licini M, Bussi AR, et al. Effects of sex and age on the growth hormone response to galanin in healthy human subjects. J Clin Endocrinol Metab 1993;76(5):1369–72.

28. Visvanathan R, Chapman IM. Undernutrition and anorexia in the older person. Gastroenterol Clin North Am 2009;38(3):393–409.

29. Matsumura T, Nakayama M, Nomura A, et al. Age-related changes in plasma orexin-A concentrations. Exp Gerontol 2002;37(8–9):1127–30.

30. Batterham RL, Cohen MA, Ellis SM, et al. Inhibition of food intake in obese subjects by peptide YY3-36. N Engl J Med 2003;349(10):941–8.

31. Flint A, Raben A, Astrup A, et al. Glucagon-like peptide 1 promotes satiety and suppresses energy intake in humans. J Clin Invest 1998;101:515–20.

32. Dempsey Daniel T, Brunicardi FC, Andersen DK, et al. Schwartz's principles of surgery, 9e. "Chapter 26. Stomach" (Chapter). Available at: http://www.accessmedicine.com/content.aspx?aID=5030324. Accessed November, 2010.

33. Rigamonti AE, Pincelli AI, Corra B, et al. Plasma ghrelin concentrations in elderly subjects: comparison with anorexic and obese patients. J Endocrinol 2002;175:R1–5.

34. Horvath TL, Diano S, Sotonyi P, et al. Minireview: ghrelin and the regulation of energy balance–a hypothalamic perspective. Endocrinology 2001;142:4163–9.

35. Toshinai K, Mondal MS, Nakazato M, et al. Upregulation of ghrelin expression in the stomach upon fasting, insulin-induced hypoglycemia, and leptin administration. Biochem Biophys Res Commun 2001;281:1220–5.

36. Lee HM, Wang G, Englander EW, et al. Ghrelin, a new gastrointestinal endocrine peptide that stimulates insulin secretion: enteric distribution, ontogeny, influence of endocrine, and dietary manipulations. Endocrinology 2002;143:185–90.
37. Hosoda H, Kojima M, Matsuo H, et al. Ghrelin and des-acyl ghrelin: two major forms of rat ghrelin peptide in gastrointestinal tissue. Biochem Biophys Res Commun 2000;279:909–13.
38. Asakawa A, Inui A, Fujimiya M, et al. Stomach regulates energy balance via acylated ghrelin and desacyl ghrelin. Gut 2005;54:18–24.
39. Murdolo G, Lucidi P, Di Loreto C, et al. Insulin is required for prandial ghrelin suppression in humans. Diabetes 2003;52:2923–7.
40. Roubenoff R, Harris TB, Abad LW, et al. Monocyte cytokine production in an elderly population: effect of age and inflammation. J Gerontol A Biol Sci Med Sci 1998;53(1):M20–6.
41. Johnson DA, Fennerty MB. Heartburn severity underestimates erosive esophagitis severity in elderly patients with gastroesophageal reflux disease. Gastroenterology 2004;126:660–4.
42. Richter JE. Gastroesophageal reflux disease in the older patient: presentation, treatment, and complications. Am J Gastroenterol 2000;95:368–73.
43. Stanghellini V. Three-month prevalence rates of gastrointestinal symptoms and the influence of demographic factors. Results from the Domestic/International Gastroenterology Surveillance Study (DIGEST). Scand J Gastroenterol 1999;34:20.
44. Spechler SJ. Epidemiology and natural history of gastro-esophageal reflux disease. Digestion 1992;51:24–9.
45. Colleen MJ, Abdulian JD, Chen YK. Gastroesophageal reflux disease in the elderly: more severe disease that requires aggressive therapy. Am J Gastroenterol 1995;90:1053–7.
46. Kim N, Lee SW, Cho SI, et al. The prevalence of and risk factors for erosive esophagitis prospective study in Korea. Aliment Pharmacol Ther 2008;27:173–85.
47. Richter JE, Falk GW, Vaezi MF. Helicobacter pylori and gastroesophageal reflux disease: the bug may not be all bad. Am J Gastroenterol 1998;93:1800–2.
48. Richter JE, Friedenberg FK. Gastroesophageal reflux disease. In: Feldman M, Friedman LS, Brandt LJ, editors. Sleisgner & Fordtram's gastrointestinal and liver disease. 9th edition. Philadelphia (PA): Elsevier/Saunder; 2010. p. 705–26.
49. Sonnenberg A. Salivary secretion in reflux esophagitis. Gastroenterology 1982;83:889–97.
50. Mattioli S, D'Ovidio F, Pilotti V, et al. Hiatus hernia and intrathoracic migration of the esophagogastric junction in gastroesophageal reflux disease. Dig Dis Sci 2003;48:1823.
51. Sontag SJ, Schnell TG, Miller TQ, et al. The importance of hiatal hernia in reflux esophagitis compared with lower esophageal sphincter pressure or smoking. J Clin Gastroenterol 1991;13:628.
52. Kahrilas PJ, Lin S, Chen J, et al. The effect of hiatus hernia on gastro-esophageal junction pressure. Gut 1999;44:476.
53. Kahrilas PJ, Shi G, Manka M, et al. Increased frequency of transient lower esophageal sphincter relaxation induced by gastric distension in reflux patients with hiatal hernia. Gastroenterology 2000;118:688.
54. Paterson WG, Kolyn DM. Esophageal shortening induced by short-term intraluminal acid perfusion: a cause for hiatus hernia? Gastroenterology 1994;107:1736.

55. Wilson LJ, Ma W, Hirschowitz BI. Association of obesity with hiatus hernia and esophagitis. Am J Gastroenterol 1999;94:262.
56. Smith AB, Dickerman RD, McGuire CS, et al. Pressure overload induced sliding hiatal hernia in power athletes. J Clin Gastroenterol 1999;28:352.
57. Thor KB, Hill RD, Mercer DD, et al. Reappraisal of the flap valve mechanism in the gastroesophageal junction: a study of a new valvuloplasty procedure in cadavers. Acta Chir Scand 1987;153:25–8.
58. Holloway RH, Penagini R, Ireland AC. Criteria for objective definition of transient lower esophageal sphincter incompetence in patients with symptomatic gastroesophageal reflux. Gut 1988;29:1020–8.
59. Salles N. Basic mechanisms of the aging gastrointestinal tract. Dig Dis 2007;25:112–7.
60. Hurwitz A. Gastric acidity in older adults. JAMA 1997;278:659–62.
61. El-Serag HB, Ergun GA, Pandolfino J, et al. Obesity increases oesophageal acid exposure. Gut 2007;56:749–55.
62. Asaka M, Sugiyama T, Nobuta A, et al. Atrophic gastritis and intestinal metaplasia in Japan: results of a large multicenter study. Helicobacter 2001;6:294–9.
63. Lasch H, Castell DO, Castell JA. Evidence for diminished visceral pain with aging. Studies using graded intraesophageal balloon distension. Am J Physiol 1997;272:G1–3.
64. Ferriolli E, Dantas RO, Oliveira RB, et al. The influence of aging on oesophageal motility after ingestion of liquids with different viscosities. Eur J Gastroenterol Hepatol 1996;8:793–8.
65. Tack J, Vantrappen G. The aging esophagus. Gut 1997;41:422–4.
66. Soergel KH, Zboralske FF, Amberg JR. Presbyesophagus esophageal motility in nonagenarians. J Clin Invest 1964;43:1472–9.
67. Ren J, Shaker R, Kusano M, et al. Effect of aging on secondary esophageal peristalsis: presbyesophagus revisited. Am J Physiol 1995;268:9772–9.
68. Lee J, Anggiansah A, Anggiansah R, et al. Effects of age on gastroesophageal junction, esophageal motility and reflux disease. Clin Gastroenterol Hepatol 2007;5:1392–8.
69. Madsen JL, Graff J. Effects of aging on gastrointestinal motor function. Age Ageing 2004;33(2):154–9.
70. Madsen JL. Effects of gender, age, and body mass index on gastrointestinal transit times. Dig Dis Sci 1992;37:1548–53.
71. Brogan A, Loreno M, Catalano F, et al. Radioisotopic assessment of gastric emptying of solids in elderly subjects. Aging Clin Exp Res 2006;18:493–6.
72. Horowitz M, Maddern GJ, Chatterton BE, et al. Changes in gastric emptying rates with age. Clin Sci 1984;67:213–8.
73. Clarkston WK, Pantano MM, Morley JE, et al. Evidence for the anorexia of aging: gastrointestinal transit and hunger in healthy elderly vs. young adults. Am J Physiol 1997;272:R242–8.
74. Shimamoto C, Hirata I, Hiraike Y, et al. Evaluation of gastric motor activity in the elderly by electrogastrography and the (13)C-acetate breath test. Gerontology 2002;48:381–6.
75. Bouras EP, Tangalos EG. Chronic constipation in the elderly. Gastroenterol Clin North Am 2009;38(3):463–80; 1997;92(1):95–8.
76. Drossman DA, Li Z, Andruzi E, et al. US householder survey of the functional gastrointestinal disorders: prevalence, sociodemography and health impact. Dig Dis Sci 1993;38:1569–80.

77. Higgins PD, Johanson JF. Epidemiology of constipation in North America: a systematic review. Am J Gastroenterol 2004;99:750–9.
78. Heaton KW, Radvan J, Cripps H, et al. Defecation frequency and timing, and stool form in the general population: a prospective study. Gut 1992;33:818–24.
79. Johanson JF, Sonnenberg A, Koch TR. Clinical epidemiology of chronic constipation. J Clin Gastroenterol 1989;11:525–36.
80. Everhart JE, Go VL, Johannes RS, et al. A longitudinal survey of self-reported bowel habits in the United States. Dig Dis Sci 1989;34:1153–62.
81. Herz MJ, Kahan E, Zalevski S, et al. Constipation: a different entity for patients and doctors. Fam Pract 1996;13(2):156–9.
82. Lembo A, Camilleri M. Chronic constipation. N Engl J Med 2003;349(14): 1360–8.
83. Rao SS, Go JT. Update on the management of constipation in the elderly: new treatment options. Clin Interv Aging 2010;5:163–71.
84. Mertz H, Naliboff B, Mayer E. Physiology of refractory chronic constipation. Am J Gastroenterol 1999;94:609–15.
85. Ashraf W, Park F, Lof J, et al. An examination of the reliability of reported stool frequency in the diagnosis of idiopathic constipation. Am J Gastroenterol 1996;91:26–32.
86. Wald A, Hinds JP, Caruana BJ. Psychological physiological characteristics of patients with severe idiopathic constipation. Gastroenterology 1989;97:932–7.
87. Rao SS. Constipation. Evaluation and treatment of colonic and anorectal motility disorders. Gastroenterol Clin North Am 2007;36(3):687–711.
88. Rao SSC, Tuteja AK, Vellema T, et al. Dyssynergic defecation: demographics, symptoms, stool patterns and quality of life. J Clin Gastroenterol 2004;38: 680–5.
89. Bharucha AE, Phillips SF. Slow transit constipation. Gastroenterol Clin North Am 2001;30:77–95.
90. Locke GR 3rd, Pemberton JH, Phillips SF. American gastroenterological association medical position statement: guidelines on constipation. Gastroenterology 2000;119(6):1761–6.
91. Melkersson M, Andersson H, Bosaeus I, et al. Intestinal transit time in constipated and non-constipated geriatric patients. Scand J Gastroenterol 1983; 18(5):593–7.
92. Evans JM, Fleming KC, Talley NJ, et al. Relation of colonic transit to functional bowel disease in older people: a population-based study. J Am Geriatr Soc 1998;46(1):83–7.
93. Meir R, Beglinger C, Dederding J, et al. Influence of age, gender, hormonal status and smoking habits on colonic transit time. Neurogastroenterol Motil 1995;7:235–8.
94. Metcalf AM, Phillips SF, Zinsmeister AR, et al. Simplified assessment of segmental colonic transit. Gastroenterology 1987;92(1):40–7.
95. Eastwood HD. Bowel transit studies in the elderly: radio-opaque markers in the investigation of constipation. Gerontol Clin (Basel) 1972;14(3):154–9.
96. Towers AL, Burgio KL, Locher JL, et al. Constipation in the elderly: influence of dietary, psychological, and physiological factors. J Am Geriatr Soc 1994;42(7): 701–6.
97. Gallagher P, O'Mahony D. Constipation in old age. Best Pract Res Clin Gastroenterol 2009;23(6):875–87.
98. Rich AJ, Lennard TW, Wilsdon JB. Hirschsprung's disease as a cause of chronic constipation in the elderly. Br Med J (Clin Res Ed) 1983;287(6407):1777–8.

99. Talley NJ, O'Keefe EA, Zinsmeister AR, et al. Prevalence of gastrointestinal symptoms in the elderly: a population-based study. Gastroenterology 1992; 102(3):895–901.

100. Rao SS, Paulson J, Saad R, et al. Assessment of colonic, whole gut and regional transit in elderly constipated and healthy subjects with novel wireless pH/pressure capsule (SmartPill). Gastroenterology 2009;136:A950.

101. Leroi AM, Berkelmans I, Denis P, et al. Anismus as a marker of sexual abuse: consequences of abuse on anorectal motility. Dig Dis Sci 1995;40:1411–6.

102. Voderholzer WA, Schatke W, Muhldorfer BE, et al. Clinical response to dietary fiber treatment of chronic constipation. Am J Gastroenterol 1997;92(1): 95–8.

103. Sonnenberg A, Koch TR. Physician visits in the United States for constipation: 1958 to 1986. Dig Dis Sci 1989;34:606–11.

104. Tzavella K, Riepl RL, Klauser AG, et al. Decreased substance P levels in rectal biopsies from patients with slow transit constipation. Eur J Gastroenterol Hepatol 1996;8:1207–11.

105. Xing JH, Soffer EE. Adverse effects of laxatives. Dis Colon Rectum 2001;44(8): 1201–9.

106. Cuppoletti J, Malinowska DH, Tewari KP, et al. SPI-0211 activates T84 cell chloride transport and recombinant human ClC-2 chloride currents. Am J Physiol Cell Physiol 2004;287(5):C1173–83.

107. Johanson JF, Drossman DA, Panas R, et al. Clinical trial: phase 2 study of lubiprostone for irritable bowel syndrome with constipation. Aliment Pharmacol Ther 2008;27(8):685–96.

108. Johanson JF, Morton D, Geenen J, et al. Multicenter, 4-week, double-blind, randomized, placebo-controlled trial of lubiprostone, a locally-acting type-2 chloride channel activator, in patients with chronic constipation. Am J Gastroenterol 2008;103(1):170–7.

109. Johanson JF, Ueno R. Lubiprostone, a locally acting chloride channel activator, in adult patients with chronic constipation: a double-blind, placebo-controlled, dose-ranging study to evaluate efficacy and safety. Aliment Pharmacol Ther 2007;25(11):1351–61.

110. Nyam DC, Pemberton JH, Ilstrup DM, et al. Long-term results of surgery for chronic constipation. Dis Colon Rectum 1997;40(3):273–9.

111. Hassan I, Pemberton JH, Young-Fadok TM, et al. Ileorectal anastomosis for slow transit constipation: long-term functional and quality of life results. J Gastrointest Surg 2006;10(10):1330–6 [discussion: 1336–7].

112. Preston DM, Lennard-Jones JE. Anismus in chronic constipation. Dig Dis Sci 1985;30:413.

113. Rao SS, Welcher KD, Leistikow JS. Obstructive defecation: a failure of rectoanal coordination. Am J Gastroenterol 1998;93:1042.

114. Tang SY. Geriatric fecal incontinence. Clin Geriatr Med 2004;20:571–87.

115. Macmillan AK, Merrie AE, Marshall RJ, et al. The prevalence of fecal incontinence in community dwelling adults: a systematic review of the literature. Dis Colon Rectum 2004;47:1341–9.

116. Whitehead W, Borrud L, Goode PS, et al. Fecal incontinence in US adults: epidemiology and risk factors. Gastroenterology 2009;137:512–7.

117. Nelson RL. Epidemiology of fecal incontinence. Gastroenterology 2004; 126(Suppl 1):S3–7.

118. Perry S, Shaw C, McGrother C, et al. Prevalence of faecal incontinence in adults aged 40 years or more living in the community. Gut 2002;50:480–4.

119. Bharucha AE, Zinsmeister AR, Locke GR, et al. Prevalence and burden of fecal incontinence: a population-based study in women. Gastroenterology 2005;129: 42–9.
120. Lam T, Kennedy M, Chen F, et al. Prevalence of faecal incontinence: obstetric and constipation risk factors – a population based study. Int J Colorectal Dis 1999;1:197–203.
121. Goode P, Burgio K, Halli A, et al. Prevalence and correlates of fecal incontinence in community-dwelling older adults. J Am Geriatr Soc 2005;53:629–35.
122. Roberts R, Jacobsen S, Reilly W, et al. Prevalence of combined fecal and urinary incontinence: a community-based study. J Am Geriatr Soc 1999;47(7):837–41.
123. Rao SSC. Practice guidelines: diagnosis and management of fecal incontinence. Am J Gastroenterol 2004;99:1585–604.
124. Mohanty S, Schulze K, Stessman M, et al. Behavioral therapy for rectal hypersensitivity. Am J Gastroenterol 2001;96:S301.
125. Bannister JJ, Abouzekry L, Read NW. Effect of aging on anorectal function. Gut 1987;28:353–7.
126. Rociu E, Stoker J, Eigkemans MJ, et al. Normal anal sphincter anatomy and age- and sex-related variations at high-spatial-resolution endoanal MR in aging. Radiology 2000;217:395–401.
127. Fox JC, Fletcher JG, Zinsmeister AR, et al. Effect of aging on anorectal and pelvic floor functions in females. Dis Colon Rectum 2006;49:1726–35.
128. Kamm MA. Obstetric damage and faecal incontinence. Lancet 1994;344:730–3.
129. Sultan AH, Kamm MA, Hudson CN, et al. Anal-sphincter disruption during vaginal delivery. N Engl J Med 1993;329:1905–11.
130. Borello-France D, Burgio KL, Richter HE, et al. Fecal and urinary incontinence in primiparous women. Obstet Gynecol 2006;108:863–72.
131. Rao SS. Pathophysiology of adult fecal incontinence. Gastroenterology 2004; 126:S14–22.
132. Haadem K, Ling L, Ferno M, et al. Estrogen receptors in the external sphincter muscle. Am J Obstet Gynecol 1991;164:609–10.
133. Laurberg S, Swash M. Effects of aging on anorectal function. Gut 1987;28: 353–7.
134. Read NW, Abouzekry L, Read MG, et al. Anorectal function in elderly patients with fecal impaction. Gastroenterology 1985;89:959–66.
135. Goligher JC. Functional results after sphincter-saving resections of the rectum. Hunterian lecture. Ann R Coll Surg Engl 1951;8:421–38.
136. Leung FW, Schnelle JR. Urinary and fecal incontinence in nursing home residents. Gastroenterol Clin North Am 2008;37:697–707.
137. Rao SS. Sleisgner & Fordtram's gastrointestinal and liver disease. 9th edition. Philadelphia (PA): Elsevier/Saunder; 2010. p. 241–58.
138. Delvaux M. Digestive health in the elderly: faecal incontinence in adults. Aliment Pharmacol Ther 2003;18(2):84–9.

Index

Note: Page numbers of article titles are in **boldface** type.

A

ABCB 4 gene mutations, intrahepatic cholestasis of pregnancy in, 338–339
Abdominal pain, in IBS, 266–267
Acupressure and acupuncture, for nausea and vomiting of pregnancy, 320
Acute fatty liver of pregnancy, 340–342
Acute intermittent porphyria, in pregnancy, 345
Adalimumab, for IBD, 408
Adefovir, for hepatitis B, 366–367
Adenomas
    colon, 416–417
    liver, 345
S-Adenosylmethionine, for intrahepatic cholestasis of pregnancy, 340
Aflatoxin, hepatocellular carcinoma related to, 435–436
Aging. *See* Older female patients.
Alanine aminotransferase, in pregnancy, 336
Alcohol consumption, colorectal cancer development and, 418
Alosetron, for IBS, 269–271
Alternative medicine, for IBS, 277–281
Alvimopan, for constipation, 457–458
Aminosalicylates, for IBD, 405
Amitriptyline, for IBS, 268–269
Anal sphincter dysfunction, fecal incontinence in, 458–459
Anemia, microangiopathic hemolytic, in HELLP syndrome, 342–344
Anorexia, in older female patients, 449–453
Antacids, for nausea and vomiting of pregnancy, 323
Antibiotics
    for IBD, 406
    for IBS, 269
Anticholinergics, for nausea and vomiting of pregnancy, 322
Antidepressants, for IBS, 268–269
Antiemetics, for nausea and vomiting of pregnancy, 321
Antigliadin antibody, in Celiac disease, 300
Antihistamines
    for intrahepatic cholestasis of pregnancy, 340
    for nausea and vomiting of pregnancy, 322, 324
    for PBC, 380–381
Antimitochondrial antibodies, in PBC, 375
Antiretroviral therapy, for hepatitis B, 360–361, 364–369
Appetite loss, in older female patients, 449–453
Aspartate aminotransferase, in pregnancy, 336

Gastroenterol Clin N Am 40 (2011) 467–479
doi:10.1016/S0889-8553(11)00047-1
0889-8553/11/$ – see front matter
gastro.theclinics.com

Moving?

Make sure your subscription moves with you!

To notify us of your new address, find your **Clinics Account Number** (located on your mailing label above your name), and contact customer service at:

Email: journalscustomerservice-usa@elsevier.com

800-654-2452 (subscribers in the U.S. & Canada)
314-447-8871 (subscribers outside of the U.S. & Canada)

Fax number: 314-447-8029

Elsevier Health Sciences Division
Subscription Customer Service
3251 Riverport Lane
Maryland Heights, MO 63043

*To ensure uninterrupted delivery of your subscription, please notify us at least 4 weeks in advance of move.

Printed and bound by CPI Group (UK) Ltd, Croydon, CR0 4YY

21/10/2024

01776965-0001